# Prostate Cancer Screening

# CURRENT CLINICAL UROLOGY

Eric A. Klein, MD, SERIES EDITOR

# Prostate Cancer Screening

## Second Edition

*Edited by*

## Donna P. Ankerst, Ph.D.

*Technical University, Garching, Germany and University of Texas
Health Science Center at San Antonio, San Antonio, TX, USA*

## Catherine M. Tangen, DrPh

*Fred Hutchinson Cancer Research Center, Seattle,
WA, USA*

## Ian M. Thompson Jr, MD

*University of Texas Health Science Center at San Antonio,
San Antonio, TX, USA*

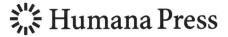 Humana Press

*Editors*
Donna P. Ankerst
Professor, Department of Mathematics
Technical University, Garching, Germany
Associate Professor, Departments
  of Urology, and Epidemiology/Biostatistics
University of Texas Health Science Center
  at San Antonio
San Antonio, TX, USA
ankerst@uthscsa.edu

Catherine M. Tangen
Member, Southwest Oncology Group
  Statistical Center
Fred Hutchinson Cancer Research Center
  Seattle, WA, USA
ctangen@fhcrc.org

Ian M. Thompson
Professor and Chair, Department of Urology
  University of Texas Health Science Center
  at San Antonio
San Antonio, TX, USA
thompsoni@uthscsa.edu

*Series Editor*
Eric A. Klein
Professor of Surgery
Cleveland Clinic Lerner College
  of Medicine
Head, Section of Urologic Oncology
Glickman Urological and
  Kidney Institute
Cleveland, OH, USA

ISBN 978-1-60327-280-3       e-ISBN 978-1-60327-281-0
DOI 10.1007/978-1-60327-281-0

Library of Congress Control Number: 2008943026

Printed on acid-free paper

springer.com

# Preface

We are entering a remarkable time in medicine. In the USA and other countries, preventive medicine and public health efforts have successfully increased life expectancy substantially; concurrently, the demographics of the post-World War II population tells us that the over-50 population will dramatically increase over the next two decades. As prostate cancer is distinctly age-related, we can anticipate a tsunami-like increase in the numbers of patients with this disease. How will we respond to this challenge over the next two decades?

Between the early 1900s and the mid-1980s, about the only strategy against this disease was a digital rectal examination (DRE) with the goal of early detection and treatment; if the disease was detected late, hormonal therapy was the mainstay of therapy. Unfortunately, systematic analyses of DRE as a screening tool found that the majority of cases detected were incurable by the time the tumor was palpable. In the case of hormonal therapy for advanced disease, 60 years after its discovery, average survival remains only about 2–3 years.

With the discovery of PSA, a remarkable marker of prostate cancer risk, and with a national enthusiastic embrace of this test, the entire approach to this disease changed. The number of diagnosed prostate cancers more than doubled and the majority of tumors detected were organ-confined and probably cured. A man's lifetime risk of prostate cancer diagnosis more than doubled from 8% in the early 1980s to almost 18% today.

When PSA first began to be used for screening in the early to mid-1980s, screening was a simple matter for the patient and doctor: If his PSA was above 4.0 ng/mL, it was *abnormal* and a biopsy was recommended. If it was below 4.0 ng/mL, it was *normal* and he was reassured that all was well.

We now know that this concept is not correct and that evaluating a man's risk of prostate cancer is considerably more complex. PSA is not *abnormal* or *normal* but reflects a range of risk with each increase in level associated with an increased level of risk. We know that a PSA value in one person with few other risk factors of prostate cancer means something completely different than the same PSA value in another man who has other risk factors that increase his risk of cancer. Clinicians can no longer say "your PSA is normal" but instead must understand how to integrate other measures of risk as well as understand when to request other screening tests. They must also understand how to explain these risks to their patients who have been accustomed to 20 years of normal/abnormal readings on their PSA slips.

Concurrent with our understanding of this has been the explosion of new biomarkers and biomeasures of prostate cancer. We discriminate between the two terms, understanding that a "biomarker" may be the measured value of a substance in a bodily fluid or other biologic sample while a "biomeasure" could include body mass index, number of affected male relatives with prostate cancer, or other observed and quantifiable values. Biomarker and biomeasure discovery has rapidly emerged as one of the primary focus areas in prostate cancer screening, with the hope of significantly improving benefits of screening through more accurate diagnosis. The translational endeavors, however, bring significant technologic, statistical methodologic, and clinical challenges.

This book incorporates a series of thoughtful and cutting-edge works from the world's experts in prostate cancer screening, ranging from the current status quo of prostate cancer screening across the globe, consensus on optimal utilization of the traditional PSA and DRE tests, cutting-edge research in new biomarkers, biomeasures and extended risk algorithms for prostate cancer, and last but not least, coverage of large ongoing international prevention and screening trials that aim to reduce prostate cancer mortality. The information will be helpful not only to the clinician who is faced with explaining risk to the patient but also to the researcher who is developing new biomarkers, to the public health and policy decision-maker who is determining how screening should be implemented, as well as to current and future members of the biomarker industry who seek methods to better develop and support markers and measures of prostate cancer.

We are indebted to our colleagues around the world who have contributed their time to this wonderful text. These are the scientists who have made and will continue to make discoveries that will impact the lives of hundreds of millions of men worldwide as they face the most common cancer in men – cancer of the prostate.

# Contents

# Contributors

SANJAI K. ADDLA, FRCS • *Department of Urology, University of Brussels, Erasme Hospital, University Clinics of Brussels, Brussels, Belgium*

DONNA P. ANKERST, PHD • *Department of Mathematics, Technical University, Garching, Germany, and Departments of Urology, and Epidemiology/Biostatistics, University of Texas Health Science Center at San Antonio, San Antonio, TX, USA*

JUSTO LORENZO BERMEJO, MD • *Division of Molecular Genetic Epidemiology, German Cancer Research Center, Heidelberg, Germany*

JOKE BEUTEN, PHD • *Department of Cellular and Structural Biology, The University of Texas Health Science Center, San Antonio, TX, USA*

AMANDA BLACK, PHD • *Early Detection Research Group, Division of Cancer Prevention and, the Cancer Prevention Fellowship Program, Office of Preventive Oncology, National Cancer Institute, Bethesda, MD, USA*

RICHARD J. BRYANT • *Lecturer in Urology, Nuffield Department of Surgery, Fellow of Balliol, University of Oxford, John Radcliffe Hospital, Oxford OX3 9DU, United Kingdom*

EDITH CANBY-HAGINO, MD, MS • *Wilford Hall Medical Center, Lackland AFB, San Antonio, TX, USA*

FELIX K.-H. CHUN, MD • *Department of Urology, University of Hamburg, Germany*

NIGEL CLEGG, PHD • *Divisions of Human Biology and Clinical Research, Fred Hutchinson Cancer Research Center, Seattle, WA, USA*

E. DAVID CRAWFORD, MD • *Division of Urology, University of Colorado School of Medicine, Denver, CO, USA*

ANTHONY V. D'AMICO, MD, PHD • *Department of Radiation Oncology, Brigham & Women's Hospital and Dana Farber Cancer Institute, Harvard Medical School, Boston, MA, USA*

BOB DJAVAN MD, PHD • *Department of Urology, University of Brussels, Erasme Hospital, University Clinics of Brussels, Brussels, Belgium*

JASON A. EFSTATHIOU, MD, PHD • *Department of Radiation Oncology, Brigham & Women's Hospital and Dana Farber Cancer Institute, Harvard Medical School, Boston, MA, USA*

RUTH ETZIONI, MD • *Fred Hutchinson Cancer Research Center, Seattle, WA, USA*

ZIDING FENG, PHD • *Fred Hutchinson Cancer Research Center, Seattle, WA, USA*

ROBERT H. GETZENBERG, PHD • *The Brady Urological Institute, Johns Hopkins Hospital, Baltimore, MD, USA*

PHYLLIS J. GOODMAN, MS • *Southwest Oncology Group Statistical Center, Fred Hutchinson Cancer Research Center, Seattle, WA, USA*

JACK GROSKOPF, PHD • *Gen-Probe Incorporated, San Diego, CA, USA*

ROBERT L. GRUBB III, MD • *Division of Urologic Surgery, Washington University, St. Louis, MO, USA*

ROMAN GULATI, MS • *Fred Hutchinson Cancer Research Center, Seattle, Washington, USA*

ALEXANDER HAESE, MD, PHD • *Department of Urology, University Clinic Hamburg-Eppendorf, Hamburg, Germany*

FC HAMDY, MD • *Nuffield Department of Surgery, Fellow of Balliol, University of Oxford, John Radcliffe Hospital, Oxford OX3 9DU, United Kingdom*

KARI HEMMINKI, MD • *Division of Molecular Genetic Epidemiology, German Cancer Research Center, Heidelberg, Germany and Center for Family and Community Medicine, Karolinska Institute, Huddinge, Sweden*

RUI HENRIQUE, MD, PHD • *Department of Pathology, Portuguese Oncology Institute – Porto, Portugal, and Department of Pathology and Molecular Immunology, Institute of Biomedical Sciences Abel Salazar (ICBAS), University of Porto, Portugal*

JAVIER HERNANDEZ, MD, MS • *Brooke Army Medical Center, Fort Sam Houston, TX, USA*

CARMEN JERÓNIMO, PHD • *Department of Genetics, Portuguese Oncology Institute – Porto, Portugal, Department of Pathology and Molecular Immunology, Institute of Biomedical Sciences Abel Salazar (ICBAS), University of Porto, Portugal, and Fernando Pessoa University School of Health Sciences, Porto, Portugal*

TERESA L JOHNSON-PAIS, PHD • *Department of Pediatrics, The University of Texas Health Science Center, San Antonio, TX, USA*

JACOB KAGAN, PHD • *Cancer Biomarkers Research Group, National Cancer Institute, USA*

PIERRE I. KARAKIEWICZ, MD • *Cancer Prognostics and Health Outcomes Unit, University of Montreal, Montreal, Quebec, Canada*

MICHAEL W. KATTAN, PHD • *Department of Quantitative Health Sciences, The Cleveland Clinic, Cleveland, OH, USA*

ERIC A. KLEIN, MD • *Cleveland Clinic Glickman Urological and Kidney Institute, Cleveland, OH, USA*

LAURENCE H. KLOTZ, MD • *Division of Urology, Sunnybrook Health Sciences Centre, University of Toronto, Toronto, ON, Canada*

EDDY S. LEMAN, PHD • *The Brady Urological Institute, Johns Hopkins Hospital, Baltimore, MD, USA*

ANGELA MARIOTTO, PHD • *Division of Cancer Control and Population Sciences, National Cancer Institute, Bethesda, MD, USA*

ROBERT K. NAM, MD • *Division of Urology, Sunnybrook Health Sciences Centre, University of Toronto, Toronto, ON, Canada*

PETER S. NELSON, MD • *Divisions of Human Biology and Clinical Research, Fred Hutchinson Cancer Research Center, Seattle, WA, USA*

DIPEN J PAREKH, MD • *Department of Urology, University of Texas at San Antonio, San Antonio, TX, USA*

ALAN W. PARTIN, MD PHD • *Department of Urology, Oncology, Johns Hopkins Medical Institutions, Baltimore, MD, USA*

AMANDA REED, MD • *Department of Urology, University of Texas at San Antonio, San Antonio, TX, USA*

HARRY RITTENHOUSE, PHD • *Gen-Probe Incorporated, San Diego, CA, USA*

JACK SCHALKEN, PHD • *Department of Urology, Radboud University Nijmegen Medical Centre, The Netherlands*

FRITZ H. SCHRÖDER, MD • *Department of Urology, Erasmus University and Academic Hospital, Rotterdam, The Netherlands*

SHAHROKH F. SHARIAT, MD • *Division of Urology, Memorial Sloan-Kettering Cancer Center, New York, NY, USA*

SUDHIR SRIVASTAVA, PHD, MPH, • *Cancer Biomarkers Research Group, National Cancer Institute, USA*

JEFFREY E. TAM, PHD • *Beckman Coulter Inc., Chaska, MN, USA*

CATHERINE M. TANGEN, DRPH • *Southwest Oncology Group Statistical Center, Fred Hutchinson Cancer Research Center, Seattle, WA, USA*

IAN M. THOMPSON, JR., MD • *Department of Urology, University of Texas Health Science Center at San Antonio, San Antonio, TX, USA*

KADEE THOMPSON, MD • *Department of Urology, University of Texas at San Antonio, San Antonio, TX, USA*

TINEKE WOLTERS, MD • *Department of Urology, Erasmus University and Academic Hospital, Rotterdam, The Netherlands*

YINGYE ZHENG, PHD • *Department of Biostatistics and Biomathematics, Fred Hutchinson Cancer Research Center, Seattle, WA, USA*

# Color Plates

PLCO screening centers: Alabama (University of Alabama, Birmingham); Michigan (Henry Ford Health System, Detroit); Colorado (University of Colorado, Denver); Hawaii (Pacific Health Research Institute, Honolulu); Wisconsin (Marshfield Clinic Research Foundation, Marshfield); Minnesota (University of Minnesota, Minneapolis); Pennsylvania (University of Pittsburgh, Pittsburgh); Utah (University of Utah, Salt Lake City); Idaho (University of Utah/Boise, Boise) (Utah Satellite Center); Missouri (Washington University, St. Louis); Washington DC (Georgetown University, Washington).

(Source: H. de Koning (2002). International Journal of Cancer 98: 268–73.)

# I TRENDS IN PROSTATE CANCER SCREENING

# 1

# Overview of US Prostate Cancer Trends in the Era of PSA Screening

*Ruth Etzioni, Roman Gulati, and Angela Mariotto*

## SUMMARY

Prostate cancer rates in the United States have changed radically over the last two decades. The introduction of prostate-specific antigen (PSA) screening impacted incidence substantially; however, in the absence of randomized clinical trials, its role in the precipitous mortality decline remains unclear. Simultaneous advances in treatment, shifting patterns of care, and changing health behaviors may also have contributed to this decline. Two veins of investigation—ecologic and modeling studies—provide insights into the benefits and costs of PSA screening, with the latter positioned to help design optimal intervention policies.

**Key Words:** PSA screening, Natural experiment, Will Rogers phenomenon, Lead time, Overdiagnosis, Ecologic studies, Surveillance modeling.

## INTRODUCTION

Prostate cancer trends in the United States have displayed great upheavals in the last two decades. Prior to the introduction of prostate-specific antigen (PSA) screening in the mid-1980s, incidence had been steadily increasing, reaching 119 per 100,000 by 1986. Then, with the introduction of PSA screening, incidence rapidly doubled, peaking at 237 per 100,000 in 1992. Following this peak, incidence declined by a dramatic 29% before

From: *Current Clinical Urology: Prostate Cancer Screening*, Edited by: D. P. Ankerst et al.
DOI 10.1007/978-1-60327-281-0_1 © Humana Press, a part of Springer Science+Business Media, LLC 2009

returning to a modest increasing trend which has more recently also been followed by a decline (1).

Meanwhile, prostate cancer mortality in the United States continues its steady march downwards, having dropped by a staggering 37% since 1992, from 39.2 per 100,000 to 24.6 per 100,000. Mortality declines have been most pronounced in men aged 65–69; in this age group mortality has declined by 46%. However, substantial declines have occurred in all age groups with a 30% drop observed in men aged 50–59 and a 33% decline for men over 80 (2).

The widespread adoption of PSA screening in the United States has dramatically increased the chance that a man will be diagnosed with prostate cancer in his lifetime. Based on prostate cancer incidence in 2002–2004, the current lifetime probability of a prostate cancer diagnosis is 17%, up from 9% in 1984–1986 (3).

The questions generated by these patterns of prostate cancer incidence and mortality strike at the heart of ongoing controversies about PSA and prostate cancer management in general. First, do the mortality declines imply that PSA screening is beneficial? In the absence of results from randomized screening trials, the natural experiment in the US population has taken center stage in the debate about the likely efficacy of screening but offers only limited conclusions. Second, how might any benefits balance out against the inevitable problems of overdetection and overtreatment, and what can we infer about these costs from incidence data? Third, what other factors are playing a role in incidence and mortality patterns? Major changes in prostate cancer management have occurred concurrently with the adoption of PSA screening including new radiation technologies, earlier use of hormonal therapies, and use of PSA to monitor for recurrent disease. The likely influence of these factors on prostate cancer trends cannot be ignored when interpreting mortality declines.

In this chapter we present an overview of prostate cancer incidence and mortality in the United States over the last quarter century. We examine disease incidence by race, age, stage, grade, and year and explain how these data may be used to make inferences about overdiagnosis and background incidence. In addition, we review screening, biopsy, and treatment trends and their potential association with mortality declines.

Many of the results that we present are based on data from the Surveillance, Epidemiology and End Results (SEER) registry of the National Cancer Institute (http://seer.cancer.gov/). This population-based registry records demographic, clinical, and survival information on all cancer cases diagnosed within 17 geographic areas in the United States (up from 9 areas in 1975), representing approximately 26% of the US population. We use data from the nine primary SEER areas over the calendar interval 1983–2005 for this review. In addition we reference data on practice patterns from the linked SEER-Medicare database (http://healthservices.cancer.gov/seermedicare/), the National Health Interview Survey (http://www.cdc.gov/nchs/nhis.htm), and several recent studies documenting changing screening and treatment practices in the United States during the PSA era (4–6).

## PROSTATE CANCER INCIDENCE IN THE UNITED STATES: 1983–2005

Figures 1, 2, 3, 4 summarize the trends in prostate cancer incidence by race, age, stage, and grade. The trends clearly show the dramatic effect of the rapid dissemination of PSA screening in the early 1990s. The incidence peak in whites occurred in 1992, one year prior to the incidence peak in blacks (Fig. 1), consistent with a slightly delayed

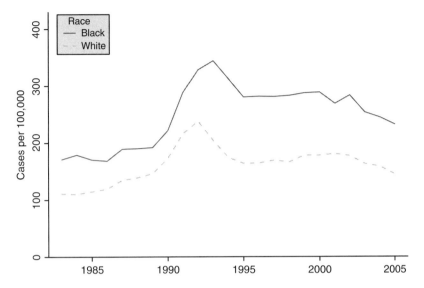

**Fig. 1.** Age-adjusted incidence for blacks and whites, 1983–2005.

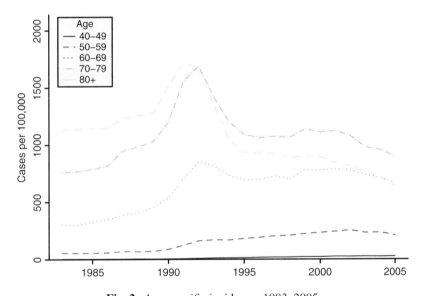

**Fig. 2.** Age-specific incidence, 1983–2005.

adoption of PSA screening in blacks relative to whites. Overall, 45% of white men and 43% of black men aged 40–84 had at least one PSA test by the year 2000 *(4)*.

The widespread adoption of PSA screening has changed the face of prostate cancer in the United States. Prostate cancer is now being detected at earlier ages and earlier stages than ever before. The trends are reflected in Figs. 2 and 3, which show annual disease incidence rates by age and SEER historic stage. Figure 5 plots annual PSA screening frequencies among blacks and whites based on the estimates of Mariotto et al. *(4)*.

While historical incidence trends showed a clear increase in prostate cancer rates with age, prostate cancers are now detected most commonly among men in their 70s, which

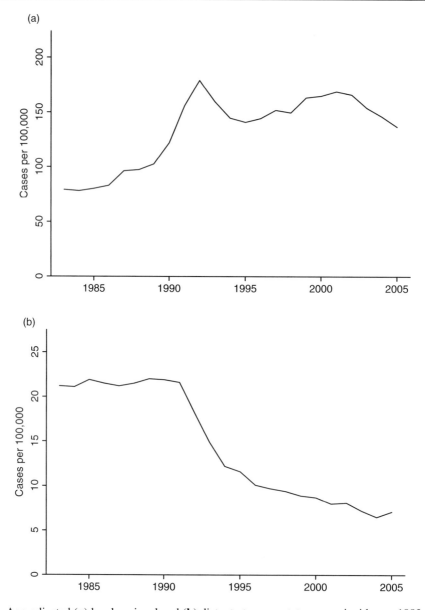

**Fig. 3.** Age-adjusted (**a**) local-regional and (**b**) distant-stage prostate cancer incidence, 1983–2005.

is also the age group most frequently tested *(4)*. Moreover, incidence among men over 80 has declined and is now approaching that of men aged 60–69. In 1985, the median age at prostate cancer diagnosis was 72; in 2004 it was 67.

Perhaps the most striking sign of the changing nature of prostate cancer in the PSA era is the decline in the frequency of distant-stage disease. Since 1990, the incidence of distant-stage prostate cancer has declined by more than 70%, from 22 per 100,000 to 6.5 per 100,000 *(1)*. It seems likely that the dramatic drop in distant-stage incidence is largely attributable to PSA screening, but a recent study modeling the stage shift associated with PSA in the United States was not able to reproduce the full decline *(7)*. The investigators concluded that other factors, including increasing public awareness of

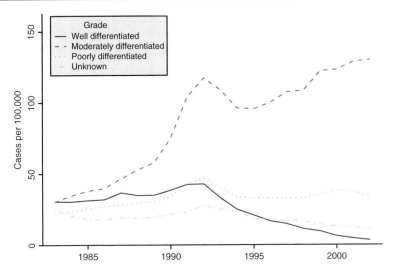

**Fig. 4.** Age-adjusted grade-specific incidence, 1983–2002.

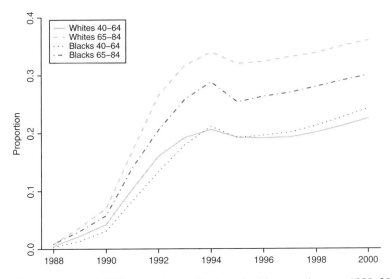

**Fig. 5.** Annual frequencies of PSA screening in black and white men by age, 1988–2000. Source Mariotto et al. *(4)*.

prostate cancer symptoms and use of PSA testing for diagnostic purposes, may also be acting to advance prostate cancer diagnosis.

The incidence of local-regional disease has correspondingly increased, but this increase consists not only of cases shifted from distant to local-regional stage at diagnosis but also of overdiagnoses—cases detected via PSA screening who would not have been diagnosed in their lifetimes in the absence of the test.

A notable characteristic of prostate tumors detected during the PSA era has been the trend toward tumors with higher Gleason grades. Initially this was thought to reflect the detection of clinically significant cancers by PSA screening. However, much of the observed shift toward higher grade tumors has been shown to be an artifact of changes in grading practices, an artifact termed the Will Rogers phenomenon *(8,9)*. Trends in grade-specific incidence are illustrated in Fig. 4 (this figure ends in 2002 due to a change in SEER coding at this time).

The clear indications that prostate cancer diagnosis is being advanced lead naturally to the following pressing questions: (a) how much earlier are prostate tumors being detected today relative to before the PSA era and (b) how many prostate tumors are being overdiagnosed and potentially overtreated?

The interval by which PSA screening advances diagnosis is called the lead time. When a new screening test is introduced in the population, the height and width of the resulting incidence peak will vary depending on the lead time (10). Given a specified pattern of screening dissemination, a longer lead time will generate a higher and wider peak in incidence than a shorter lead time. Thus, the population incidence under screening can be informative about the lead time. The lead time, in turn, is closely linked with the frequency of overdiagnosis; a screening test with a relatively lengthy lead time will be associated with a relatively high likelihood of overdiagnosis, and conversely.

Several studies have estimated the lead time associated with PSA screening using data on trends in prostate cancer incidence in the United States (11–13). Etzioni et al. (11) showed that lead times of approximately 5 and 7 years on average were consistent with observed incidence trends in whites and blacks over age 65; corresponding over-diagnosis frequencies were 29% for whites and 44% for blacks. Building on this work, Telesca et al. (13) formally estimated the lead times to be 6.3 years and 7.7 years on average among whites and blacks, respectively, over age 50. These studies assumed that disease incidence would have remained constant over time had PSA screening not been adopted, and the resulting estimates pertain to the entire population of screen-detected cases, including those overdiagnosed by PSA screening. The higher lead times among blacks are consistent with the observation that incidence rates in blacks do not drop as much as incidence rates in whites after peaking in the early 1990s. A recent study (14) compared three different models for estimating lead time based on US prostate cancer incidence in men aged 40–84 and found average lead times among screen-detected, non-overdiagnosed cases to be between 5.4 and 6.9 years with corresponding overdiagnosis frequencies ranging from 20 to 40%. These estimates are lower than those estimated in other populations and in other settings, such as the Rotterdam section of the European Randomized Study of Screening for Prostate Cancer (15). Draisma et al. (14) discuss reasons for the difference.

In summary, PSA screening has clearly left its mark on prostate cancer incidence patterns in the United States. The trends are consistent with tumors being detected an average of 5–7 years earlier than they would have been in the absence of screening. In addition to the large peak in incidence observed in the early 1990s due to rapid adoption of PSA screening, a subsequent, smaller peak has become apparent in recent years and this is likely due to the use of extended (10–12 core) biopsy protocols which began in the late 1990s and is now standard practice in the United States. In the next section, we discuss the implications of incidence changes for mortality and explore other changes in patterns of care that might also be acting to reduce prostate cancer deaths.

## PROSTATE CANCER MORTALITY IN THE UNITED STATES: 1983–2005

Figure 6 summarizes trends in prostate cancer mortality by age and race. Joinpoint analysis of these data (2) reveals that prostate cancer mortality has declined by 35% since its peak in 1992, 36% in whites and 31% in blacks (the latter decline measured

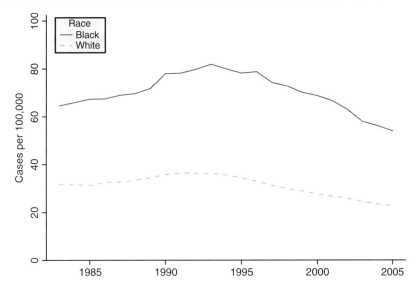

**Fig. 6.** Age-adjusted prostate cancer mortality by race, 1983–2005 *(2)*. Regression lines and annual percent change (APC) are calculated using the Joinpoint *(30)* method (http://srab.cancer.gov/joinpoint/).

from 1993, since this was the year in which the death rate peaked among blacks). Although mortality has been declining in other major cancers since the early 1990s, the annual declines in prostate cancer are among the largest in magnitude. From 1995 to 2005, prostate cancer mortality for both whites and blacks declined by an average of 4.1% per year *(2)*. These figures clearly suggest a degree of success in controlling the disease.

Perhaps even more striking than the mortality trends are the trends in survival rates among men with prostate cancer. The latest figures from SEER cite a 5-year relative survival of 99% among prostate cancer cases diagnosed in 2000, up from 78% among men diagnosed in 1986. However, it is important to recognize that improvements in relative and cause-specific survival rates do not reflect true increases in life expectancy since survival rates among men diagnosed during the PSA era can be greatly inflated by overdiagnosis and lead time. In addition, the relative survival calculated by SEER is based on excess deaths observed among prostate cancer cases relative to deaths among age-matched men in the US population. Since more than half of the prostate cancer cases detected today are identified through PSA screening and since men undergoing screening tend to be healthier than age-matched population controls *(16)*, today's prostate cancer cases represent a relatively healthy cohort, yielding a correspondingly lower number of excess deaths when compared against the general population and a correspondingly higher relative survival. Therefore, comparison of relative survival across different calendar intervals is not a valid indicator of the true increase in life expectancy among prostate cancer cases.

In the absence of results from randomized controlled trials regarding the efficacy of PSA screening, population data have become the primary source of information on the likely benefits of PSA screening. Although many have speculated that there must be a causal association between the rise in screening and the fall in mortality, formal analysis has been challenging, not least because cancer registry data do not include a variable indicating whether a prostate cancer case was diagnosed by routine screening or not. Studies that have attempted to make formal inferences from the population data in the PSA era generally fall into one of the two categories: ecologic and modeling studies.

In ecologic analysis, prostate cancer death rates are compared across geographic regions in which screening utilization varies. The analysis goal is to determine whether the areas with higher screening frequencies have greater mortality declines than those with lower screening frequencies.

Most ecologic analyses conducted to date have yielded negative results. For example, in the United States, an ecologic study comparing prostate cancer mortality in the Seattle and Connecticut SEER registries was highly influential in fueling skepticism about the efficacy of the test (17). The study found that the PSA testing rate from 1987 to 1990 in Seattle was five times that in Connecticut, but mortality due to prostate cancer was almost identical in the two areas by 1997. However, a further analysis (18) that included all nine core SEER areas found that the differences in annual PSA testing frequencies between Seattle and Connecticut were essentially confined to the first few years of the PSA era and that between 1991 and 1996 the proportions of men tested in the two areas were fairly similar. Moreover, even the SEER areas with the lowest frequencies of PSA screening had substantial numbers of men tested. For example, from 1991 to 1996, the SEER areas with lowest PSA use had about 30% of eligible men tested each year on average, and those with the highest PSA use had about 45% of eligible men tested. This study therefore concluded that differences in the PSA use across SEER areas may not have been sufficient to produce noticeable differences in disease-specific mortality, particularly in light of variation in other patterns of care across areas.

Among the other changes in prostate cancer patterns of care, the most significant has probably been the initial treatment of primary tumors. Even before the PSA era, the introduction of nerve-sparing surgical techniques for radical prostatectomy had led to a dramatic increase in the frequency of surgery as primary treatment for the disease. From 1983 to 1987 the fraction of local-regional cases who received therapy with curative intent (surgery or radiation) was 43% (1); by 1991 it was close to 70% (6) (Fig. 7). In addition, radiation therapies have evolved enormously since the 1980s, with the development of novel technologies for delivering higher doses of radiation without substantially increasing morbidity. Finally, the use of hormonal therapies as adjuvant to primary radiation therapies has increased dramatically (5,19) following randomized trials (20) that showed a significant advantage to be associated with combination therapy in locally advanced cases. The combination of increased aggressive therapy in the 1980s, increased intensity of radiation therapies in the 1990s, and the addition of hormonal therapies as adjuvant to radiation therapy could have produced a substantial reduction in prostate cancer mortality during the PSA era. Acknowledging this possibility, Albertsen (21), in an editorial titled *The Prostate Cancer Conundrum* states that "The recent decline in prostate cancer mortality rates suggests that some treatment is having an impact. Whether this is the result of the early use of androgen withdrawal therapy or whether this is the result of widespread use of surgery or radiation remains to be determined."

The fact that trends in disease-specific death rates are a complex product of screening and treatment changes over time makes it extremely challenging to determine how much of the mortality decline may be attributed to any single intervention such as screening. To assess the likely contribution of PSA screening to mortality trends, several models of

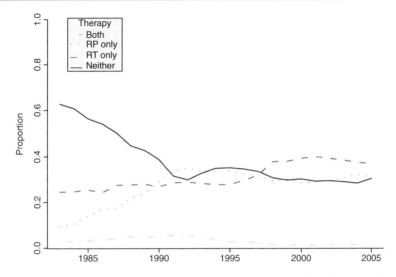

**Fig. 7.** Proportion of local-regional diagnoses selecting specified initial therapy, 1983–2005.

screening in the population setting have been developed. These models are referred to as surveillance models because they aim to replicate surveillance data reflecting cancer trends in the population.

Surveillance models provide a quantitative link between the frequency of screening in the population and the number of lives plausibly saved by early detection. The results of these models indicate that PSA screening plausibly explains a significant fraction but not all the drop in mortality. For example, a simple early model suggested that the initial downturn in mortality could have been wholly attributed to PSA screening only under an implausibly short-average lead time (about 3 years) *(22)*. A more extensive version of this model projected mortality trends through 2000 in the absence and in the presence of PSA screening and estimated that by the year 2000 PSA screening could account for approximately 45% of the difference between mortality projected in the absence of screening and observed mortality *(23)*. A second model estimated that PSA screening could account for as much as 70% of the difference between observed mortality and mortality projected in the absence of screening *(12,23)*. Both models superimpose observed screening trends on an underlying model of disease natural history. This produces a shift in the distribution of stage at diagnosis in the population. The mortality declines projected by the models arise from the assumption that a case shifted by screening to an earlier stage at diagnosis has a corresponding shift in expected disease-specific survival.

Rather than using population screening patterns to generate a stage shift, Feuer et al. *(24)* directly investigated the implications of the observed decline in distant-stage incidence for mortality trends. Assuming that each case not diagnosed in distant-stage represented a case shifted to local-regional stage by screening, and that each such case would have a corresponding shift in disease-specific survival, their model projected mortality declines of 18% from 1990 to 1999 among whites, whereas the observed mortality decline was 21%. This model is not completely comparable with the aforementioned models *(12,23)*, however, because its results assume that mortality would have remained at the level observed in 1992 in the absence of screening, whereas both aforementioned models project that mortality would have increased beyond the level observed in 1992 in the absence of screening.

Taken together, the models of PSA screening, stage-specific incidence, and prostate cancer mortality consistently suggest a positive role for early detection under the fundamental assumption that stage shift equals survival shift. However, they also leave room for benefits of treatment and potentially also for the effects of other interventions such as early detection of recurrent disease due to PSA monitoring or even behavioral changes that may have acted to reduce disease-specific mortality.

## DISCUSSION

This review of prostate cancer trends before and during the PSA era tells the story of a historical shift in the United States in the way the disease is detected and treated *(25)*. Not only are tumors being diagnosed earlier by a combination of PSA screening and extended core biopsy, but also treatments previously reserved for metastatic tumors are now being used fairly routinely as adjuvant and neoadjuvant therapies for localized disease.

While population cancer trends have the potential to be highly informative about the benefits and costs of interventions as implemented in the population setting, it can be extremely challenging to interpret incidence and mortality patterns correctly. In the case of prostate cancer, there are many different factors to consider. In addition to screening and treatment, changes over time in epidemiologic exposures or health behaviors may be sufficient to impact population disease trends. For instance, obesity, which showed a substantial increase in frequency between 1980 and 2000 in the United States, has been linked with higher incidence of poorly differentiated prostate tumors and shorter disease-specific survival following diagnosis *(26–28)*.

Isolating the impact of any single factor on disease trends requires excellent data on patterns of care and a valid analytic approach. A major issue in determining the likely impact of PSA screening is that dissemination of the test was not tracked in real time. Thus, our current best picture of the spread of PSA screening in the US population is based on a reconstruction of screening frequencies using information from a year 2000 population survey and medical claims data. Even now, information on how the test is actually being used, including criteria for biopsy referral and the frequency of biopsy, is not systematically collected. It is likely that these have changed over time as our knowledge of disease natural history in relation to PSA has evolved.

Making inferences about intervention impact based on population disease trends requires a valid analytic model. We have discussed ecologic studies and surveillance modeling approaches to assess the impact of PSA screening on mortality. We are concerned that ecologic analysis may have limited utility for quantitative inference in the case of PSA screening because of the potential for variation in other patterns of care across geographic areas. Ecologic analyses are easily misinterpreted, particularly if they are negative *(29)*.

Surveillance modeling is an alternative approach that quantitatively links patterns of care in the population with disease incidence and mortality trends. Because such models invariably rest on a variety of assumptions, it is critical for these assumptions to be clearly stated and the model limitations clearly understood. Ideally, several models should be developed and compared to increase confidence that the model results are robust. This is the objective of the Cancer Intervention and Surveillance Modeling

Network of the National Cancer Institute (http://cisnet.cancer.gov/), which is currently sponsoring three independent prostate cancer modeling groups to quantify the effects of screening and treatment changes on prostate cancer mortality trends in the United States.

In conclusion, the trends in prostate cancer mortality in the United States clearly show that something is working in the management of the disease. The results of the ongoing randomized screening trials in the United States and Europe will shed important light on the likely role of PSA screening but will almost certainly raise a host of new questions about designing optimal screening policies. The challenge for the future will be to clarify how the trial results translate into the population setting and ultimately to devise population strategies for disease control that balance the benefits with the inevitable costs.

**Acknowledgements**   Research supported by Cancer Intervention and Surveillance Modeling Network, National Cancer Institute, grant number U01-CA88160.

# REFERENCES

1. Surveillance, Epidemiology, and End Results (SEER) Program (www.seer.cancer.gov) SEER*Stat Database: Incidence—SEER 9 Regs Limited-Use, Nov 2006 Sub (1973–2005), National Cancer Institute, DCCPS, Surveillance Research Program, Cancer Statistics Branch, released April 2008, based on the November 2007 submission.
2. Surveillance, Epidemiology, and End Results (SEER) Program (www.seer.cancer.gov) SEER*Stat Database: Mortality—All COD, Public-Use With State, Total U.S. (1969–2005), National Cancer Institute, DCCPS, Surveillance Research Program, Cancer Statistics Branch, released April 2008. Underlying mortality data provided by NCHS (www.cdc.gov/nchs).
3. Surveillance, Epidemiology, and End Results (SEER) Program (www.seer.cancer.gov). Prevalence database: "US Estimated Complete Prevalence Counts on 1/1/2005". National Cancer Institute, DCCPS, Surveillance Research Program, Statistical Research and Applications Branch, released April 2008, based on the November 2007 SEER data submission.
4. Mariotto, A., Etzioni, R., Krapcho, M., and Feuer, E. J. (2007) Reconstructing prostate-specific antigen (PSA) testing patterns among black and white men in the US from Medicare claims and the National Health Interview Survey *Cancer* **109,** 1877–86.
5. Cooperberg, M. R., Grossfeld, G. D., Lubeck, D. P., and Carroll, P. R. (2003) National practice patterns and time trends in androgen ablation for localized prostate cancer *J Natl Cancer Inst* **95,** 981–9.
6. Zeliadt, S., Potosky, A., Etzioni, R., Ramsey, S., and Penson, D. (2004) Racial disparity in primary and adjuvant treatment for nonmetastatic prostate cancer: SEER-Medicare trends 1991 to 1999 *Urology* **64,** 1171–6.
7. Etzioni, R., Gulati, R., Falcon, S., and Penson, D. (2008) Impact of PSA screening on the incidence of advanced stage prostate cancer in the US: A surveillance modeling approach *Med Decis Making* **28**(3), 323–31.
8. Albertsen, P. C., Hanley, J. A., Barrows, G. H., Penson, D. F., Kowalczyk, P. D., Sanders, M. M., and Fine, J. (2005) Prostate cancer and the Will Rogers phenomenon *J Natl Cancer Inst* **97,** 1248–53.
9. Thompson, I. M., Canby-Hagino, E., and Lucia, M. S. (2005) Stage migration and grade inflation in prostate cancer: Will Rogers meets Garrison Keillor *J Natl Cancer Inst* **97,** 1236–7.
10. Feuer, E. J., and Wun, L. M. (1992) How much of the recent rise in breast cancer incidence can be explained by increases in mammography utilization? A dynamic population model approach *Am J Epidemiol* **136,** 1423–36.
11. Etzioni, R., Penson, D. F., Legler, J. M., Di Tommaso, D., Boer, R., Gann, P. H., and Feuer, E. J. (2002) Overdiagnosis due to prostate-specific antigen screening: Lessons from U.S. prostate cancer incidence trends *J Natl Cancer Inst* **94,** 981–90.
12. Tsodikov, A., Szabo, A., and Wegelin, J. (2006) A population model of prostate cancer incidence *Stat Med* **25,** 2846–66.
13. Telesca, D., Etzioni, R., and Gulati, R. (2008) Estimating Lead Time and Overdiagnosis Associated with PSA Screening from Prostate Cancer Incidence Trends *Biometrics* **64,** 10–9.

14. Draisma, G., Etzioni, R., Tsodikov, A., Mariotto, A., Wever, E., Gulati, R., Feuer, E., and De Koning, H. J. (2008, Submitted for publication) Reconciling Differing Estimates of Lead Time and Overdiagnosis Due to PSA Screening: Results from the Cancer Intervention and Surveillance Modeling Network *J Natl Cancer Inst*.
15. Draisma, G., Boer, R., Otto, S. J., Van Der Cruijsen, I. W., Damhuis, R. A., Schröder, F. H., and De Koning, H. J. (2003) Lead times and overdetection due to prostate-specific antigen screening: Estimates from the European Randomized Study of Screening for Prostate Cancer *J Natl Cancer Inst* **95,** 868–78.
16. Weiss, N. S., and Rossing, M. A. (1996) Healthy screened bias in epidemiologic studies of cancer incidence *Epidemiology* **7,** 319–22.
17. Lu-Yao, G., Albertsen, P. C., Stanford, J. L., Stukel, T. A., Walker-Corkery, E. S., and Barry, M. J. (2002) Natural experiment examining impact of aggressive screening and treatment on prostate cancer mortality in two fixed cohorts from Seattle area and Connecticut *BMJ* **325,** 740.
18. Shaw, P. A., Etzioni, R., Zeliadt, S. B., Mariotto, A., Karnofski, K., Penson, D. F., Weiss, N. S., and Feuer, E. J. (2004) An ecologic study of prostate-specific antigen screening and prostate cancer mortality in nine geographic areas of the United States *Am J Epidemiol* **160,** 1059–69.
19. Zeliadt, S. B., Potosky, A. L., Etzioni, R., Ramsey, S. D., and Penson, D. F. (2004) Racial disparity in primary and adjuvant treatment for nonmetastatic prostate cancer: SEER-Medicare trends 1991 to 1999 *Urology* **64,** 1171–6.
20. Bolla, M., Collette, L., Blank, L., Warde, P., Dubois, J. B., Mirimanoff, R. O., Storme, G., Bernier, J., Kuten, A., Sternberg, C., Mattelaer, J., Lopez Torecilla, J., Pfeffer, J. R., Lino Cutajar, C., Zurlo, A., and Pierart, M. (2002) Long-term results with immediate androgen suppression and external irradiation in patients with locally advanced prostate cancer (an EORTC study): A phase III randomised trial *Lancet* **360,** 103–6.
21. Albertsen, P. C. (2003) The prostate cancer conundrum *J Natl Cancer Inst* **95,** 930–1.
22. Etzioni, R., Legler, J. M., Feuer, E. J., Merrill, R. M., Cronin, K. A., and Hankey, B. F. (1999) Cancer surveillance series: Interpreting trends in prostate cancer—Part III: Quantifying the link between population prostate-specific antigen testing and recent declines in prostate cancer mortality *J Natl Cancer Inst* **91,** 1033–9.
23. Etzioni, R., Tsodikov, A., Mariotto, A., Szabo, A., Falcon, S., Wegelin, J., Ditommaso, D., Karnofski, K., Gulati, R., Penson, D. F., and Feuer, E. (2008) Quantifying the role of PSA screening in the US prostate cancer mortality decline *Cancer Causes Control* **19,** 175–81.
24. Feuer, E. J., Mariotto, A., and Merrill, R. (2002) Modeling the impact of the decline in distant stage disease on prostate carcinoma mortality rates *Cancer* **95,** 870–80.
25. Cooperberg, M. R., Lubeck, D. P., Meng, M. V., Mehta, S. S., and Carroll, P. R. (2004) The Changing Face of Low-Risk Prostate Cancer: Trends in Clinical Presentation and Primary Management *J Clin Oncol* **22,** 2141–9.
26. Kristal, A. R., and Gong, Z. (2007) Obesity and prostate cancer mortality *Future Oncol* **3,** 557–67.
27. Gong, Z., Agalliu, I., Lin, D. W., Stanford, J. L., and Kristal, A. R. (2007) Obesity is associated with increased risks of prostate cancer metastasis and death after initial cancer diagnosis in middle-aged men *Cancer* **109,** 1192–202.
28. Gong, Z., Neuhouser, M. L., Goodman, P. J., Albanes, D., Chi, C., Hsing, A. W., Lippman, S. M., Platz, E. A., Pollak, M. N., Thompson, I. M., and Kristal, A. R. (2006) Obesity, diabetes, and risk of prostate cancer: results from the prostate cancer prevention trial *Cancer Epidemiol Biomarkers Prev* **15,** 1977–83.
29. Etzioni, R., and Feuer, E. (In Press) Learning from international studies of prostate cancer mortality: A cautionary tale *Lancet Oncol*.
30. Kim, H. J., Fay, M. P., Feuer, E. J., and Midthune, D. N. (2000) Permutation tests for joinpoint regression with applications to cancer rates *Stat Med* **19,** 335–51.

# 2

# Trends in Prostate Cancer Screening: Overview of the UK

*Richard J. Bryant and Freddie C. Hamdy*

## CONTENTS

## SUMMARY

There is a continuing lack of evidence that screening for prostate cancer results in a significant improvement in survival and/or quality of life of men with the disease. Moreover, there is a growing concern that the introduction of a national prostate cancer screening programme might result in over-diagnosis of men with "clinically insignificant" or "indolent" prostate cancer who could be harmed by unnecessary treatments. To date, systematic screening for prostate cancer has not been introduced as a public health policy in the United Kingdom, and the rate of opportunistic prostate-specific antigen (PSA) testing remains low compared to countries in Western Europe and in the USA. The UK Department of Health guidelines recommend that when an asymptomatic man requests PSA testing, he should be counselled regarding the controversies and uncertainties surrounding prostate cancer screening and treatment, and PSA testing should proceed only once he is able to make a fully informed decision. Several randomised controlled trials are in progress in Europe and the UK and will shed new light on whether or not PSA-based screening for prostate cancer offers more benefit than harm. Until such data become available, the responsibility of the urological community at large is to inform appropriately men who are seeking screening and to prevent over-diagnosis and over-treatment of this common but ubiquitous malignancy.

**Key Words:** Prostate cancer, Screening, United Kingdom, Prostate-specific antigen (PSA).

Prostate cancer is an important health problem in the UK. In 2004 there were almost 35,000 new cases of prostate cancer diagnosed and each year around 10,000 men die from this disease alone *(1)*. It is now the most commonly diagnosed male malignancy

From: *Current Clinical Urology: Prostate Cancer Screening*, Edited by: D. P. Ankerst et al.
DOI 10.1007/978-1-60327-281-0_2 © Humana Press, a part of Springer Science+Business Media, LLC 2009

and the second most common cause of male cancer related death in the UK. The incidence has increased during the late 1980s and 1990s, as in many other Western countries, largely as a result of prostate-specific antigen (PSA) testing. The mortality rate from prostate cancer peaked in the early 1990s in the UK and the age-adjusted mortality rate has subsequently declined over the last 15 years for reasons that as yet remain unclear *(2)*. This reduction in prostate cancer mortality since 1992 has been less pronounced in the UK compared with the USA *(3)*. The US reduction coincided with the widespread uptake of PSA testing in that country, but whilst this might indicate an early effect of initial screening rounds on men with more aggressive but asymptomatic disease, there is still no conclusive evidence to support the concept that PSA-based screening decreases prostate cancer-specific mortality *(4)*. The recent differences between the USA and UK in rates of decline in prostate cancer-related mortality may also be attributable to other factors such as different approaches to detection or prostate cancer treatment.

Proponents of PSA-based prostate cancer screening in the UK include members of the general public, the media, and the medical profession, however, at present, the merits of introducing a national prostate cancer screening programme in the UK are unclear, and the evidence to support such a programme remains insufficient. In the absence of robust data from randomised controlled trials (RCTs) indicating a survival benefit for men who undergo prostate cancer screening compared with men who do not, it would be inappropriate to introduce such a programme on a national scale. The situation appears somewhat different in the USA, where the American Urological Association and the American Cancer Society both recommend screening men over the age of 50 for prostate cancer. In order for a disease to qualify for a screening programme it should meet several criteria as defined by Wilson and Jungner *(5)* (Table 1). These valid principles have so far guided the debate on the introduction of a national prostate cancer screening programme in the UK.

The aim of any "screening" programme is to use an appropriate test to identify cases, within a population at risk, before clinical symptoms or signs are present, rather than the disease being diagnosed at a later and more advanced stage when symptoms or signs have become apparent. In the case of cancer, the assumption is that either the malignancy or a precursor lesion may be detectable during a "latent" period prior to clinical

Table 1
**Wilson and Jungner Criteria for Mass Screening for Any Disease**

1   The condition is an important health problem
2   There is adequate knowledge of the natural history of the condition, with a recognised latency period or early symptomatic stage
3   There is a simple, safe, acceptable, precise, and validated screening test
4   There is an agreed policy on the further diagnostic intervention
5   There is an effective treatment or intervention
6   There are evidence-based policies covering who to treat and how to treat
7   There is evidence from high-quality RCTs that screening reduces mortality or morbidity
8   There is evidence that the complete screening programme (i.e. test, diagnostic procedures, treatment/intervention) is clinically, socially, and ethically acceptable
9   There is evidence that overall benefit from the screening programme outweighs the physical and psychological harm

manifestation. The over-riding aim of any population-based screening programme is to reduce cancer morbidity and mortality caused by the disease, based on the premise that early diagnosis and treatment improves both prognosis and survival. Prostate cancer may be detected at an early stage in men by performing a serum PSA test followed by a prostate biopsy, and patients with organ-confined prostate cancer may be cured by either radical prostatectomy or radical radiotherapy. Because of significant lead-times to the development of life-threatening disease, and the recognised stage-migration caused by screening, many cancers are not likely to cause harm to men who harbour the disease. "Over-diagnosis" and subsequent "over-treatment" of disease which does not need to be cured could therefore prevail as a consequence of systematic screening, in the absence of tests which can discriminate between potentially harmful and clinically insignificant cancers.

Current experience and controversies surrounding prostate cancer screening in the UK are discussed below.

## WHAT HAPPENED IN THE UK SINCE THE INTRODUCTION OF PSA TESTING?

A small scale study of screening acceptability was performed in the UK in the late 1980s, which demonstrated that men in the community will attend for PSA testing if invited (6). As PSA testing became widely available in the following years, the Department of Health discouraged the use of PSA testing for prostate cancer screening, until the late 1990s. In 1995, the Health Technology Assessment (HTA) programme commissioned two systematic reviews of the literature, which clearly stated that there was insufficient evidence to recommend mass-screening for prostate cancer as a public health policy (7,8). The reviews recommended that urgent research into screening and treatment of prostate cancer should be undertaken in the form of large RCTs. Subsequently, HTA issued a call for primary research in this area, and commissioned the feasibility phase of the ProtecT (*Pro*state *te*sting for *c*ancer and *T*reatment) study, followed by the full trial in 2001 (9,10). The ProtecT study is currently the largest randomised controlled trial of treatment effectiveness in prostate cancer worldwide. The feasibility phase demonstrated that screening was acceptable amongst British men, and that the majority agreed to be randomised to a three-arm trial of active monitoring, radical prostatectomy, and 3-D conformal radiotherapy. The main trial started in 2001, and aims to test 130,000 asymptomatic men aged 50–70 years over a period of 5 years. Of those, 1,800 patients with clinically localised prostate cancer will be randomised to active monitoring, radical prostatectomy, or radiotherapy. The primary end-point will be survival at 10 years, with a number of secondary end-points including detailed quality of life analyses. The study has been extended through further support from Cancer Research, UK and the Department of Health to include the evaluation of case-finding. This effectively converted the ProtecT study into the intervention arm of a clustered randomised trial of screening. Recruitment to the study is near completion, and results will become available within the next decade, at the same time as the other much awaited screening studies in Europe and the USA.

By the year 2000, the UK Department of Health recommended that if a man requested PSA testing to be screened for prostate cancer, careful counselling should be given regarding the uncertainties surrounding the diagnosis and treatment of the disease, and

PSA testing should be performed only after the man is fully informed and able to make such a decision.

Despite the absence of a proven benefit from PSA-based prostate cancer screening recent years have seen a modest rise in the number of men undergoing ad hoc PSA-test screening in the UK. A study in England and Wales suggests that the annual rate of PSA testing in men aged 45–84 years without a previous prostate cancer diagnosis is approximately 6% (11), which remains low compared to rates of testing in Western Europe and in the USA where a recent estimate suggested testing rates of over 25% in men aged 50–75 years (12). A recent pilot study of screening in a younger age group of men between 45 and 49 years embedded in the UK ProtecT study not only showed a lower uptake of testing in these men compared with the older population, albeit in the context of an RCT, but also demonstrated that clinically significant cancers occur in these younger men (13).

The "lead-time" for a cancer is the length of time by which the date of diagnosis is advanced through screening from the date it would have been diagnosed clinically. For prostate cancer the lead-time using PSA testing ranges from 5 to 14 years depending on the grade and stage of the disease (14–18). The decline in mortality seen in the UK since the early 1990s is therefore unlikely to be attributable to PSA testing as the effect has appeared too early, given the long lead-time involved in the progression of prostate cancer. For instance, only a small proportion of men with early stage prostate cancer would be predicted to die from this malignancy over the next 20 years in the absence of screening even when treated conservatively (19). Although PSA testing became widespread in the USA in the late 1980s and early 1990s, the reduction in mortality occurred too quickly to be attributed to early detection alone (20,21), whilst the reduced mortality seen in the UK coincided with a period where PSA testing and aggressive treatment for prostate cancer was considerably more limited. It is likely that hitherto unidentified factors other than increased detection and radical treatment of early-stage prostate cancer account for the decline in prostate cancer mortality witnessed in the UK since the early 1990s. This has been particularly apparent in men aged 55–74 years but has also been witnessed to a lesser degree in men aged over 75 years. Potential explanations for this reduction in prostate cancer-specific mortality since the early 1990s include increasingly radical therapy amongst younger men with localised or screen-detected low-volume disease, effects of stage migration, and more widespread use of medical androgen suppressing therapies and aggressive treatment of early locally advanced disease.

Current knowledge of the natural history of prostate cancer is limited to clinically diagnosed cases, whilst very little is known of the natural history of cases of screen-detected prostate cancer, although this is likely to improve in the near future following the results of randomised clinical trials on both sides of the Atlantic (22,23). Given that clinically detected prostate cancer often remains indolent or progresses very slowly and thereby may be considered "clinically insignificant", it is likely that a substantial proportion of men in the UK who may be found to have screen-detected prostate cancer would never develop clinically significant disease. A recent study suggests that over half of all men eligible for expectant management are actually over-treated in the USA (24). Indeed, it is likely that many men in the UK with screen-detected prostate cancer would die of competing morbidity, and it has been estimated that only around one in eight cases of screen-detected prostate cancer would cause mortality if left untreated (25). Prostate cancer screening would primarily detect organ-confined disease, and it is presently difficult to differentiate between indolent organ-confined cases, which could undergo active surveillance, and high-risk or potentially aggressive cases which would merit active intervention *(26)*.

Despite the persistent lack of evidence, recent guidelines from the UK National Institute for Clinical Excellence (NICE) recommend that men with low-risk prostate cancer should first be offered active surveillance, a view contested by the British Association of Urological Surgeons, which recommends that men with perceived low-risk disease should be explained the uncertainties around treatment, and offered active surveillance alongside radical interventions in order to make an informed decision regarding management of their disease *(27)*. It is hoped that improved risk stratification, based on novel biomarkers in clinical samples, may enable improved targeting of radical treatment to those men with organ-confined prostate cancer at risk of rapid progression. The development of a "molecular signature" for risk stratification of prostate cancer cases is warranted in combination with nomograms, which together may enable more accurate risk assessment of clinically localised disease in the future *(28)*.

A screening test should ideally have a high sensitivity, specificity, positive predictive value, and negative predictive value. The level of serum PSA used as a threshold to separate cases of the disease from men without prostate cancer is controversial. For instance, the Prostate Cancer Prevention Trial demonstrated that a significant proportion of asymptomatic men with a PSA less than 4 ng/mL may harbour a prostate cancer detectable by prostate biopsy *(29)*. There is therefore no PSA threshold below which an asymptomatic man can be told confidently that he does not have prostate cancer, and furthermore, no test can reliably differentiate "indolent" from clinically significant disease, making reliable treatment decisions difficult to reach. Paradoxically, a raised PSA test does not necessarily mean that the individual has prostate cancer, whilst a "low" PSA value does not eliminate the possibility of an underlying prostate cancer *(30,31)*, and the debate regarding the use of PSA testing in the UK as a screening tool must also consider the acceptability of performing large numbers of prostate biopsies, a substantial proportion of which will not detect a malignancy. A reduction in the PSA threshold used to trigger a prostate biopsy would increase both the number of cancers detected and the negative biopsy rate, and this may result in the PSA test being unacceptable in the context of a screening programme as demonstrated by Roddam et al. *(32)*, on behalf of the UK Prostate Cancer Risk Management Group. Lowering the PSA threshold to 2 ng/mL would increase the number of referrals from 110 to 230 per 1,000 men tested with an increase in the cancer-detection rate from 3.6% to 5.8% in the UK. As the extra cancers detected are likely to be clinically localised, with no evidence that their treatment improves the outcome of the disease, such changes do not appear to be justified at present. Two large RCTs investigating the effects of prostate cancer screening are currently in progress in Europe (ERSPC) and in the USA. (the Prostate, Lung, Colon and Ovary trial) and their results are eagerly awaited *(22,23)*.

There is a paucity of studies investigating the psychological impact of repeat testing and biopsies for prostate cancer, the anxiety generated by the suspicion of cancer diagnosis, and the associated cost to society. The appropriate course of action in men with a raised PSA who are not found to have prostate cancer on an initial biopsy remains unclear, and must be taken into consideration in the prostate cancer screening debate.

The UK health providers have consistently taken the view that evidence of treatment effectiveness in screen-detected prostate cancer and benefits of screening must be

provided first, in order to inform public health policy. Very few RCTs have been performed to directly compare the outcomes of the various treatment options for men with
organ-confined prostate cancer. An important study in Scandinavia comparing "watchful waiting" with radical prostatectomy for early-stage prostate cancer demonstrated for
the first time a survival benefit and a reduced rate of disease progression for men undergoing surgery *(33)*, however, the majority of cases in this study were not representative
of screen-detected disease. It is hoped that the UK ProtecT trial described earlier in
this chapter, and the US Prostate Cancer Intervention Versus Observation Trial (PIVOT)
comparing radical prostatectomy with expectant management for all-cause mortality
*(34)*, will inform clinicians and public health policy-makers of the effectiveness of these
treatments for screen-detected localised disease.

Today, the likelihood of harm from prostate cancer screening outweighs the prospect
of benefit, leading to the inescapable conclusion that screening remains unjustified outside randomised trials investigating its effects. These longstanding dilemmas are being
resolved through large robust RCTs supported by governments and funding institutions
in the UK and elsewhere, the results of which are awaited eagerly in order to inform
public health policy.

## REFERENCES

1. Cancer Research UK Statistics http://info.cancerresearchuk.org/cancerstats/types/prostate/incidence/
2. Hussain, S., Gunnell, D., Donovan, J., McPhail S., Hamdy F., Neal D., Albertsen P., Verne J.,
   Stephens P., Trotter C., and Martin, R.M. (2008) Secular trends in prostate cancer mortality, incidence
   and treatment: England and Wales, 1975–2004 *BJU Int* **101**, 547–55.
3. Collin, S.M., Martin, R.M., Metcalfe, C., Gunnell, D., Albertsen, P.C., Neal, D., Hamdy, F.,
   Stephens, P., Lane, J.A., Moore, R., and Donovan, J. (2008) Prostate-cancer mortality in the US and
   UK in 1975–2004: an ecological study *Lancet Oncol* **9**, 445–52.
4. Ilic, D., O'Connor, D., Green, S., and Wilt, T. (2006) Screening for prostate cancer *Cochrane Database
   Syst Rev* **3**, CD004720.
5. Wilson, J.M., and Jungner, Y.G. (1968) Principles and practice of mass screening for disease *Bol Oficina
   Sanit Panam* **65**, 281–393.
6. Chadwick, D.J., Kemple, T., Astley, J.P., MacIver, A.G., Gillatt, D.A., Abrams, P., and Gingell, J.C.
   (1991) Pilot study of screening for prostate cancer in general practice *Lancet* **338**, 613–6.
7. Chamberlain, J., Melia, J., Moss, S., and Brown, J. (1997) The diagnosis, management, treatment and
   costs of prostate cancer in England and Wales *Health Technol Assess* **1(3):i–vi**, 1–53.
8. Selley, S., Donovan, J., Faulkner, A., Coast, J., and Gillatt, D. (1997) Diagnosis, management and
   screening of early localised prostate cancer *Health Technol Assess* **1(2):i**, 1–96.
9. Donovan, J.L., Hamdy, F.C., Neal, D.E., Peters, T., Oliver, S., Brindle, L., Jewell, D., Powell, P., Gillatt,
   D., Dedman, D., Mills, N., Smith, M., Noble, S., and Lane, A. (2003) Prostate testing for cancer and
   treatment (ProtecT) feasibility study *Health Technol Assess* **7**, 1–88
10. Donovan, J., Mills, N., Smith, M., Brindle, L., Jacoby, A., Peters, T., Frankel, S., Neal, D., and Hamdy,
    F. (2002) Quality improvement report: Improving design and conduct of randomised trials by embed-
    ding them in qualitative research: ProtecT (prostate testing for cancer and treatment) study *BMJ* **325**,
    766–70.
11. Melia, J., Moss, S., and Johns, L. (2004) Rates of prostate-specific antigen testing in general practice
    in England and Wales in asymptomatic and symptomatic patients: a cross-sectional study *BJU Int* **94**,
    51–6.
12. Scales, C.D. Jr., Curtis, L.H., Norris, R.D., Schulman, K.A., Albala, D.M., and Moul, J.W. (2006)
    Prostate specific antigen testing in men older than 75 years in the United States *J Urol* **176**, 511–4.
13. Lane, J.A., Howson, J., Donovan, J., Goepel, J., Dedman, D., Down, L., Turner, E., Neal, D., and
    Hamdy, F.C. (2007) Prostate cancer detection in an unselected young population: experience of the
    ProtecT study*BMJ* **335**, 1139–43.
14. Draisma, G., Boer, R., Otto, S.J., van der Cruijsen, I.W., Damhuis, R.A., Schröder, F.H., and de
    Koning, H.J. (2003) Lead times and overdetection due to prostate-specific antigen screening: estimates

from the European Randomized Study of Screening for Prostate Cancer *J Natl Cancer Inst* **95**, 868–78.

15. Brant, L.J. and Sheng, S.L. (2003) Screening for prostate cancer by using random-effects models *Royal Statist Soc* **166**, 51–62.

16. Auvinen, A., Maattanen, L., Stenman, U.H., Tammela, T., Rannikko, S., Aro, J., Juusela, H., and Hakama, M. (2002) Lead-time in prostate cancer screening (Finland) *Cancer Causes Control* **13**, 279–85.

17. Stenman, U.H., Hakama, M., Knekt, P., Aromaa, A., Teppo, L., and Leinonen, J. (1994) Serum concentrations of prostate specific antigen and its complex with alpha 1-antichymotrypsin before diagnosis of prostate cancer *Lancet* **344**, 1594–8.

18. Lilja, H., Ulmert, D., and Vickers, A.J. (2008) Prostate-specific antigen and prostate cancer: prediction, detection and monitoring *Nat Rev Cancer* **8**, 268–78.

19. Albertsen, P.C., Hanley, J.A, and Fine, J. (2005) 20-year outcomes following conservative management of clinically localized prostate cancer *JAMA* **293**, 2095–101.

20. Oliver, S.E., Gunnell, D., and Donovan, J.L. (2000) Comparison of trends in prostate-cancer mortality in England and Wales and the US *Lancet* **355**, 1788–9.

21. Shibata, A., and Whittemore, A.S. (2001) Re: Prostate cancer incidence and mortality in the United States and the United Kingdom *J Natl Cancer Inst* **93**, 1109–10.

22. de Koning, H.J., Auvinen, A., Berenguer Sanchez, A., Calais da Silva, F., Ciatto, S., Denis, L., Gohagan, J.K., Hakama, M., Hugosson, J., Kranse, R., Nelen, V., Prorok, P.C., and Schröder, F.H. European Randomized Screening for Prostate Cancer (ERSPC) Trial; International Prostate Cancer Screening Trials Evaluation Group. (2002) Large-scale randomized prostate cancer screening trials: program performances in the European Randomized Screening for Prostate Cancer trial and the Prostate, Lung, Colorectal and Ovary cancer trial *Int J Cancer* **97**, 237–44.

23. Roobol, M.J., and Schroder, F.H. (2003) European Randomized Study of Screening for Prostate Cancer: achievements and presentation *BJU international* **92**, 117–22.

24. Miller, D.C., Gruber, S.B., Hollenbeck, B.K., Montie, J.E., and Wei, J.T. (2006) Incidence of initial local therapy among men with lower-risk prostate cancer in the United States *J Natl Cancer Inst* **98**, 1134–41.

25. McGregor, M., Hanley, J.A., Boivin, J.F., and McLean, R.G. (1998) Screening for prostate cancer: estimating the magnitude of overdetection *CMAJ* **159**, 1368–72.

26. Eisenberger, M., and Partin, A. (2004) Progress toward identifying aggressive prostate cancer *N Engl J Med* **351**, 180–1.

27. Graham, J., Baker, M., Macbeth, F., and Titshall, V. (2008) Guideline Development Group. Diagnosis and treatment of prostate cancer: summary of NICE guidance *BMJ* **336**, 610–2.

28. Steyerberg, E.W., Roobol, M.J., Kattan, M.W., van der Kwast, T.H., de Koning, H.J., and Schröder, F.H. (2007) Prediction of indolent prostate cancer: validation and updating of a prognostic nomogram *J Urol.* **177**, 107–12.

29. Thompson, I.M., Pauler, D.K., Goodman, P.J., Tangen, C.M., Lucia, M.S., Parnes, H.L., Minasian, L.M., Ford, L.G., Lippman, S.M., Crawford, E.D., Crowley, J.J., and Coltman, C.A. Jr. (2004) Prevalence of prostate cancer among men with a prostate-specific antigen level < or =4.0 ng per milliliter *N Engl J Med* **350**, 2239–46.

30. Kranse, R., Beemsterboer, P., Rietbergen, J., Habbema, D., Hugosson, J., and Schroder, F.H. (1999) Predictors for biopsy outcome in the European Randomized Study of Screening for Prostate Cancer (Rotterdam region) *The Prostate* **39**, 316–22.

31. Schroder, F.H., van der Cruijsen-Koeter, I., de Koning H.J., Vis, A.N., Hoedemaeker, R.F., and Kranse, R. (2000) Prostate cancer detection at low prostate specific antigen *J Urol* **163**, 806–12.

32. Roddam, A.W., Hamdy, F.C., Allen, N.E., and Price, C.P. (2007) The impact of reducing the prostate-specific antigen threshold and including isoform reflex tests on the performance characteristics of a prostate-cancer detection programme *BJU Int* **100**, 514–7.

33. Bill-Axelson, A., Holmberg, L., Ruutu, M., Häggman, M., Andersson, S.O., Bratell, S., Spångberg, A., Busch, C., Nordling, S., Garmo, H., Palmgren, J., Adami, H.O., Norlén, B.J., and Johansson, J.E. (2005) Scandinavian Prostate Cancer Group Study No. 4. Radical prostatectomy versus watchful waiting in early prostate cancer *N Engl J Med* **352**, 1977–84.

34. Wilt, T.J., and Brawer, M.K. (1997) The Prostate Cancer Intervention Versus Observation Trial (PIVOT) *Oncology (Williston Park)* **11**, 1133–9.

# 3 Trends in Prostate Cancer Screening: Canada

*Robert K. Nam and Laurence H. Klotz*

CONTENTS

## SUMMARY

In Canada, prostate cancer is the most common male malignancy and the third most common cause of cancer death in males. Within a publicly funded healthcare system, government guidelines do not support prostate cancer screening with prostate-specific antigen (PSA), despite national primary care and specialist groups taking a more favorable position. Current surveys among patients and physicians indicate that the practice of prostate cancer screening is widespread. This has translated into temporal trends in the national incidence rates for prostate cancer which are similar to other constituencies which employ widespread screening. Methods of prostate cancer screening mainly consist of PSA, the free:total PSA ratio, and digital rectal examination (DRE). Nomograms based on Canadian-based cohorts are being used and evaluated in the context of a prostate cancer screening program. Factors such as age, ethnicity, family history of prostate cancer, and urinary symptoms are being incorporated in PSA evaluations to assess an individual's risk for prostate cancer.

**Key Words:** Prostate cancer, Screening, PSA, Nomogram, Canada.

From: *Current Clinical Urology: Prostate Cancer Screening*, Edited by: D. P. Ankerst et al.
DOI 10.1007/978-1-60327-281-0_3 © Humana Press, a part of Springer Science+Business Media, LLC 2009

## THE STATE OF PROSTATE CANCER IN CANADA

Prostate cancer is a large public health burden in Canada. It is the most common male malignancy, and is the third most common cause of cancer deaths in males *(1)*. It was estimated for 2007 that 22,300 new cases would be diagnosed and 4,300 would die from the disease *(1)*.

The incidence of prostate cancer rose in the early 1980s largely due to the advent of transurethral resection of the prostate (TURP) for benign prostatic hyperplasia (BPH) (Fig. 1). This minimally invasive technique increased the volume of prostate surgery which increased the rate of incidental, sub-clinical prostate cancer from the prostate specimens removed by TURP. The incidence, subsequently, sharply rose by 1987 with

**Age-Standardized Incidence Rates (ASIR) for Selected Cancers, Males, Canada, 1978-2007**

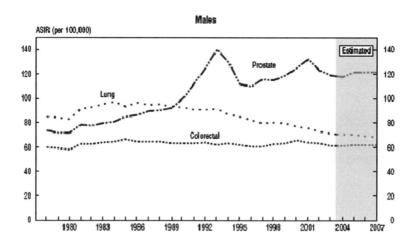

**Age-Standardized Mortality Rates (ASMR) for Selected Cancers, Males, Canada, 1978-2007**

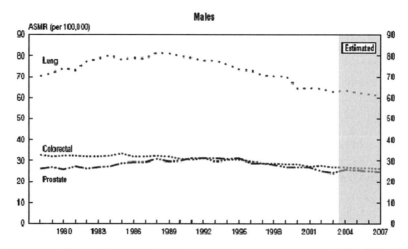

**Fig. 1.** Age-standardized incidence and mortality rates for prostate cancer, 1978–2007, Canada.

the introduction of serum prostate-specific antigen (PSA) level as a new screening instrument for prostate cancer *(2)* and peaked by 1993 (Fig. 1). The drop after 1993 was likely due to the harvest effect of prior identification of prevalent cases of cancer.

Although this has paralleled US trends in prostate cancer incidence, a second peak in incidence occurred in 2001 which was not seen in the USA. The reason for this is unclear. A possible explanation is a wave of intensified screening after a well-known Canadian public figure was diagnosed with clinically localized prostate cancer and underwent surgery for treatment in early 2001 *(1)*. The Right Honorable Mr. Allan Rock was the current Minister of Health for the federal government and his diagnosis and treatment was highly publicized *(1)*. He further spoke openly at many prostate cancer academic and continuing education events.

Beginning in 1978, prostate cancer mortality rates rose, but more slowly than incidence rates. In the 1990s, prostate cancer was the second leading cause of death, but recently, dropped to the third most common cause after colon cancer (Fig. 1). This is due to a drop in mortality rates of 2.7% per year between 1994 and 2003 *(1)*. This has been attributed to a combination of earlier detection and improved treatment for prostate cancer *(1)*. However, given the long natural history of prostate cancer progression from early diagnosis to metastasis over 15–20 years *(3)*, and given that this drop began relatively soon after PSA screening was introduced, this observation may not be a reflection of the effects of PSA screening directly improving mortality rates for patients diagnosed with early stage prostate cancer.

Rather, it may be due to the harvesting of the prevalent cases of patients with subclinical, locally advanced or metastatic prostate cancer discovered by PSA screening. From controlled clinical trials, early or immediate treatment regimens among patients with locally advanced or metastatic prostate cancer have been shown to improve mortality rates compared to other regimens that treat only when patients develop clinical symptoms of prostate cancer progression *(4–6)*. Although these studies were not conducted at the time, it is likely that physicians initiated immediate treatment at the time of diagnosis, which could have improved mortality rates within this time period. Continued drops in annual mortality rates over the next 10 years would be required to demonstrate positive effects of a PSA screening program for the detection of early stage prostate cancer.

## PRACTICE GUIDELINES FOR PROSTATE CANCER SCREENING

### *Government Guidelines*

The Canadian healthcare system consists of publicly funded, provincially based, health insurance plans governed by the federal Canada Health Act of 1984. This law essentially guarantees all citizens health coverage regardless of medical history, personal income, or standard of living. Thus, many policies and guidelines are issued by provincial and federal taskforces that have significant cost implications.

There are no formal screening programs for prostate cancer promoted by the federal or provincial governments. The Canadian Task Force on Preventive Health Guidelines mandated by Health Canada (2004) – an agency of the federal government – does not recommend screening for prostate cancer using PSA, based on its low-predictive value and the known risk of adverse effects associated with therapies of unproven effectiveness *(7)*. Similar guidelines have been published by the provinces, including Ontario,

Saskatchewan, Alberta, and British Columbia *(8)*. These publications do not specifically state the methodology with which these conclusions were based nor was there any transparency in how the guidelines were arbitrated or who the members of the committees were.

## THE COLLEGE OF FAMILY PHYSICIANS OF CANADA
## AND THE CANADIAN UROLOGICAL ASSOCIATION

In Canada, all patients who desire to undergo PSA testing must be assessed by a primary care physician (or family physician). Patients cannot self-order a PSA test at a laboratory or self-refer to a specialist. In 2004, after a MEDLINE-based literature review, Pickles et al. on behalf of the College of Family Physicians of Canada, concluded that indirect evidence suggests that all men older than 45 years with at least a 10-year life expectancy should be informed of the potential benefits and drawbacks of PSA screening so they can make an informed decision on whether to have the test *(9)*.

In 1994, the Canadian Urological Association (CUA) published a consensus statement on the use of PSA for prostate cancer screening *(10)*. Within this statement, prostate cancer screening was recommended after the risks and benefits are discussed with the patient. Further, the CUA strongly advocated that the PSA testing be universally available and that funding be provided to cover its costs.

Thus, a schism exists between government policies that pay for healthcare and physician organizations that provide healthcare in regards to PSA screening. None of these policies or statements are mandatory or governed by regulation within the healthcare system and the decision as to whether to undergo PSA screening is left with the individual patient and physician. Nevertheless, it is Canada's centralized, government-funded health insurance system that poses some particular challenges with respect to PSA screening. Canadian provincial ministries of health tend to look skeptically at large-scale screening programs, leery of the cost implications, and do not fund PSA screening programs. As a monopoly, they face no competition with respect to funding care. Patients who believe that PSA should be funded have nowhere to go. Government panels have emphasized the absence of randomized trials showing a mortality reduction, and the risks of morbidity and overtreatment. Increasingly, this issue has become politicized, with prostate cancer support groups overwhelmingly demanding that PSA screening be funded.

## CURRENT PROSTATE CANCER SCREENING PRACTICES

Despite these recommendations, the practice of prostate screening with PSA is widespread across Canada based on surveys from both patients and physicians. Based on a nationwide survey, up to 67% of men between 40 and 79 years reported that they underwent a PSA test for prostate cancer screening purposes in 2000/01 *(8)*. This has increased up to 75.7% from the same survey in 2005/6 *(11)*. This survey was administered by Statistics Canada, an agency of the federal government legislated to collect census data. Data on PSA screening were obtained from Statistics Canada's 2000/01 and 2005/06 Canadian Community Health Survey (CCHS) which surveys over 130,000 people using a multistage stratified cluster design for sampling the population *(8)*.

These results are consistent with physician attitudes toward prostate cancer screening. From a provincial survey of 264 physicians in Ontario, 63% ordered a PSA test for prostate cancer screening purposes *(12)*. Also, from a national survey among urologists from the CUA, 87% believed that men should undergo PSA testing for prostate cancer screening *(13)*.

These surveys are also supported by age-specific prostate cancer incidence rates. Since the introduction of PSA screening, incidence rates of prostate cancer for all age groups have increased. After 1993, incidence rates dropped due to the harvest effect of detecting all prevalent cases of prostate cancer. However, when examining specific age groups, the 50–59-year-old age groups continued to rise steadily after 1993, whereas the rates for older age groups subsided (Fig. 2). Further, after 1993, the incidence rate of prostate cancer among the 80+ year group had the greatest decline. These data suggest that the introduction of PSA testing led to more diagnoses in younger men – the target screening population, compared to older men, particularly the 80+ year age group – the non-target screening group.

Thus, despite federal and provincial guidelines not recommending prostate cancer screening strategies, the practice is very common among physicians and widely accepted among men. However, it is important to observe that a key basis of the government recommendations was that there was no level one evidence that treatment for patients with early stage prostate cancer improved survival. With the recent publication of a randomized study showing improved overall and prostate cancer-specific mortality with surgery compared to men who did not undergo surgery (watchful waiting) *(14)*, future government-based guidelines warrant modification.

Differences between Canadian and US health care systems have resulted in a some-what different perspective on PSA screening. In Canada, PSA testing is one of the few tests that patients are required to pay for out of pocket, and this represents a psychological barrier for many patients. Patient support groups in Canada view funding of PSA testing as a major priority for provincial health care systems.

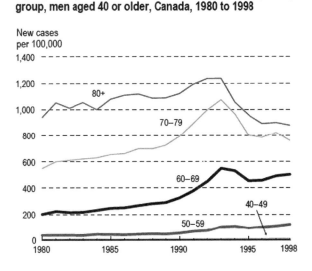

**Fig. 2.** Age-specific prostate cancer incidence rates, 1980–1998, Canada.

## SCREENING INSTRUMENTS

The main instruments used for prostate cancer screening in Canada are serum PSA levels and DRE. The only adjunct serological test that is readily available is free-PSA measurements to calculate the free:total PSA ratio. Other PSA-based tests including complexed-PSA *(15)*, pro-PSA *(16)*, and human kallikrien-2 (hK2) *(17)* are not widely available for commercial use in Canada. Serum insulin-like growth factor-1 (IGF-1) is commercially available, but has not been used for prostate cancer detection. IGF-1 levels have been shown to be associated with the future development of prostate cancer, but it is not predictive of cancer at the time of biopsy *(18)*. It has been argued that high IGF-1 levels are a risk factor for prostate cancer and not a tumor marker, analogous to the relationship between cholesterol levels and heart disease. This is consistent with our observation that serum IGF-1 levels are positively associated with pre-neoplastic lesions of the prostate, including high-grade prostatic intraepithelial neoplasia *(19)*. Future studies that establish whether high IGF-1 levels are a risk factor for prostate cancer would be of interest, since this would have chemo-preventative implications.

Recent studies have now demonstrated that PSA alone cannot accurately predict new cases of prostate cancer because of the low proportion of cancer to normal prostate volume among incident cases *(20,21)*. Abnormal PSA levels cannot reliably distinguish patients with prostate cancer from those with benign prostatic hyperplasia *(2)*, and a high rate of prostate cancer is present among men considered to have normal PSA levels *(21)*. Further, a proportion of patients diagnosed with prostate cancer through a PSA screening program have non-aggressive forms that do not require any treatment *(22,23)*.

From the Prostate Cancer Prevention Trial (PCPT), the performance characteristics of PSA and DRE for prostate cancer detection among men in the placebo arm of the study (which is reflective of a screening population) was low with an area under the curve (AUC) of 0.68 for the receiver operating characteristic (ROC) curve *(24)*. To improve upon the accuracy, age, ethnicity, family history of prostate cancer, and previous prostate biopsy information were incorporated into a predictive model among these men *(25)*.

## NOMOGRAM SCREENING INSTRUMENTS FROM CANADIAN DATA

Similar to the USA, predictive models that attempt to improve the predictive ability of PSA to detect prostate cancer have been used in Canada. Karakiewicz et al. developed a nomogram model to predict prostate cancer risk among men who underwent a biopsy for an abnormal PSA level ($>4.0$ ng/mL) from cohorts from Canada and Germany *(26)*. Predictor variables used in the model were age, PSA, free:total PSA ratio, and DRE and resulting AUCs ranged from 0.69 to 0.77 for various sub-groups *(26)*.

It has been well established that other risk factors including ethnicity and family history of prostate cancer are also important predictors for prostate cancer. We have previously shown that incorporating established risk factors for prostate cancer in a multivariable model can significantly improve the positive predictive value of PSA *(27,28)*. By combining a panel of predictive variables in a statistical model, including age, ethnicity, family history of prostate cancer, and prostate volume, we were able to improve the positive predictive value of PSA to detect prostate cancer *(27)*.

To construct a model that considers all risk factors and tumor markers for prostate cancer, we developed a nomogram prostate cancer risk assessment instrument based on 3,108 men who underwent a prostate biopsy in Ontario (Fig. 3) *(29)*. Predictor variables

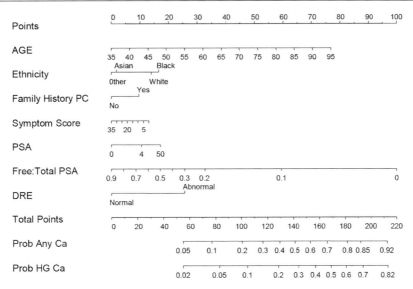

**Fig. 3.** Nomogram instrument for assessing individual prostate cancer risk. The nomogram is used by first locating a patient's position for each predictor variable on its horizontal scale and then a point value is assigned according to the Points scale (*top axis*). Point values are summed for each variable and the total points are located on the Total Points scale (*bottom axis*). This corresponds to a probability value for having prostate cancer or aggressive prostate cancer. Symptom score is measured by total AUA symptom score. PSA is measured in ng/mL. Free:total PSA is measured by ratios (PC = prostate cancer; DRE = digital rectal examination; Ca = cancer; HG = high grade).

included age, ethnicity, family history of prostate cancer, the presence of urinary symptoms, total PSA, free:total PSA, and DRE. We also included a subset of men consisting of volunteers with normal PSA levels who underwent a prostate biopsy. We did not include prostate volume in the model, but rather used urinary obstructive symptoms as a surrogate measure. These factors can be easily and non-invasively determined at the time of screening.

Of the 3,108 men, 1,304 (42.0%) were found to have prostate cancer (median number of needle cores=8). Among the 408 men with a normal PSA (<4.0 ng/mL), 99 (24.3%) had prostate cancer. The AUC for the nomogram was 0.74 (95% confidence interval (C.I.): 0.71–0.81) for predicting prostate cancer and 0.77 (95% C.I.: 0.74–0.81) for high-grade prostate cancer (defined as Gleason Score 7 or more). This was significantly greater than the AUC of the model that only considered the conventional screening methods PSA and DRE (0.62, 95% C.I.: 0.58–0.66 for any cancer; 0.69, 95% C.I.: 0.65–0.73 for high-grade cancer).

From the ROC analysis, risk factors including age, ethnicity, family history of prostate cancer, symptoms, and free:total PSA ratio contributed significantly more predictive information than PSA and DRE. If PSA and DRE were removed from the nomogram model, the incremental AUC drop was only 0.010 (Table 1). However, if we removed all of the other risk factors (age, ethnicity, family history of prostate cancer, and the presence of urinary symptoms) the incremental AUC drop was 0.082 (Table 1). Each of the risk factors alone including age, ethnicity, family history of prostate cancer, and LUTS were the same or better than PSA when comparing the incremental drop in the AUC. Significant predictors for the presence of high-grade cancer were age, DRE, PSA, and free:total PSA ratio (Table 2).

Table 1
AUC Analysis of Nomogram Variables for Each Predictor Variable in Predicting
Any Cancer. The Contribution of Each Factor is Examined by their Drop in AUC
if Removed from the Overall Model

| Factors | Incremental drop in AUC |
|---|---|
| | AUC for PC = 0.74 (95% CI: 0.71–0.81) (n=3,108) |
| Conventional screening: | |
|   PSA | 0.001 |
|   DRE | 0.009 |
| Total drop in AUC: | 0.010 |
| Additional nomogram Factors: | |
|   Age | 0.016 |
|   Ethnic background | 0.001 |
|   Family history | 0.001 |
|   LUTS | 0.001 |
|   Free:total PSA ratio | 0.063 |
| Total drop in AUC: | 0.082 |

The advantage of this nomogram is that clinicians can assess prostate cancer risk on an individual basis and make management decisions. For example, for a patient with a PSA < 4.0 ng/mL with other risk factors for prostate cancer, a biopsy may be justified based on the nomogram. In contrast, if the nomogram predicts a low chance for having aggressive prostate cancer for an older patient with a high-PSA level, then it would be reasonable for the patient to forego a biopsy. The exact probability cut-off for undergoing or foregoing a biopsy would be left with the treating physician and patient, and should be individualized.

Another aspect of this study is the construction of a nomogram that can predict the presence of aggressive forms of prostate cancer (Gleason Score 7 or more). Based on a large population-based survey, Albertsen et al. showed that patients with low-grade cancer (Gleason Score 6 or less) have significantly fewer life years lost from prostate cancer, compared to patients with high-grade cancers (3). However, many experts would agree that patients with prostate cancer of Gleason Score 7 or more require aggressive treatment (3,30).

Currently, this nomogram is being evaluated as a screening instrument for prostate cancer detection in a multi-institutional study across Canada. This instrument provides important information for physicians and patients in assessing an individual's risk for prostate cancer and we have made it available for the general public at *http://prostaterisk.ca.*

## CANADIAN UROLOGISTS: PRACTICE PATTERNS AT INITIAL AND REPEAT PROSTATE BIOPSY

A survey of Canadian urologists who conduct prostate biopsies performed in 1998 revealed that 62.9% perform a sextant pattern at initial biopsy (31). It is likely that a higher number of needle cores are obtained today, since it is well established that at least 8–12 needle cores are needed at the time of initial biopsy (32).

Table 2
Comparison of Factors Between Patients with Aggressive Cancer and Non-aggressive Cancer

| Factor | Non-aggressive prostate cancer Gleason Score 6 or less (n=553) | Aggressive prostate cancer Gleason Score 7 or more (n=751) | p-Value |
|---|---|---|---|
| Median age (years) | 64.3 (mean: 64.3) (range: 42.7–88.5) | 67.2 (mean: 67.0) (range: 41.3–93.8) | < 0.0001 |
| Family history of PC | | | |
| Absent | 458 (41.9%) | 635 (58.1%) | 0.40 |
| Present | 95 (45.0%) | 116 (55.0%) | |
| Ethnicity | | | |
| Asian | 16 (39.0%) | 25 (61.0%) | 0.48 |
| Caucasian | 474 (43.2%) | 623 (56.8%) | |
| Black | 55 (39.3%) | 85 (60.7%) | |
| Other | 8 (30.8%) | 18 (69.2%) | |
| LUTS | | | |
| Absent | 317 (41.9%) | 440 (58.1%) | 0.65 |
| Present | 236 (43.1%) | 311 (56.9%) | |
| DRE | | | |
| No nodule | 445 (47.8%) | 486 (52.2%) | < 0.0001 |
| Nodule | 108 (29.0%) | 265 (71.0%) | |
| Median PSA (ng/mL) | 6.50 (mean: 7.7) (range: 0.3–45.0) | 8.35 (mean: 11.2) (range: 0.6–48.7) | < 0.0001 |
| Free:total PSA ratio | 0.14 (mean: 0.16) (range: 0.007–0.9) | 0.10 (mean: 0.12) (range: 0.02–0.9) | < 0.0001 |

The pattern of practice of repeat prostate biopsy is erratic, since there are no established standards in place. Patients who undergo a repeat biopsy after an initial negative biopsy have cancer detection rates between 10% and 30% (33–39). This is primarily due to error with random sampling at the initial biopsy.

We showed that among men with an initial negative biopsy in Ontario, 33% undergo a repeat biopsy within 1 year, and approximately 25% have cancer (40). Of the cancers detected at repeat biopsy, 31% were of high grade. Factors that increased the likelihood for having a repeat biopsy were initial histology of prostatic intraepithelial neoplasia or atypia and PSA level. However, only initial histology and age were predictors for cancer at repeat biopsy (40).

Similar to nomograms developed to assess prostate cancer risk at initial biopsy, nomograms that identify men at increased risk for prostate cancer at repeat biopsy have been developed (41). Based on a study of 343 US men, factors including age, DRE, number of needle cores, PSA, PSA velocity, and family history of prostate cancer were evaluated. Similar to our Canadian-based study, PSA was not a predictor for prostate cancer at repeat biopsy and the strongest predictor was initial histology *(41)*.

## CONCLUSIONS

Differences between Canadian and US health care systems have resulted in a somewhat different perspective on PSA screening. Regulatory and provincial health insurance plans have not supported the development of formal PSA screening programs, and PSA as a screening test remains unfunded in most constituencies. Nonetheless, ad hoc PSA screening is widespread across the country. Mortality reductions similar to that seen in other screened constituencies have occurred. Enthusiasm for prostate cancer screening and early detection remains high. Research into new biomarkers and risk nomograms is ongoing in Canada for initial and repeat prostate biopsy in the context of a prostate cancer screening program.

## REFERENCES

1. Canadian Cancer Statistics 2007. Toronto: National Cancer Institute of Canada; 2007.
2. Stamey TA, Yang N, Hay R, McNeal JE, Freiha FS, Redwine E. Prostate-specific antigen as a serum marker for adenocarcinoma of the prostate. New Engl J Med 1987;317:909–15.
3. Albertsen PC, Fryback DG, Storer BE, Kolon TF, Fine J. Long-term survival among men with conservatively treated localized prostate cancer. JAMA 1995;274:626–31.
4. Bolla M, Collette L, Blank L, et al. Long-term results with immediate androgen suppression and external irradiation in patients with locally advanced prostate cancer (an EORTC study): a phase III randomised trial. Lancet 2002;360:103–6.
5. Immediate versus deferred treatment for advanced prostatic cancer: initial results of the Medical Research Council Trial. The Medical Research Council Prostate Cancer Working Party Investigators Group. Br J Urol 1997;79:235–46.
6. Messing EM, Manola J, Sarosdy M, Wilding G, Crawford ED, Trump D. Immediate hormonal therapy compared with observation after radical prostatectomy and pelvic lymphadenectomy in men with node-positive prostate cancer. N Engl J Med 1999;341:1781–8.
7. Canada H. Progress Report on Cancer Control in Canada. 2004 [cited; Available from: http://www.phac-aspc.gc.ca/publicat/prccc-relccc/pdf/F244_HC_Cancer_Rpt_English.pdf].
8. Gibbons L, Waters C. Prostate cancer – testing, incidence, surgery and mortality. Health Reports 2003;14:9–18.
9. Pickles T. Current status of PSA screening. Early detection of prostate cancer. CAN Fam physician 2004;50:57–63.
10. Ramsey EW. Early detection of prostate cancer. Recommendations from the Canadian Urological Association. CAN J Oncol 1994;4 Suppl 1:82–5.
11. Canada S. Canadian Community Health Survey (CCHS), Cycle 3.1. 2007 [cited; Available from: http://www.statcan.ca/english/concepts/health/cycle3_1/index.htm].
12. Bunting PS, Goel V, Williams JI, Iscoe NA. Prostate-specific antigen testing in Ontario: reasons for testing patients without diagnosed prostate cancer. CMAJ 1999;160:70–5.
13. Ramsey EW, Elhilali M, Goldenberg SL, et al. Practice patterns of Canadian urologists in benign prostatic hyperplasia and prostate cancer. Canadian Prostate Health Council. J Urol 2000;163:499–502.
14. Bill-Axelson A, Holmberg L, Ruutu M, et al. Radical prostatectomy versus watchful waiting in early prostate cancer. N Engl J Med 2005;352:1977–84.
15. Partin AW, Brawer MK, Bartsch G, et al. Complexed prostate specific antigen improves specificity for prostate cancer detection: results of a prospective multicenter clinical trial. J Urol 2003;170:1787–91.
16. Catalona WJ, Bartsch G, Rittenhouse HG, et al. Serum pro-prostate specific antigen preferentially detects aggressive prostate cancers in men with 2 to 4 ng/ml prostate specific antigen. J Urol 2004;171(6 Pt 1):2239–44.

17. Nam RK, Diamandis EP, Toi A, et al. Serum human glandular kallikrein-2 (hK2) protease levels predict the presence of prostate cancer among men with elevated prostate-specific antigen. J Clin Oncol 2000;18:1036–42.

18. Pollak M. Insulin-like growth factors and prostate cancer. Epidemiol Rev 2001;23:1–8.

19. Nam RK, Trachtenberg J, Jewett MA, et al. Serum insulin-like growth factor-I levels and prostatic intraepithelial neoplasia: a clue to the relationship between IGF-I physiology and prostate cancer risk. Cancer Epidemiol Biomarkers Prev 2005;14:1270–3.

20. Stamey TA, Caldwell M, McNeal JE, Nolley R, Hemenez M, Downs J. The prostate specific antigen era in the United States is over for prostate cancer: what happened in the last 20 years? J Urol 2004;172(4 Pt 1):1297–301.

21. Thompson IM, Pauler DK, Goodman PJ, et al. Prevalence of prostate cancer among men with a prostate-specific antigen level < or =4.0 ng per milliliter. N Engl J Med 2004;350:2239–46.

22. Albertsen PC, Hanley JA, Gleason DF, Barry MJ. Competing risk analysis of men aged 55 to 74 years at diagnosis managed conservatively for clinically localized prostate cancer. JAMA 1998;280:975–80.

23. Barry MJ, Albertsen PC, Bagshaw MA, et al. Outcomes for men with clinically nonmetastatic prostate carcinoma managed with radical prostatectomy, external beam radiotherapy, or expectant management. Cancer 2001;91:2302–14.

24. Thompson IM, Ankerst DP, Chi C, et al. Operating characteristics of prostate-specific antigen in men with an initial PSA level of 3.0 ng/ml or lower. JAMA 2005;294:66–70.

25. Thompson IM, Ankerst DP, Chi C, et al. Assessing prostate cancer risk: results from the Prostate Cancer Prevention Trial. J Natl Cancer Inst 2006;98:529–34.

26. Karakiewicz PI, Benayoun S, Kattan MW, et al. Development and validation of a nomogram predicting the outcome of prostate biopsy based on patient age, digital rectal examination and serum prostate specific antigen. J Urol 2005;173:1930–4.

27. Nam RK, Toi A, Trachtenberg J, et al. Making Sense of PSA: Improving its Predictive Value Among Patients Undergoing Prostate Biopsy. J Urol 2006;175:489–94.

28. Nam RK, Toi A, Klotz LH, et al. Nomogram Prediction for Prostate Cancer and Aggressive Prostate Cancer at Time of Biopsy: Utilizing All Risk Factors and Tumour Markers for Prostate Cancer. Can J Urol 2006;13(Supplement 2):2–10.

29. Nam RK, Toi A, Klotz LH, et al. Assessing Individual Risk for Prostate Cancer. J Clin Oncol 2007;25:3582–88.

30. Catalona WJ. Management of cancer of the prostate. New Engl J Med 1994;331:996–1004.

31. Fleshner N, Rakovitch E, Klotz L. Differences between urologists in the United States and Canada in the approach to prostate cancer. J Urol 2000;163:1461–6.

32. Presti JC, Jr., Chang JJ, Bhargava V, Shinohara K. The optimal systematic prostate biopsy scheme should include 8 rather than 6 biopsies: results of a prospective clinical trial. J Urol 2000;163:163–6.

33. Keetch DW, Catalona WJ, Smith DS. Serial prostatic biopsies in men with persistently elevated serum prostate specific antigen values. J Urol 1994;151:1571–4.

34. Rietbergen JB, Kruger AE, Hoedemaeker RF, Bangma CH, Kirkels WJ, Schroder FH. Repeat screening for prostate cancer after 1-year follow up in 984 biopsied men: clinical and pathological features of detected cancer. J Urol 1998;160(6 Pt 1):2121–5.

35. Durkan GC, Greene DR. Elevated serum prostate specific antigen levels in conjunction with an initial prostatic biopsy negative for carcinoma: who should undergo a repeat biopsy? BJU Int 1999;83:424–8.

36. Hayek OR, Noble CB, de la Taille A, Bagiella E, Benson MC. The necessity of a second prostate biopsy cannot be predicted by PSA or PSA derivatives (density or free:total ratio) in men with prior negative prostatic biopsies. Curr Opin Urol 1999;9:371–5.

37. Djavan B, Zlotta A, Remzi M, et al. Optimal predictors of prostate cancer on repeat prostate biopsy: a prospective study of 1,051 men PG. J Urol 2000;163:1144–8; discussion 1148–9.

38. Borboroglu PG, Comer SW, Riffenburgh RH, Amling CL. Extensive repeat transrectal ultrasound guided prostate biopsy in patients with previous benign sextant biopsies. J Urol 2000;163:158–62.

39. Roehl KA, Antenor JA, Catalona WJ. Serial biopsy results in prostate cancer screening study. J Urol 2002;167:2435–9.

40. Nam RK, Toi A, Trachtenberg J, et al. Variation in patterns of practice in diagnosing screen-detected prostate cancer. BJU Int 2004;94:1239–44.

41. Lopez-Corona E, Ohori M, Scardino PT, Reuter VE, Gonen M, Kattan MW. A nomogram for predicting a positive repeat prostate biopsy in patients with a previous negative biopsy session. J Urol 2003;170(4 Pt 1):1184–8; discussion 8.

# 4

# Trends in Prostate Cancer Screening – Overview of Europe

*Sanjai K. Addla and Bob Djavan*

**CONTENTS**

## SUMMARY

Prostate cancer is the most common cancer diagnosed in men in the western world. Historically, a quarter of patients have presented with metastatic incurable disease, resulting in significant morbidity and mortality. Since the introduction and regular usage of prostate-specific antigen (PSA) in clinical practice over the last two decades, a significant shift in the stage of prostate cancer at diagnosis towards earlier stages has been seen. This, along with more favourable histological features, has facilitated treatments with a curative intent. There are concerns regarding diagnosis of indolent disease and overtreatment of screen-detected malignancies, with suggestions that screening causes more harm than good. This has prompted studies looking at the efficacy of prostate cancer screening in decreasing the mortality from prostate cancer at an acceptable price in terms of quality of life and costs. Currently there are two large randomized screening studies on either side of the Atlantic nearing completion. Over the next few years these studies will hopefully provide the incontrovertible evidence required either to initiate or refute the need for mass population screening programmes for prostate cancer. Against this background we discuss the present

From: *Current Clinical Urology: Prostate Cancer Screening*, Edited by: D. P. Ankerst et al.
DOI 10.1007/978-1-60327-281-0_4 © Humana Press, a part of Springer Science+Business Media, LLC 2009

state of knowledge based on European screening trials and make a case for screening, and also present evidence to the contrary.

**Key Words:** Prostate cancer, Screening, Europe, PSA.

## PROSTATE CANCER IN EUROPE

According to estimates for 2006, prostate cancer was the most frequently diagnosed cancer in European men *(1)*, with an estimated 345,900 new cases diagnosed, accounting for 20.3% of the entire cancer load in men. During the same year prostate cancer was estimated to be the cause of death in 87,400 patients, accounting for 9.2% of cancer deaths in men. Studying the trends in incidence and mortality from carcinoma of the prostate (CaP) between 1978 and 1994 in the European Union, Vercelli et al. noted a mean difference percent (MD%) increase per year of +3.2 in Finland and England, and +5.7 in the Netherlands. In Central Europe, very high MD%s, ranging between +8.4 in France and +16.6 in Austria, were noted *(2)*. These estimates indicate a significant cancer burden with important public health ramifications. Prostate cancers trends worldwide and especially in the USA were replicated in Europe, with peak prostate cancer-specific mortality reached in 1993. This peak of 15.7/100,000 lowered to 14.1/100,000 by 1999 *(3)*. Age-standardized analysis for each subsequent age group of men from 50 years and over showed a larger decrease in mortality in the elderly population *(3)*.

The exact cause for the rise and fall in mortality from CaP is open to debate *(4)*. This trend has been attributed to the introduction of prostate-specific antigen (PSA) into clinical practice, causing an increase in the incidence, diagnosis, and subsequent treatment of cases during the early curable stage, thus leading to a fall in mortality *(5)*. However, the sharp rise and fall in the mortality trends very soon after the introduction of PSA is at odds with the long natural history of prostate cancer as has been known from long-term ($\geq 20$ years) studies of conservatively managed localized CaP patients *(6)*. Another argument in favour of PSA screening not being the only reason for this change in incidence is the findings of similar trends of rise and fall of prostate cancer mortality from countries such as the UK, which have a very low level of opportunistic screening for CaP using PSA *(7)*. Another theory is that a proportion of the rising and falling pool of diagnosed patients in the 1990s might have been mislabelled as dying of prostate cancer *(8)*. Nevertheless, the fact that prostate cancer is a major health problem with significant associated morbidity and mortality satisfies the first requirement of the criteria for mass screening *(9)*.

## SCREENING IN EUROPE

Screening is defined as "a public health service in which members of a defined population, who do not necessarily perceive they are at risk of, or are already affected by a disease or its complications, are asked a question or offered a test, to identify those individuals who are more likely to be helped than harmed by further tests or treatment to reduce the risk of a disease or its complications"*(10)*. The primary requisites from this definition for screening point towards a test to diagnose the disease with the objective of identifying individuals who would benefit from the diagnosis rather than being brought to harm.

The European Association of Urology guidelines for 2007 regarding prostate cancer screening state that "At the present time, there is lack of evidence to support or disregard widely adopted population-based screening programmes for early detection of CaP aimed at all men, in a given population" *(11)*. Similar views have been expressed by the Advisory Committee on Cancer Prevention in the European Union *(12)* and the World Health Organisation regional office for Europe *(13)* that mass screening should not be supported prior to the availability of data from randomized trials.

## PROSTATE CANCER SCREENING STUDIES

Current information available regarding prostate cancer disease status and screening in Europe is principally from two studies: The Tyrol Prostate Cancer Demonstration Project *(14,15)* (Tyrol Study) and the European Randomized Screening for Prostate Cancer (ERSPC) Study *(16)*, in particular, the Rotterdam section. Contrasts of contemporary screening trials in Europe are provided in Table 1.

### *The Tyrol Prostate Cancer Demonstration Project (Tyrol Study)*

Since 1993 this prospective early prostate cancer detection programme has been carried out in the Federal State of Tyrol (one of the nine Federal states of the Republic of Austria) using PSA testing as the screening tool. The objective of the Tyrol Study was to evaluate the effectiveness of a well-controlled programme of early detection and treatment on prostate cancer mortality, by comparing Tyrol, where PSA testing was freely available, with the rest of Austria, where it was not introduced *(14,15)*. The Tyrol Study is a non-randomized study of the effect of screening in a natural experiment setting.

### *European Randomized Screening for Prostate Cancer (ERSPC) Study*

The ERSPC is a large, multi-centre, randomized controlled screening trial that aims to show or exclude a decrease in prostate cancer mortality of at least 20% in men randomized to a screening arm compared to men in the control arm. From 1992 to 2001, seven countries in Europe recruited 163,126 men aged 55–69 years. With an assumed 25% intervention effect in men actually screened and a 20% contamination rate, the trial is expected to reach a power of 0.86 in 2008 *(16,17)*. The Rotterdam and Goteborg sections of the ERSPC are the more extensively studied groups, with interim analysis of several aspects of prostate cancer screening already published.

### *Pilot Randomized Screening Study (Norrkoping, Sweden) (Norrkoping Study)*

This randomized pilot study was initiated in 1987 with the objectives of investigating the organisational, psychological, and economic consequences of screening. All men aged 50–69 years in the city of Norrkoping in 1987 were identified and every sixth man was randomized to the study group (total 1,494), with the remaining 7,532 men acting as the control. The initial two rounds of screening assessment only involved digital rectal examination (DRE), but for the third and fourth rounds of screening (1993 and 1996, respectively), DRE was combined with PSA, with abnormal DRE or PSA $\geq$ 4 ng/ml triggering prostate aspiration biopsies *(18)*. The clinical consequences of screening after

Table 1
European Screening Studies

| Study name | Study methodology | Study commenced | Expected finish date | Screening tests | Schedule |
|---|---|---|---|---|---|
| Norrkoping Study (18) | Feasibility study of randomized screening | 1987 | Results published in 2004 | Only DRE between 1987 and 1993 ; DRE + PSA $\geq$ 4 ng/ml from 1993 | Screening every 3 years |
| Tyrol Study (14,15) | Non-randomized natural experimental study | 1993 | Results published in 2001 and updated in 2008 | Age-referenced PSA along with percentage-free PSA; artificial neural network used since 1996 to determine the need for biopsy | Screening every 3 years |
| ERSPC Study (16) | Randomized screening study | 1992 | Results expected 2008–2010 | PSA $\geq$ 3.0 only trigger for biopsy since 1997 | Swedish arm – 2 yearly, other centres every 4 years |

a 15-year follow-up have been reported. This study was not powered to analyse the difference in the cancer-specific mortality between the two arms.

## SCREENING METHODS

The ideal screening test is minimally invasive, easily available and performed, acceptable to the general population, and accurate, and has a significant influence on the outcome of the disease, such as the mortality rate. Currently, there is no diagnostic test for CaP available that would satisfy all of the above requirements. The methods that have been studied in a European setting and found to be useful as a screening tool are discussed below.

### *Prostate-Specific Antigen and Its Derivatives*

While the PSA test is simple and safe, the dilemma of the precise cut-off levels that trigger biopsy in a screened patient remains unobtainable following the results of the Prostate Cancer Prevention Trial *(19)*.

In the Tyrol Study, initially age-referenced PSA values (>2.5 ng/ml for 40–49 years; >3.5 ng/ml for 50–59 years; >4.5 ng/ml for 60–69 years, and >6.6 ng/ml for 70–79 years) *(20)* were used in combination with percentage-free PSA levels of <22% as criteria for recommending biopsy. After October 1995, the PSA levels for considering biopsy were lowered (>1.25 ng/ml for 40–49 years; >1.75 ng/ml for 50–59 years; >2.25 ng/ml for 60–69 years, and >3.25 ng/ml for 70–79 years) along with percentage-free PSA levels of <18%. Since March 1996, artificial neural networks incorporating total and free PSA, age, DRE, and *trans*-rectal ultra sound scan (TRUS) have been used. PSA velocity has also been added to this combination since 2005, with the aim of improving the specificity of the screening tests.

At the outset of the ERSPC trial, PSA ≥ 4.0 ng/ml and/or an abnormal DRE or TRUS was used as an indication for biopsy. Since February 1997, the PSA threshold of ≥3.0 ng/ml is the only trigger for biopsy *(17)*.

It is estimated that using the PSA threshold values of 2.6 ng/ml and 4.1 ng/ml for referral to biopsy (and assuming biopsy is 100% sensitive and specific), the sensitivity for detecting all cancers is 40.5% and 20.5%, increasing to 78.9% and 50.9% for Gleason ≥ 8 prostate cancers, respectively; the specificity for the same values of PSA for all cancers is estimated to be 81.1% and 93.8% and for Gleason ≥ 8 prostate cancers, 75.1% and 89.1%, respectively *(21,22)*. Using a PSA threshold ≥ 4.0 ng/ml, the estimated number needed to screen (NNS) to detect one cancer is 50–77 in men in their 50s; 21–30 for men in their 60s and 11 for men in their 70s *(23)*. These figures look favourable when compared to the NNS for other malignancies like colorectal and cervical malignancies with established screening programmes. Using the proportional incidence method and studying the interval cancers in the ERSPC, the sensitivity of screening in ERSPC is calculated to be 80% in the screened population *(24)*.

Derivatives of PSA in the form of free to total PSA ratio (*F/T* ratio, percent-free PSA), PSA velocity *(25)*, PSA density, and PSA density of the transitional zone have been studied, but none have been found to be useful as a principal screening tool. They have been utilized for studying indications for re-biopsy and stratifying patients for differentiating between indolent and significant cancers. The *F/T* PSA ratio has been shown to increase the specificity of total serum PSA in the PSA range between 4.0 and

10.0 ng/ml, but not significantly *(26)*. The combination of PSA less than 3.0 ng/ml and *F/T* PSA ratio greater than 18% has been used to define a population at very low risk of cancer of the prostate, in whom the screening intervals could be prolonged *(27)*. PSA density of the transition zone has been shown to enhance the specificity of serum PSA in the 4.0–10 ng/ml range. PSA density of the transition zone was more effective in prostates greater than 30 cc and percent-free PSA in prostates less than 30 cc. The combination of percent-free PSA with PSA density of the transition zone further increased prostate cancer prediction *(28)*.

## *Digital Rectal Examination (DRE)*

Efficacy of DRE findings has been evaluated both as a screening tool and also for determining the screening interval and follow-up in men with an elevated PSA ($\geq$ 3.0 ng/ml) and negative biopsy. After the first screening round of the ERSPC Study, DRE was not used because of its low-positive predictive value (PPV), ranging between 4% and 11% in men with PSA levels of <3.0 ng/ml, increasing from 33% to 83% in men with PSA levels of 3.0–9.9 ng/ml *(29,30)*. DRE findings have also been shown not to be of much use in determining the follow-up of patients with elevated PSA and negative biopsies. On comparing patients with abnormal versus normal DRE in the first screening round who were followed over a period of 8 years with two screening rounds of biopsy, there were no differences in the overall, significant or interval cancer diagnoses *(31)*.

## SCHEDULE OF SCREENING

The screening interval period varied in the different studies, mainly determined by the CaP burden particular to each region and the evolving knowledge about natural history and estimated lead time of screen-detected CaP. In the Tyrol and Norrkoping studies it was triennial, in the Goteborg branch of the ERSPC biennial, and in remaining centres of ERSPC every 4 years. The interval cancers (ICs) detected in the screening arm give an indication regarding the adequacy of the screening interval.

In the Norrkoping Study, 49.4% of the cancers detected in the screening arm were interval cancers. The possible reason for this high IC with 3 year screening intervals compared to 20.2% noted with the 4-year screening schedule of the ERSPC might be due to the methodology of screening, which was only based on DRE during the first two rounds of screening, implying inadequacy of DRE as a single screening tool.

In the first round of screening of the Rotterdam section of the ERSPC, 17,226 men were randomized between screening and control arms (8,350 vs. 8,876) with 91.9% of the men in the screening arm undergoing full screening *(32)*. Over the following 4-year period, prostate cancers detected in the control arm over the following 4-year period and between screening rounds in the screened arm were identified by the linkage to the Dutch National Cancer Registry. The rate of IC relative to the number of cancers in the control group was 18.5% (25/135). The sensitivity of the screening protocol was 79.8% when considering all IC cases diagnosed, and 85.5% when considering IC diagnosed in the men who underwent full screening investigations (biopsy). The low-IC detection rate suggests the adequacy of the methods used as well as the screening interval *(32)*. Comparison of ICs diagnosed using a 2- versus 4-year screening schedule in the ERSPC found no difference in either the incidence of IC or diagnosis of aggressive IC *(33)*.

Based on current evidence from the European trials use of the PSA cut-off $\geq 3.0$ ng/ml as the sole screening tool with a 4-year screening cycle seems to have sensitivity and specificity expected of a screening trial.

## ADVANTAGES OF PROSTATE CANCER SCREENING

Information about the efficacy of CaP screening for improving the outcome of patients can be ascertained by comparing the characteristics of cancers detected in the screened population and controls. Comparison of characteristics of cancers detected in each of the screening rounds gives an indication of the immediate effects of screening on down-staging of the disease. Though the main objective of a decrease in cancer-specific mortality with screening has not been demonstrated conclusively to date in any randomized study, the pattern of variation in parameters that determine the natural course of disease should provide information for making informed judgments at the present time. Parameters that have been extensively studied as prognostic markers in the management of prostate cancer are PSA at diagnosis, Gleason grade, and clinical stage *(34)*. Much of the information available on this disease migration comes from the Rotterdam section of the ERSPC trial *(35)*.

### *PSA at Diagnosis*

Comparing the PSA levels at diagnosis in the screened and control population, the ERSPC trial showed a mean (median) PSA of 9.6 ng/ml (5.2 ng/ml) in the screened arm compared to 73.8 ng/ml (11.6 ng/ml) in the control arm. In the screened arm, half of the cancers had a PSA between 4 and 10 ng/ml, whereas in the control arm half of the cancers had a PSA > 10 ng/ml. The mean (median) PSA value decreased with each screening round, from 10.5 ng/ml (5.7 ng/ml) in the first round to 5.7 ng/ml (4.3 ng/ml) in the second and to 4.5 ng/ml (4.0 ng/ml) in the third *(35)*.

### *Grade Migration*

A favourable shift in the Gleason score patterns was seen in the screened arm which improved further with each screening round. In the first round of screening, 36.2% of cancers in the screened arm had Gleason score $\geq 7$ compared to more than half (55%) in the control arm. The incidence of Gleason $\geq 7$ cancers further decreased significantly with each subsequent round of screening, to 22.3% and 12.5%, respectively, in the next two rounds *(35)*.

### *Stage Migration*

There was a significantly favourable stage distribution in the screening compared to control population. In the first round of screening 78.6% of the cancers in the screening arm were staged $\leq$ T2 compared to 58.9% in the control arm *(35)*. In the second screening round 95.5% of the cancers were $\leq$T2 with only one case of metastatic disease being diagnosed in the screening arm after the first round of prevalence screening. Similar results have been noted in the Norrkoping Study with more than half the cancers (56.5%) being localized (T1-2, N0/Nx, M0) compared to around a quarter (26.7%) in the control group *(18)*.

### Decrease in Diagnosis of Metastatic Disease

There was a decrease in the number of cases that were detected with metastasis in the screened compared to the control population in the ERSPC (0.6% vs. 8%). Taking into account the number of men randomized, the incidence of distant metastasis was five times more common in the control arm compared to the screening arm *(35)*. Similar trends of decreased detection of cases with metastasis in the screened group have been reported from the Norrkoping Study *(18)* and also from the Goteborg branch of ERSPC *(36)*.

## Curative Treatment

In view of the lower stage of disease at diagnosis, more cancers in the screened population could be treated with curative intent. In the ERSPC trial, 81.9% of patients in the screening arm and 54.7% of the patients in the control arm were offered curative treatment *(37)*. Pathological analysis of radical prostatectomy specimens revealed a higher proportion of cases with Gleason grade $\geq$ 7 (53.5% vs. 34.6%) with a significantly larger tumour volume (3.9 ml vs. 1.0 ml) in the control arm compared to the screening arm *(37)*.

## Decreased Cancer-Specific Mortality

To date no randomized population screening data are available that have shown a decrease in cancer-specific mortality following screening for prostate cancer. In the non-randomized Tyrol Study, the estimated cancer deaths in Tyrol in 2005 were 54% (95% confidence interval [CI] 34–69%) lower than expected, compared with only 29% (95% CI: 22–35%) lower than expected in the rest of Austria *(15)*. This was attributed to free availability of PSA testing since 1993 in the Tyrol region along with good standardized management of the diagnosed malignancy. From 1993 onwards investigators found a yearly reduction in the mortality rate of 7.3% (95% CI: 5.1–9.5%) in Tyrol compared to 3.2% (95% CI: 2.6–3.8%) in rest of Austria. However, the Tyrol Study was a non-randomized natural experimental study where all patients diagnosed with cancers had been offered treatment with either curative or palliative intent, depending on the stage at diagnosis. Among the patients with localized disease (T1-2), 89.3% underwent radical prostatectomy, 10.4% had radiotherapy, and only 0.3% were managed with watchful waiting. These figures are in contrast to 10% of the patients in the ERSPC being managed by active surveillance policy following the first round of screening, which increased to 22% in the second round *(24)*. In the Norrkoping Study, which was a randomized trial, though there was evidence suggesting a lower cancer-specific mortality in the screened arm, this was not found to be statistically significant *(18)*. The ERSPC and its planned combined analysis with the Prostate, Lung, Colorectal, and Ovary cancer trial (PLCO trial) *(38)* should provide the conclusive evidence regarding the change in cancer-specific mortality with prostate cancer screening.

## DISADVANTAGES OF SCREENING

### Overdiagnosis and Lead Time

Prostate cancer incidence has increased dramatically since the introduction of PSA into clinical practice *(39)*. In the ERSPC trial the cumulative incidence has been noted to be 7.5% in the screening arm and 2.2% in the control arm. In many years the incidence is 15.9 and 4.2 per 1,000 in the screened and control population, respectively *(37)*. It has been well known for many years that a patient with prostate cancer is more likely to die with prostate cancer rather than from it *(40)*. This has been used as one of the definitions of overdetection; where the probability of overdetection is equal to the probability of dying of other causes during the lead time *(41)*. Lead time is defined as the amount of time, in years, between cancer detection and either clinical diagnosis in the absence of screening or death by any other cause *(42)*. The mean estimated lead time in the ERSPC trial with regular screening is between 9.9 and 13.3 years. Draisma et al. estimated that screening at 4 yearly intervals from the age of 55 to 67 would detect 70% of all clinically relevant cancers. However, it would also diagnose clinically irrelevant or indolent cancers in 41 per 1,000 men, corresponding to an overdetection rate of 48% (range 44–55%). Extending the screening to the age of 75 would detect 95% of all clinically relevant cancers but would increase the overdetection rate to >60% *(42)*.

### *Diagnosis of Indolent Disease*

Indolent prostate cancer is defined as a pathological organ confined cancer with a tumour volume of ≤0.5 cc without any Gleason grade 4 or 5 *(43)*. It is estimated that up to half of the patients in the ERSPC trial undergoing radical prostatectomy might have indolent disease *(44)*. The diagnosis of indolent cancer was significantly higher in the screening arm compared to the control arm patients who underwent radical prostatectomy (27% vs. 11.4%). There was a significant decrease in tumour volume noted at diagnosis from the first to second round of screening with 33% of radical prostatectomy specimens from first round and 43% from second round showing minimal prostate cancer *(24)*. However, the exact extent of overdiagnosis and detection of indolent disease in treated screened populations is still not clear. In the Tyrol Study, using the Epstein criteria *(45)*, the estimated overdiagnosis is reported to be as low as 8.7%, with a finding of insignificant cancer in radical prostatectomy specimens of only 19.7% in the low-PSA group (PSA 2–4 ng/ml) and 17.6% in the high-PSA group (PSA 4–10 ng/ml) *(15)*.

### *Morbidity from Diagnostic Investigations*

The morbidity associated with prostate cancer screening arises from the invasive nature of the TRUS biopsy which has to be performed in about one out of five volunteers (21%) *(24)*. With the introduction of local anaesthetic infiltration and prophylactic antibiotics, the morbidity has improved, but still remains significant *(46)*. In the ERSPC Study, haematuria lasting longer than 3 days and haematospermia were present in 22.6% and 50.4% of patients, respectively, and 3.5% of the patients developed a mild fever. The risk of retention of urine and hospitalization were found to be low (0.4%) *(46,47)*.

### *Morbidity of Treatment*

The morbidity of treating prostate cancer with any of the available treatment modalities is significant and is known to be related to the quality of treatment provided *(48)*. Following radical prostatectomy, 80–90% of patients report erectile dysfunction and up to half complain of urinary incontinence. The complications associated with radiotherapy are more related with bowel dysfunction (30–35%) and impotence (approximately 50%). However, in the Tyrol Study, in which 1765 radical prostatectomies were performed between 1988 and 2005, at 1 year follow-up, 95.1% of patients were continent with erectile function maintained in 78.9% of men aged $< 65$ yrs *(15)*. There is evidence to indicate that with the availability of minimal invasive surgery and robotic technology, the morbidity associated with radical prostatectomy is improving *(49,50)*.

## SUMMARY

There is a clear evidence to suggest that population-based screening for CaP results in the diagnosis of cancer at a lower grade, stage, and PSA level, with more patients being eligible for treatment with a curative intent. Whether this leads to a decrease in cancer-specific mortality is still not clear. Though screening leads to invasive investigations in a significant proportion of patients (20%), patient compliance appears to be high, ranging between *75%* and *90%*, thus indicating the acceptability of the process *(18,24)*.

In view of the potential risk of overdiagnosis and overtreatment, screening-mediated improvements in disease status need to be properly quantified, so that patients can make an informed judgment when offered screening. The decrease in diagnosis of metastatic disease in the ERSPC (Goteborg branch) with screening provides a very good example to illustrate this point. There was a statistically significant relative risk reduction of diagnosis of metastatic prostate cancer by almost 50% in the screening arm compared to control, but the absolute numbers were very small. In that study the chance of being alive for 10 years without being diagnosed with metastatic prostate cancer in the screening arm was 99.76% compared to 99.53% in the control arm, with a 1.8-fold increase in diagnosis of CaP in the screening arm *(36)*.

## CONCLUSIONS

Whilst screening has the potential to save lives or improve the quality of life, whether this happens with prostate cancer is still open to debate *(4)*. The objectives of screening are best summarized by a statement from the UK screening advisory committee: "Screening has important ethical differences from clinical practice, as the health service is targeting apparently healthy people, offering to help individuals to make better informed choices about their health *(10)*." There is already evidence of this happening in the ERSPC, where with a better understanding of the natural history of CaP, an increasing percentage of patients are deciding on clinical surveillance as the treatment option *(24)*.

## REFERENCES

1. Ferlay J, Autier P, Boniol M, Heanue M, Colombet M, Boyle P. Estimates of the cancer incidence and mortality in Europe in 2006. Ann Oncol 2007; 18(3):581–92.
2. Vercelli M, Quaglia A, Marani E, Parodi S. Prostate cancer incidence and mortality trends among elderly and adult Europeans. Crit Rev Oncol Hematol 2000; 35(2):133–44.
3. Levi F, Lucchini F, Negri E, Boyle P, La Vecchia C. Leveling of prostate cancer mortality in Western Europe. Prostate 2004; 60(1):46–52.
4. Schroder FH, Albertsen P. Open to debate. The motion: there is evidence that prostate cancer screening does more good than harm. Eur Urol 2006; 50(2):377–380.
5. Hankey BF, Feuer EJ, Clegg LX, Hayes RB, Legler JM, Prorok PC et al. Cancer surveillance series: interpreting trends in prostate cancer – part I: Evidence of the effects of screening in recent prostate cancer incidence, mortality, and survival rates. J Natl Cancer Inst 1999; 91(12):1017–1024.
6. Albertsen PC, Hanley JA, Fine J. 20-year outcomes following conservative management of clinically localized prostate cancer. JAMA 2005; 293(17):2095–2101.

7. Boyle P, d'Onofrio A, Maisonneuve P, Severi G, Robertson C, Tubiana M et al. Measuring progress against cancer in Europe: has the 15% decline targeted for 2000 come about? Ann Oncol 2003; 14(8):1312–25.

8. Feuer EJ, Merrill RM, Hankey BF. Cancer surveillance series: interpreting trends in prostate cancer – part II: Cause of death misclassification and the recent rise and fall in prostate cancer mortality. J Natl Cancer Inst 1999; 91(12):1025–1032.

9. Wilson JM, Jungner YG. [Principles and practice of mass screening for disease]. Bol Oficina Sanit Panam 1968; 65(4):281–393.

10. UK National Screening Committee. Second report of the UK National Screening Committee. Available at www.nsc.nhs.uk. 2004. Ref Type: Internet Communication

11. Heidenreich A, Aus G, Bolla M, Joniau S, Matveev VB, Schmid HP et al. EAU guidelines on prostate cancer. Eur Urol 2008; 53(1):68–80.

12. Recommendations on cancer screening in the European Union. Advisory Committee on Cancer Prevention. Eur J Cancer 2000; 36(12):1473–1478.

13. Davidson P., Gabby J. Should mass screening for prostate cancer be introduced at the national level? Copenhagen, WHO Regional Office for Europe (Health Evidence Network report 2004). 2004. Ref Type: Internet Communication

14. Bartsch G, Horninger W, Klocker H, Reissigl A, Oberaigner W, Schonitzer D et al. Prostate cancer mortality after introduction of prostate-specific antigen mass screening in the Federal State of Tyrol, Austria. Urology 2001; 58(3):417–424.

15. Bartsch G, Horninger W, Klocker H, Pelzer A, Bektic J, Oberaigner W et al. Tyrol Prostate Cancer Demonstration Project: early detection, treatment, outcome, incidence and mortality. BJU Int 2008; 101(7):809–16.

16. de Koning HJ, Liem MK, Baan CA, Boer R, Schroder FH, Alexander FE. Prostate cancer mortality reduction by screening: power and time frame with complete enrollment in the European Randomised Screening for Prostate Cancer (ERSPC) trial. Int J Cancer 2002; 98(2):268–273.

17. Schroder FH, Denis LJ, Roobol M, Nelen V, Auvinen A, Tammela T et al. The story of the European Randomized Study of Screening for Prostate Cancer. BJU Int 2003; 92 Suppl 2:1–13.:1–13.

18. Sandblom G, Varenhorst E, Lofman O, Rosell J, Carlsson P. Clinical consequences of screening for prostate cancer: 15 years follow-up of a randomised controlled trial in Sweden. Eur Urol 2004; 46(6):717–723.

19. Thompson IM, Pauler DK, Goodman PJ, Tangen CM, Lucia MS, Parnes HL et al. Prevalence of prostate cancer among men with a prostate-specific antigen level < or =4.0 ng per milliliter. N Engl J Med 2004; 350(22):2239–2246.

20. Oesterling JE, Jacobsen SJ, Chute CG, Guess HA, Girman CJ, Panser LA et al. Serum prostate-specific antigen in a community-based population of healthy men. Establishment of age-specific reference ranges. JAMA 1993; 270(7):860–864.

21. Crawford DE, Abrahamsson PA. PSA-based Screening for Prostate Cancer: How Does It Compare with Other Cancer Screening Tests? Eur Urol 2008; 54(2):262–273.

22. Thompson IM, Ankerst DP, Chi C, Lucia MS, Goodman PJ, Crowley JJ et al. Operating characteristics of prostate-specific antigen in men with an initial PSA level of 3.0 ng/ml or lower. JAMA 2005; 294(1):66–70.

23. Harris R, Lohr KN. Screening for prostate cancer: an update of the evidence for the U.S. Preventive Services Task Force. Ann Int Med 2002; 137(11):917–929.

24. Postma R, Schroder FH, van Leenders GJ, Hoedemaeker RF, Vis AN, Roobol MJ et al. Cancer detection and cancer characteristics in the European Randomized Study of Screening for Prostate Cancer (ERSPC) – Section Rotterdam. A comparison of two rounds of screening. Eur Urol 2007; 52(1):89–97.

25. Ciatto S, Bonardi R, Lombardi C, Zappa M, Gervasi G, Cappelli G. Analysis of PSA velocity in 1666 healthy subjects undergoing total PSA determination at two consecutive screening rounds. Int J Biol Markers 2002; 17(2):79–83.

26. Bangma CH, Kranse R, Blijenberg BG, Schroder FH. The value of screening tests in the detection of prostate cancer. Part II: Retrospective analysis of free/total prostate-specific analysis ratio, age-specific reference ranges, and PSA density. Urology 1995; 46(6):779–784.

27. Tornblom M, Norming U, Adolfsson J, Becker C, Abrahamsson PA, Lilja H et al. Diagnostic value of percent free prostate-specific antigen: retrospective analysis of a population-based screening study with emphasis on men with PSA levels less than 3.0 ng/mL. Urology 1999; 53(5):945–950.

28. Djavan B, Zlotta AR, Byttebier G, Shariat S, Omar M, Schulman CC et al. Prostate specific antigen density of the transition zone for early detection of prostate cancer. J Urol 1998; 160(2):411–418.

29. Schroder FH, van dC-K, I, de Koning HJ, Vis AN, Hoedemaeker RF, Kranse R. Prostate cancer detection at low prostate specific antigen. J Urol 2000; 163(3):806–812.

30. Schroder FH, van der MP, Beemsterboer P, Kruger AB, Hoedemaeker R, Rietbergen J et al. Evaluation of the digital rectal examination as a screening test for prostate cancer. Rotterdam section of the European Randomized Study of Screening for Prostate Cancer. J Natl Cancer Inst 1998; 90(23):1817–1823.

31. Gosselaar C., Roobol M.J., van den Bergh RCN., Wolters T., Schroder FH. Digital Rectal Examination and the Diagnosis of Prostate Cancer-a study Based on 8 Years and Three Screenings within the European Randomized Study of Screening for Prostate Cancer (ERSPC),Rotterdam. Eur Urol 2009; 55(1):139–147.

32. van der Cruijsen-Koeter IW, van der Kwast TH, Schroder FH. Interval carcinomas in the European Randomized Study of Screening for Prostate Cancer (ERSPC)-Rotterdam. J Natl Cancer Inst 2003; 95(19):1462–1466.

33. Roobol MJ, Grenabo A, Schroder FH, Hugosson J. Interval cancers in prostate cancer screening: comparing 2- and 4-year screening intervals in the European Randomized Study of Screening for Prostate Cancer, Gothenburg and Rotterdam. J Nat Cancer Inst 2007; 99(17):1296–1303.

34. Kattan MW. A nomogram for predicting 10-year life expectancy in men with prostate cancer after definitive therapy. Nat Clin Pract Urol 2008; 5(3):138–139.

35. van der Cruijsen-Koeter IW, Vis AN, Roobol MJ, Wildhagen MF, de Koning HJ, van der Kwast TH et al. Comparison of screen detected and clinically diagnosed prostate cancer in the European randomized study of screening for prostate cancer, section Rotterdam. J Urol 2005; 174(1):121–125.

36. Aus G, Bergdahl S, Lodding P, Lilja H, Hugosson J. Prostate cancer screening decreases the absolute risk of being diagnosed with advanced prostate cancer – results from a prospective, population-based randomized controlled trial. Eur Urol 2007; 51(3):659–664.

37. Postma R, van Leenders AG, Roobol MJ, Schroder FH, van der Kwast TH. Tumour features in the control and screening arm of a randomized trial of prostate cancer. Eur Urol 2006; 50(1):70–75.

38. de Koning HJ, Auvinen A, Berenguer SA, Calais dS, Ciatto S, Denis L et al. Large-scale randomized prostate cancer screening trials: program performances in the European Randomized Screening for Prostate Cancer trial and the Prostate, Lung, Colorectal and Ovary cancer trial. Int J Cancer 2002; 97(2):237–244.

39. Vercelli M, Quaglia A, Marani E, Parodi S. Prostate cancer incidence and mortality trends among elderly and adult Europeans. Crit Rev Oncol Hematol 2000; 35(2):133–144.

40. Carter HB, Piantadosi S, Isaacs JT. Clinical evidence for and implications of the multistep development of prostate cancer. J Urol 1990; 143(4):742–746.

41. Etzioni R, Penson DF, Legler JM, di Tommaso D, Boer R, Gann PH et al. Overdiagnosis due to prostate-specific antigen screening: lessons from U.S. prostate cancer incidence trends. J Natl Cancer Inst 2002; 94(13):981–990.

42. Draisma G, Boer R, Otto SJ, van dC, I, Damhuis RA, Schroder FH et al. Lead times and overdetection due to prostate-specific antigen screening: estimates from the European Randomized Study of Screening for Prostate Cancer. J Natl Cancer Inst 2003; 95(12):868–878.

43. Epstein JI, Walsh PC, Carmichael M, Brendler CB. Pathologic and clinical findings to predict tumor extent of nonpalpable (stage T1c) prostate cancer. JAMA 1994; 271(5):368–374.

44. Steyerberg EW, Roobol MJ, Kattan MW, van der Kwast TH, de Koning HJ, Schroder FH. Prediction of indolent prostate cancer: validation and updating of a prognostic nomogram. J Urol 2007; 177(1):107–112.

45. Epstein JI, Chan DW, Sokoll LJ, Walsh PC, Cox JL, Rittenhouse H et al. Nonpalpable stage T1c prostate cancer: prediction of insignificant disease using free/total prostate specific antigen levels and needle biopsy findings. J Urol 1998; 160(6 Pt 2):2407–2411.

46. Raaijmakers R, Kirkels WJ, Roobol MJ, Wildhagen MF, Schrder FH. Complication rates and risk factors of 5802 transrectal ultrasound-guided sextant biopsies of the prostate within a population-based screening program. Urology 2002; 60(5):826–830.

47. Rietbergen JB, Kruger AE, Kranse R, Schroder FH. Complications of transrectal ultrasound-guided systematic sextant biopsies of the prostate: evaluation of complication rates and risk factors within a population-based screening program. Urology 1997; 49(6):875–880.

48. Madalinska JB, Essink-Bot ML, de Koning HJ, Kirkels WJ, van der Maas PJ, Schroder FH. Health-related quality-of-life effects of radical prostatectomy and primary radiotherapy for screen-detected or clinically diagnosed localized prostate cancer. J Clin Oncol 2001; 19(6):1619–1628.

49. Rozet F, Jaffe J, Braud G, Harmon J, Cathelineau X, Barret E et al. A direct comparison of robotic assisted versus pure laparoscopic radical prostatectomy: a single institution experience. J Urol 2007; 178(2):478–482.
50. Chabert CC, Merrilees DA, Neill MG, Eden CG. Curtain dissection of the lateral prostatic fascia and potency after laparoscopic radical prostatectomy: a veil of mystery. BJU Int 2008; 101(10):1285–1288.

# II PROSTATE-SPECIFIC ANTIGEN

# 5

# Evolution of Prostate-Specific Antigen for Screening

*Javier Hernandez and Edith Canby-Hagino*

## SUMMARY

Prostate-specific antigen (PSA) is one of the most widely applied screening tests in current medical practice. Its widespread use has had a tremendous impact on all aspects of the management of prostate cancer. PSA screening has led to a stage migration to more organ-confined cancers at the time of diagnosis and is temporally associated with a decrease in prostate cancer mortality. However, PSA screening is imperfect and remains controversial. In this chapter we review the history of the discovery, initial studies, and subsequent widespread application of PSA screening. Initial studies were limited by the lack of applicability to all ethnic groups, upper limits of normal determined with incomplete ascertainment of disease status among study participants, and obsolete biopsy techniques. Various modifications of PSA-based screening have been adopted clinically without sufficient validation. More recent studies have elucidated the non-dichotomous nature of PSA as well as the contribution of other factors to the overall risk for prostate cancer. We await the results of large-scale clinical trials that will more clearly define the impact of PSA screening on prostate cancer mortality as well as the discovery and validation of additional prognostic biomarkers.

**Key Words:** PSA, PSA density, Screening, Prostate cancer risk.

From: *Current Clinical Urology: Prostate Cancer Screening*, Edited by: D. P. Ankerst et al.
DOI 10.1007/978-1-60327-281-0_5 © Humana Press, a part of Springer Science+Business Media, LLC 2009

# INTRODUCTION

Prostate-specific antigen (PSA) is a member of the human kallikrein gene family and a 33-kDa serine protease secreted by the prostatic epithelium and the epithelial lining of the periurethral glands. Its most important physiologic function is the lique-faction of the seminal coagulum to allow release of spermatozoa *(1)*. During the early 1970s, several investigators independently reported the earliest discoveries of a tissue-specific antigen called gamma-seminoprotein which is present in the human prostate and in seminal plasma *(2–5)*. Several years later, Sensabaugh isolated and character-ized gamma-seminoprotein from human seminal plasma while searching for a potential marker that could be used in the investigation of rape crimes *(6)*. In 1979, Wang isolated and purified an antigen from prostate tissue that was determined to be prostate-specific in nature *(7)*. This protein was confirmed to be identical to the gamma-seminoprotein previously identified by other investigators *(8)*.

Once PSA was determined to be prostate-specific, its potential as a marker for prostate cancer was investigated. Immunohistochemical studies identified the presence of PSA in both primary and metastatic prostatic neoplasms, but not in non-prostatic neoplasms *(9)*. Its utility as a serum marker for prostate cancer was proposed when investigators identified elevated levels of serum PSA in men with prostate cancer, com-pared to men without prostate cancer, men with non-prostatic malignancies, women with malignancies, and healthy women *(10)*.

Since its initial discovery and eventual widespread clinical application PSA has had a tremendous impact on all aspects of the management of prostate cancer to include detection, staging, and monitoring of the disease. In spite of the fact that PSA-based screening has resulted in a downward stage migration to more organ-confined cancers at the time of diagnosis, and is temporally associated with a decrease in prostate cancer mortality, PSA screening remains controversial. While we await results from clinical trials evaluating the efficacy of PSA screening, multiple investigators have attempted to define the optimal levels of serum PSA or its derivatives to use as a threshold for recommending a prostate biopsy. Many of these studies have limitations which limit the applicability of specific threshold PSA levels to the general population. In this chapter we present a historical perspective on the evolution of screening for prostate cancer, with particular emphasis on the design of the initial studies evaluating the role of PSA in the detection of this disease.

## INITIAL EXPERIENCE WITH PSA AS A TUMOR MARKER AND A SCREENING TOOL

Prior to the introduction of PSA, serum prostatic acid phosphatase (PAP) was used as a marker for prostate cancer. Because of its low sensitivity in localized disease, however, PAP is not suitable for prostate cancer screening *(11)*. The improved sensitivity of PSA over PAP for localized prostate cancer sparked the initial interest in PSA as a potential screening tool *(12,13)*.

Widespread use of PSA in the clinical setting began around the mid-1980s with early experience leading to several important clinical implications. Investigators noted that the PSA fall after hormonal therapy correlated with response to the treatment *(13–15)*. Additionally, a rising PSA after treatment predicted disease recurrence *(13,16,17)*. It was also noted that, after a radical prostatectomy, PSA should be undetectable, otherwise, prostate cancer will generally recur *(13,16,17)*. Finally, many of these early investigators cautioned against using PSA for screening due to a substantial overlap in PSA values between patients with and without cancer and the resulting poor test specificity *(13,18,19)*.

The results of the first large-scale studies of PSA screening among healthy men appeared in the late 1980s and early 1990s *(20–24)*. These studies examined men volunteering for screening *(20–22,24)* as well as men seen within general urologic practice *(23)*. It is important to understand that the populations being screened had never been examined with a sensitive screening test before. Prostate cancer detection rates with digital rectal examination (DRE) alone range between 0.8% *(25)* and 1.4% *(26)*. When staged pathologically following radical prostatectomy, approximately two-thirds of these patients had extraprostatic disease *(25)*. Thus, in the case of a disease with a relatively high prevalence such as prostate cancer, the introduction of a screening test with even a slightly improved sensitivity in an effectively unscreened population would lead to an increased rate of disease detection. This phenomenon was observed in the late 1980s to early 1990s when PSA screening dramatically increased across the USA *(27–29)*.

Five initial reports of PSA screening set the stage for widespread test adoption: those of Wang, Cooner, Brawer, Catalona, and Stamey *(20–24,30)*. In retrospect, the design for these various studies interfered significantly with the assessment of PSA for prostate cancer screening. Some of the limitations included lack of applicability to all ethnic groups, limited ascertainment of disease status among study participants, and obsolete biopsy techniques (e.g., <6–12 cores), among others. Few of these authors performed biopsies to ascertain cancer status of patients with low-PSA levels. Some authors did not include DRE as part of the evaluation for men with a 'normal' PSA. Some of these same investigators subsequently described relatively high-cancer detection rates among men with abnormal DRE and PSA levels less than 4.0 ng/ml *(31)*.

Although the serum PSA testing was initially approved for disease monitoring after diagnosis, widespread screening began following dissemination of the results from the initial screening series *(32)*. With increasing experience, it became recognized that patients diagnosed by screening most often had clinically organ-confined disease, about one man in four with a PSA level over 4.0 ng/ml had cancer on biopsy, and that PSA levels were associated with the risk of the disease. In one of the largest screening series, Catalona evaluated 10,251 men undergoing PSA screening as well as 266 men without a PSA determination who had a prostate biopsy for an abnormal DRE *(33)*. Cancer detection rates among screened men with PSA levels of 4.1–9.9 ng/ml and 10 ng/ml or greater were 27% and 59% during initial screening, and 42% and 41% with serial screening, respectively. A critical limitation of this study was that none of the 8,727 men with a PSA equal or less than 4.0 ng/ml underwent a prostate biopsy. Another limitation of this study was that patients with a PSA level over 4.0 ng/ml with a normal DRE and transrectal ultrasound (TRUS) did not undergo biopsy.

With the general acceptance of PSA screening and almost universal acceptance of an upper limit of normal of 4.0 ng/ml, investigators sought to address issues related to the performance characteristics of this test and propose modifications in order to improve PSA as a screening tool. Using similar study designs as those initially conducted (annual examinations with PSA and DRE; biopsy if either one is abnormal; no biopsy if both normal), various investigators proposed the following modifications.

### (a) Age-adjusted PSA

PSA increases with age *(34,35)*. Based on these findings, a lower upper limit of normal should be used for younger men versus a higher upper limit for older men. This modification was meant to improve sensitivity in younger men and specificity in older men.

## Effect of Ethnicity

PSA performance varies by ethnicity. Most investigators have found higher PSA values among African American men *(36–38)*, although some have not *(39)*. Presumably, by decreasing the upper limit of normal in African American men, test sensitivity would be increased.

## PSA Velocity

An increasing PSA level over time is often seen in men who are later diagnosed with prostate cancer *(40,41)*. Some investigators have suggested that an annual increase of 0.75 ng/ml year should prompt a biopsy, regardless of PSA level. More recently, some studies have explored the impact of age on PSA velocity thresholds for recommending a prostate biopsy *(42,43)* in addition to prognostic implications of PSA velocity *(44,45)*.

## PSA Density

As higher levels of PSA are seen in men with larger prostates, some investigators have suggested correcting PSA for prostate size to improve test specificity in large glands and sensitivity in smaller glands *(46)*. Others have not confirmed the utility of PSA density *(47,48)*.

## PSA Isoforms

A substantial fraction of circulating PSA is bound to plasma proteins. The proportion that is unbound (ratio of free-to-total PSA) has been found to be inversely associated with the risk of prostate cancer *(49–51)*. Other PSA isoforms have been related to the risk of prostate cancer detection *(52,53)*.

## FINDINGS OF THE PROSTATE CANCER PREVENTION TRIAL AND PROSTATE CANCER SCREENING IN MEN WITH LOW-PSA LEVELS

The Prostate Cancer Prevention Trial (PCPT) was the first large-scale study to ascertain prostate cancer status in study participants across the full range of PSA values. Recent reports from the PCPT have challenged the notion of considering a PSA value of 4.0 ng/ml as the upper limit of normal for recommending a prostate biopsy *(54)*. In an analysis of 2,950 PCPT participants randomized to the study's placebo group and who never had a PSA greater than 4.0 ng/ml or an abnormal digital rectal examination (DRE), the investigators found that PSA levels between 0 and 4.0 ng/ml were associated with a positive predictive value between 6.6 and 26.9%. Within this PSA range 14.9% of men with cancer had high-grade disease, with this rate reaching 25% among men with a

PSA between 3.1 and 4.0 ng/ml. Other series have reported on the rates of prostate can-cer detection at low-PSA levels. In 332 men with a normal DRE and a PSA between 2.6 and 4.0 ng/ml, Catalona found prostate cancer in 22% *(49)*. One Japanese study found no difference in cancer detection between men with PSA levels of 2.0–4.0 ng/ml and those with PSA levels of 4.1–10.0 ng/ml *(55)*. Prostate cancer was diagnosed in 23.6% of both groups.

In the absence of better prognostic markers, these studies raise the question of the clinical significance of cancers detected among men with low-PSA levels. However, a number of series suggest that a substantial number of the tumors in this population may be consequential. Among 129 men with PSA values less than 2.0 ng/ml undergoing radical cystoprostatectomy for invasive bladder cancer of whom 30 had an incidental diagnosis of prostate cancer, Ward found that 60% of the prostate cancers were clinically significant when defined as volume more than 0.5 cc, presence of Gleason's 4 or 5 disease, stage pT3, positive margins, more than three tumor foci, or adverse ploidy status or proliferation index *(56)*. Screening investigations both in Chicago and Tyrol, Austria have reported similar high rates of clinically significant tumors among men with low PSA *(57,58)*. Notably, in one series of 82 patients treated for metastatic disease, four patients had PSA levels < 2.0 ng/ml *(59)*.

## CONTRIBUTION OF OTHER FACTORS

In addition to identifying prostate cancer risk at low levels of PSA, the PCPT was also able to rebuke or validate other factors that have been proposed to increase risk for prostate cancer. In multivariate analysis of the 5,519 men in the placebo group who underwent prostate biopsies, higher PSA level, family history of prostate cancer, and abnormal digital rectal exam were associated with increased risk of prostate cancer diagnosis. A previous negative biopsy was associated with reduced risk of prostate cancer diagnosis *(60)*.0 It is interesting to note that PSA veloc-ity did not contribute to an increased likelihood of cancer diagnosis. Age at biopsy did not contribute to overall prostate cancer risk, but was found to be predictive of increased risk of high-grade (Gleason score $\geq$ 7) prostate cancer. African American race was also associated with increased risk for high-grade disease. These findings were developed into a risk calculator, which can be found on the worldwide web at www.compass.fhcrc.org/edrnnci/bin/calculator/main.asp.

The performance of the risk calculator was subsequently validated in a group of 446 men who had undergone prostate biopsy, serum PSA, and digital rectal exams, derived from a larger prospective prostate disease screening cohort in South Texas *(61)*. Using the PCPT risk calculator, the area under the ROC curve (AUC) for this cohort was 65.5%, compared to an AUC of 70.2% in the original PCPT risk calculator publication. Although smaller, this group was more racially and ethnically diverse than the PCPT cohort, supporting generalizability of this calculator to a diverse population.

Other factors may also impact the accuracy of PSA as a predictor of prostate cancer risk. Long-term treatment with 5-alpha reductase inhibitors will result in reduction of serum PSA, and PCPT demonstrated a 2.5-fold reduction in PSA in men treated with finasteride over the 7-year duration of the study *(62)*. A similar effect is seen with dutas-teride *(63)*. In response to this reduction, urologists typically lower by a factor of 2 their threshold for recommending prostate biopsies in men treated with 5-alpha reductase inhibitors. During PCPT, PSA levels were adjusted by a factor of 2, and later by 2.3 in men receiving finasteride to ensure that equal numbers of biopsies were performed in the finasteride and placebo arms. In the PCPT, PSA actually demonstrated increased sensitivity for the detection of prostate cancer, with increased area under the ROC curve when compared to men in the placebo group *(64)*. Finasteride also increases the sensitivity of DRE for the detection of prostate cancer *(65)*. It is not known whether enhancement of PSA and/or DRE sensitivity will be seen with dutasteride therapy, but multiplication of PSA by a factor of 2 in men treated with dutasteride does yield comparable rates of cancer detection compared to men on placebo (for whom PSA is not adjusted), with a PSA threshold for biopsy of 4 ng/ml *(63)*.

## CONCLUSION

Ultimately, the decision to screen for prostate cancer rests with the patient and his health care provider, after careful consideration of the merits of prostate cancer diagnosis in the context of a man's risk factors for the disease, health status, and expected longevity. PSA as a screening test for prostate cancer is not likely to disappear any time soon, as it remains the most sensitive predictor of prostate cancer risk. Ideally, the results of ongoing large-scale screening studies such as the National Cancer Institute's Prostate, Lung, Colorectal, and Ovarian Cancer (PLCO) Screening Trial and the Tyrol prostate cancer screening project will provide other clinical parameters that can be incorporated with PSA in order to identify men who are most likely to benefit from diagnosis and treatment.

## REFERENCES

1. Lilja H. (1985) A kallikrein-like serine protease in prostatic fluid cleaves the predominant seminal vesicle protein *J Clin Invest* **76**,1899–903.
2. Ablin RJ, Soanes WA, Bronson P, et al. (1970) Precipitating antigens of the normal human prostate. *J Reprod Fertil* **22**,573–4.
3. Ablin RJ, Bronson P, Soanes WA, et al. (1970) Tissue- and species specific antigens of normal human prostatic tissue. *J Immunol* **104**,1329–39.
4. Hara M, Koyanagi Y, Inoue T, et al. (1971) Some physico-chemical characteristics of "$\gamma$ – seminoprotein", an antigenic component specific for human seminal plasma. *JPN J Leg Med* **25**,322–4.
5. Li TS, Beling CG. (1973) Isolation and characterization of two specific antigens of human seminal plasma. *Fertil Steril* **24**,134–44.
6. Sensabaugh GF, Crim D. (1978) Isolation and characterization of a semen-specific protein from human seminal plasma: A potential new marker for semen identification *J Forensic Sci* **23**,106–15.
7. Wang MC, Valenzuela LA, Murphy GP, et al. (1979) Purification of a human prostate specific antigen *Invest Urol* **17**,159–63.
8. Wang MC, Papsidero LD, Chu TM. (1994) Prostate-specific antigen, p30, gamma-seminoprotein, and E1 *Prostate* **24**,107–10.
9. Nadji M, Tabei SZ, Castro A, Chu TM, Murphy GP, Wang MC, Morales AR. (1981) Prostatic-specific antigen: an immunohistologic marker for prostatic neoplasms *Cancer* **48**,1229–32.
10. Kuriyama M, Wang MC, Papsidero LD, Killian CS, Shimano T, Valenzuela L, Nishiura T, Murphy GP, Chu TM. (1980) Quantitation of prostate-specific antigen in serum by a sensitive enzyme immunoassay *Cancer Res* **40**,4658–62.
11. Gutman AB, Gutman EB. (1938) An "acid" phosphatase occurring in the serum of patients with metastasizing carcinoma of the prostate gland *J Clin Invest* **17**, 473–8.
12. Seamonds B, Whitaker MS, Yang N, Shaw LM, Anderson K, Bollinger JR. (1986) Evaluation of prostate-specific antigen and prostatic acid phosphatase as prostate cancer markers *Urology* **28**,472–9.
13. Stamey TA, Yang N, Hay AR, McNeal JE, Freiha FS, Redwine E. (1987) Prostate-specific antigen as a serum marker for adenocarcinoma of the prostate *N Engl J Med* **317**,909–16.

14. Ferro M, Gillatt D, Symes M, Smith P. (1989) High-dose intravenous estrogen therapy in advanced prostatic carcinoma. Use of serum prostate-specific antigen to monitor response. *Urology* **34**,134–8.

15. Hudson M, Bahnson R, Catalona W. (1989) Clinical use of prostate specific antigen in patients with prostate cancer. *J Urol* **142**,1011–7.

16. Oesterling JE, Chan DW, Epstein JI, Kimball AW, Jr., Bruzek DJ, Rock RC, Brendler CB, Walsh PC. (1988) Prostate specific antigen in the preoperative and postoperative evaluation of localized prostatic cancer treated with radical prostatectomy *J Urol* **139**,766–72.

17. Lange PH, Ercole CJ, Lightner DJ, Fraley EE, Vessella R. (1989) The value of serum prostate specific antigen determinations before and after radical prostatectomy *J Urol* **141**,873–9.

18. Guinan P, Bhatti R, Ray P. (1987) An evaluation of prostate specific antigen in prostatic cancer *J Urol* **137**,686–9.

19. Barak M, Mecz Y, Lurie A, Gruener N. (1989) Evaluation of prostate-specific antigen as a marker for adenocarcinoma of the prostate *J Lab Clin Med* **113**,598–603.

20. Brawer MK, Beatie J, Wener MH, Vessella RL, Preston SD, Lange PH. (1993) Screening for prostatic carcinoma with prostate specific antigen: results of the second year *J Urol* **150**,106–9.

21. Brawer MK, Chetner MP, Beatie J, Buchner DM, Vessella RL, Lange PH. (1992) Screening for prostatic carcinoma with prostate specific antigen *J Urol* **147**,841–5.

22. Terris MK, Stamey TA. (1993) Utilization of polyclonal serum prostate specific antigen levels in screening for prostate cancer: a comparison with corresponding monoclonal values. *Brit J Urol* **73**,61–4.

23. Cooner WH, Mosley BR, Rutherford CL, Beard JH, Pond HS, Terry WJ, Igel TC, Kidd DD. (1990) Prostate cancer detection in a clinical urological practice by ultrasonography, digital rectal examination and prostate specific antigen. *J Urol* **143**,1146–52.

24. Catalona W, Smith D, Ratliff T, Dodds K, Coplen D, Yuan J, Petros J, Andriole G. (1991) Measurement of prostate-specific antigen in serum as a screening test for prostate cancer. *N Engl J Med* **324**,1156–61.

25. Thompson IM, Ernst JJ, Gangai MP, Spence CR. (1984) Adenocarcinoma of the prostate: results of routine urological screening. *J Urol* **132**,690–2.

26. Chodak GW, Schoenberg HW. (1984) Early detection of prostate cancer by routine screening. *JAMA* **252**,3261–4.

27. Farkas A, Schneider D, Perrotti M, Cummings K, Ward W. (1998) National trends in the epidemiology of prostate cancer, 1973 to 1994: evidence for the effectiveness of prostate-specific antigen screening. *Urology* **52**,444–8; discussion 8–9.

28. Mettlin C, Murphy G, Babaian R, Chesley A, Kane R, Littrup P, Mostofi F, Ray P, Shanberg A, Toi A. (1996) The results of a five-year early prostate cancer detection intervention. Investigators of the American Cancer Society National Prostate Cancer Detection Project. *Cancer* **77**,150–9.

29. Jacobsen S, Katusic S, Bergstralh E, Oesterling J, Ohrt D, Klee G, Chute C, Lieber M. (1995) Incidence of prostate cancer diagnosis in the eras before and after serum prostate-specific antigen testing. *JAMA* **274**,1445–9.

30. Wang TY, Kawaguchi TP. (1986) Preliminary evaluation of measurement of serum prostate-specific antigen level in detection of prostate cancer *Ann Clin Lab Sci* **16**,461–6.

31. Carvalhal GF, Smith DS, Mager DE, Ramos C, Catalona WJ. (1999) Digital rectal examination for detecting prostate cancer at prostate specific antigen levels of 4 ng./ml. or less. *J Urol* **161**,835–9.

32. Potosky AL, Miller BA, Albertsen PC, Kramer BS. (1995) The role of increasing detection in the rising incidence of prostate cancer. *JAMA* **273**,548–52.

33. Catalona WJ, Smith DS, Ratliff TL, Basler JW. (1993) Detection of organ-confined prostate cancer is increased through prostate-specific antigen-based screening *JAMA* **270**,948–54.

34. Oesterling JE, Jacobsen SJ, Chute CG, Guess HA, Girman CJ, Panser LA, Lieber MM. (1993) Serum prostate-specific antigen in a community-based population of healthy men. Establishment of age-specific reference ranges *JAMA* **270**,860–4.

35. Gustafsson O, Mansour E, Norming U, Carlsson A, Tomblom M, Nyman CR. (1998) Prostate-specific antigen (PSA), PSA density and age-adjusted PSA reference values in screening for prostate cancer – a study o randomly selected population of 2,400 men. *Scand J Urol Nephrol* **32**,373–7.

36. Moul JW, Sesterrhenn IA, Connelly RR, Srivastava S, Mostofi F, McLeod DG. (1995) Prostate-specific antigen values at the time of prostate cancer diagnosis in African-American men. *JAMA* **274**,1277–81.

37. Eastham JA, Whatley T, Crow A, Venable DD, Sartor O. (1998) Clinical characteristics and biopsy specimen features in African-American and white men without prostate cancer. *J Natl Cancer Inst* **90**,756–60.

38. Abdalla I, Ray P, Vaida F, Vijayakumar S. (1999) Racial differences in prostate-specific antigen levels and prostate-specific antigen densities in patients with prostate cancer. *Am J Clin Oncol* **22**,537–41.

39. McCammon KA, Schellhammer PF, Wright GL, Lynch DF. (1996) Age specific PSA levels in African Americans. *J Urol* **155**,426, abstract 61.
40. Carter HB, Pearson JD, Metter EJ, Brant LJ, Chan DW, Andres R, Fozard JL, Walsh PC. (1992) Longitudinal evaluation of prostate-specific antigen levels in men with and without prostate disease. *JAMA* **267**,2215–20.
41. Carter HB, Pearson JD, Waclawiw Z, Metter EJ, Chan DW, Guess HA, Walsh PC. (1995) Prostate-specific antigen variability in men without prostate cancer: effect of sampling interval on prostate-specific antigen velocity *Urology* **45**,591–6.
42. Moul JW, Sun L, Hotaling JM, Fitzsimons NJ, Polascik TJ, Robertson CN, Dahm P, Anscher MS, Mouraviev V, Pappas PA, Albala DM. (2007) Age adjusted prostate specific antigen and prostate specific antigen velocity cut points in prostate cancer screening *J Urol* **177**,499–503; discussion -4.
43. Loeb S, Roehl KA, Catalona WJ, Nadler RB. (2007) Prostate specific antigen velocity threshold for predicting prostate cancer in young men *J Urol* **177**,899–902.
44. Carter HB, Ferrucci L, Kettermann A, Landis P, Wright EJ, Epstein JI, Trock BJ, Metter EJ. (2006) Detection of life-threatening prostate cancer with prostate-specific antigen velocity during a window of curability *J Natl Cancer Inst* **98**,1521–7.
45. D'Amico AV, Hui-Chen M, Renshaw AA, Sussman B, Roehl KA, Catalona WJ. (2006) Identifying men diagnosed with clinically localized prostate cancer who are at high risk for death from prostate cancer *J Urol* **176**,S11–5.
46. Benson MC, Whang IS, Olsson CA, McMahon DJ, Cooner WH. (1992) The use of prostate specific antigen density to enhance the predictive value of intermediate levels of serum prostate specific antigen *J Urol* **147**,817–21.
47. Brawer MK, Aramburu EA, Chen GL, Preston SD, Ellis WJ. (1993) The inability of prostate specific antigen index to enhance the predictive the value of prostate specific antigen in the diagnosis of prostatic carcinoma *J Urol* **150**,369–73.
48. Catalona WJ, Richie JP, deKernion JB, Ahmann FR, Ratliff TL, Dalkin BL, Kavoussi LR, MacFarlane MT, Southwick PC. (1994) Comparison of prostate specific antigen concentration versus prostate specific antigen density in the early detection of prostate cancer: receiver operating characteristic curves *J Urol* **152**,2031–6.
49. Catalona WJ, Smith DS, Ornstein DK. (1997) Prostate cancer detection in men with serum PSA concentrations of 2.6 to 4.0 ng/ml and benign prostate examination: Enhancement of specificity with free PSA measurement. *JAMA* **277**,1452–5.
50. Partin AW, Catalona WJ, Southwick PC, Subong EN, Gasior GH, Chan DW. (1996) Analysis of percent free prostate-specific antigen (PSA) for prostate cancer detection: influence of total PSA, prostate volume, and age *Urology* **48**,55–61.
51. Partin AW, Brawer MK, Bartsch G, Horninger W, Taneja SS, Lepor H, Babaian R, Childs SJ, Stamey T, Fritsche HA, Sokoll L, Chan DW, Thiel RP, Cheli CD. (2003) Complexed prostate specific antigen improves specificity for prostate cancer detection: results of a prospective multicenter clinical trial *J Urol* **170**,1787–91.
52. Catalona WJ, Bartsch G, Rittenhouse HG, Evans CL, Linton HJ, Amirkhan A, Horninger W, Klocker H, Mikolajczyk SD. (2003) Serum pro prostate specific antigen improves cancer detection compared to free and complexed prostate specific antigen in men with prostate specific antigen 2 to 4 ng/ml *J Urol* **170**,2181–5.
53. Mikolajczyk SD, Marker KM, Millar LS, Kumar A, Saedi MS, Payne JK, Evans CL, Gasior CL, Linton HJ, Carpenter P, Rittenhouse HG. (2001) A truncated precursor form of prostate-specific antigen is a more specific serum marker of prostate cancer *Cancer Res* **61**,6958–63.
54. Thompson IM, Pauler DK, Goodman PJ, Tangen CM, Lucia MS, Parnes HL, Minasian LM, Ford LG, Lippman SM, Crawford ED, Crowley JJ, Coltman CA Jr. (2004) Prevalence of prostate cancer among men with a prostate-specific antigen level < or=4.0 ng per milliliter. *N Engl J Med* **350**, 2239–46.
55. Kobayashi T, Nishizawa K, Ogura K, Mitsumori K, Ide Y. (2004) Detection of prostate cancer in men with prostate-specific antigen levels of 2.0 to 4.0 ng/ml equivalent to that in men with 4.1 to 10. ng/ml in a Japanese population. *Urology* **63**,727–31.
56. Ward JF, Bartsch G, Sebo TJ, Pinggera G-M, Blute ML, Zincke H. (2004) Pathologic characterization of prostate cancers with a very low serum prostate specific antigen (0–2 ng/mL) incidental to cysto-prostatectomy: is PSA a useful indicator of clinical significance? *Urol Oncol: Seminars and Original Investigations* **22**,40–7.
57. Sokolof MH, Yang XJ, Fumo M, Mhoon D, Brendler C. (2004) Characterizing prostatic adenocarcinomas in men with a serum prostate specific antigen level of <4.0 ng/mL. *BJU Int* **93**,499–502.

58. Horninger W, Berger AP, Rogatsch H, Gschwendtner A, Steiner H, Niescher M, Klocker H, Bartsch G. (2004) Characteristics of prostate cancers detected at low PSA levels *Prostate* **58**,232–7.
59. Nishio R, Furuya Y, Nagakawa O, Fuse H. (2003) Metastatic prostate cancer with normal level of serum prostate-specific antigen. *Int Urol Nephrol* **35**,189–92.
60. Thompson IM, Ankerst DP, Chi C, Goodman PJ, Tangen CM, Lucia MS, Feng Z, Parnes HL, Coltman CA, Jr. (2006) Assessing prostate cancer risk: results from the Prostate Cancer Prevention Trial *J Natl Cancer Inst* **98**,529–34.
61. Parekh DJ, Ankerst DP, Higgins BA, Hernandez J, Canby-Hagino E, Brand T, Troyer DA, Leach RJ, Thompson IM. (2006) External validation of the Prostate Cancer Prevention Trial risk calculator in a screened population *Urology* **68**,1152–5.
62. Etzioni RD, Howlader N, Shaw PA, Ankerst DP, Penson DF, Goodman PJ, Thompson IM. (2005) Long-term effects of finasteride on prostate specific antigen levels: results from the prostate cancer prevention trial *J Urol* **174**,877–81.
63. Andriole GL, Marberger M, Roehrborn CG. (2006) Clinical usefulness of serum prostate specific antigen for the detection of prostate cancer is preserved in men receiving the dual 5alpha-reductase inhibitor dutasteride *J Urol* **175**,1657–62.
64. Thompson IM, Chi C, Ankerst DP, Goodman PJ, Tangen CM, Lippman SM, Lucia MS, Parnes HL, Coltman CA, Jr. (2006) Effect of finasteride on the sensitivity of PSA for detecting prostate cancer *J Natl Cancer Inst* **98**,1128–33.
65. Thompson IM, Tangen CM, Goodman PJ, Lucia MS, Parnes HL, Lippman SM, Coltman CA, Jr. (2007) Finasteride improves the sensitivity of digital rectal examination for prostate cancer detection *J Urol* **177**,1749–52.

# 6

# The Performance Characteristics of Prostate-Specific Antigen for Prostate Cancer Screening

*Ian M. Thompson, Jr. and Donna P. Ankerst*

CONTENTS

## SUMMARY

When considering the application of a screening test for any disease, it is extremely important to understand how the performance characteristics of a test will affect its usefulness to a patient as well as to society. This chapter defines and interprets the key operating characteristics for prostate-specific antigen (PSA), the ubiquitous marker used for prostate cancer screening. Results from the Prostate Cancer Prevention Trial, which broke previously held conceptions about how to use PSA, and potential biases that affect many current studies of the performance characteristics of PSA are reviewed.

**Key Words:** Prostate-specific antigen, Sensitivity, Specificity, Verification bias, Spectrum bias.

To a man or his physician who is considering prostate cancer as a potential threat to life, there are a host of considerations that must be included in the decision-making of *when* to begin screening, *if* to screen, *what* screening tests to employ, and *how* to

From: *Current Clinical Urology: Prostate Cancer Screening*, Edited by: D. P. Ankerst et al.
DOI 10.1007/978-1-60327-281-0_6 © Humana Press, a part of Springer Science+Business Media, LLC 2009

interpret those tests. In the idealized setting, a healthy man who desires to avoid morbidity or death due to prostate cancer would expect his physician to offer him testing that would identify the presence of a tumor that has a high risk of causing suffering or death at such a time in the tumor's growth that a treatment could be initiated that would curtail progression of the disease. Unfortunately, for a variety of reasons that have been discussed at length in this text, this goal is not simple but is extraordinarily complex when applied to prostate cancer screening.

## BACKGROUND: PERFORMANCE CHARACTERISTICS OF A SCREENING TEST

When considering the application of a screening test for any disease, it is extremely important to understand how the performance characteristics of a test will affect its usefulness to a patient as well as to society. The most commonly used measures that are included in this assessment are sensitivity, specificity, and positive and negative predictive values. To understand what these measures mean and how they are calculated, we simply need to consider the four possible outcomes if we apply a screening test in seeking a disease. Table 1 shows these four outcomes and how we define them.

Sensitivity, specificity, and positive and negative predictive values refer to the four possible rates from the table. Sensitivity and specificity consider accuracy within the groups of disease present and absent. Sensitivity is the fraction of test positives among those with disease present, specificity the fraction of test negatives among those with disease absent. Alternatively, positive predictive value and negative predictive value refer to accuracy within the groups that test positive and negative: positive predictive value is the fraction of diseased individuals among those that test positive and negative predictive value is the fraction of non-diseased individuals among those that test negative. Because sensitivity and specificity have as denominator the true disease status and count among those the test result, they are referred to as retrospective measures. Positive and negative value, on the other hand, condition on test result and look forward to disease outcome. Hence they are referred to as prospective measures.

The implications of these measures for a patient and for society are vastly different. For example, a 60-year-old man whose brother just died of prostate cancer whose primary concern is to not have the same fate, may be most interested in test *sensitivity*: he wants, at all costs, to know if he has prostate cancer and to find it as early as possible. Conversely, to a health care system that is trying to apportion resources in the most efficient manner, including avoiding unnecessary and costly prostate biopsies in men who do not have cancer, test *specificity* may be an important consideration. Positive predictive value may be a very important term to a physician who is recommending

Table 1
Four Outcomes for a Disease and Screening Test

|  |  | *Test* | |
|  |  | *Positive* | *Negative* |
| Disease | Present | True positive | False negative |
|  | Absent | False positive | True negative |

a prostate biopsy to an at-risk man: communicating a 40% risk of prostate cancer on biopsy (*positive predictive value*) may be a very effective way to explain the rationale for a biopsy. On the other hand, explaining to the first man above whose only risk factor is family history of disease, that his risk of prostate cancer is only 3% and that a biopsy is therefore probably not necessary at this time (*negative predictive value*) can be a very helpful concept for both physician and patient.

It is for these reasons, both for patients and physicians as well as for health policy experts that a full understanding of the performance characteristics of a cancer screening test such as prostate-specific antigen (PSA) is extremely important. Unfortunately, until now, these characteristics have been extremely elusive and, even now, data are forthcoming that do not properly describe these values. As noted in the chapter on *PSA screening* by Canby-Hagino and Hernandez, one reason for this has been the changes in how PSA was applied: initially systematically excluding patients with PSA values less than 4.0 ng/mL from a biopsy, later lowering this threshold. As discussed below these practices influence measures of performance characteristics of PSA away from their "true" intrinsic values.

## BIASES IN ASSESSMENT OF PERFORMANCE CHARACTERISTICS IN BIOMARKER STUDIES

### *Verification Bias*

A leading reason for the difficulty in assessment of PSA-performance characteristics in many studies, including current ones, is biases in how the study population undergoing prostate biopsy is selected. To demonstrate, we assume for illustration purposes only, estimates of the distribution of PSA and rates of positive biopsy by stratum of PSA reported in the Prostate Cancer Prevention Trial (PCPT) as reflective of true population rates *(1)*. The illustration is not wholly unrealistic since the PCPT was the first study with required prostate cancer verification for all participants regardless of PSA or digital rectal exam (DRE) status, i.e., prostate cancer prevalence was assessed even in the full range of PSA values less than 4.0 ng/mL. The PCPT population, however, was generally older and healthier (required PSA ≤ 3.0 ng/mL and normal DRE at entry of the 7-year study) than the general US population *(2)*.

The second through fourth columns of Table 2 summarize numbers of men with PSA values in specific ranges and of these, numbers with cancers as would be expected in a random sample of 100 men from the PCPT population. Under assumption that PCPT rates are the same as for the general population and that prostate biopsy is 100% specific and sensitive for prostate cancer, the sample in these columns arises from an unbiased study since it includes random representative individuals from the true population, all with biopsy performed independently of PSA level. In this sample 21 of the 100 men (21.0%) have prostate cancer and the rate of prostate cancer decreases as PSA decreases: 45.5%, 26.1%, and 15.2% for PSA > 4, between 2.1 and 4.0, and ≤ 2.0 ng/mL, respectively.

For the sample in the second through fourth columns of Table 2 the values of sensitivity, specificity, and positive and negative predictive values (NPV, PPV) for the PSA cutoffs 2.0 and 4.0 ng/mL are listed under the "Unbiased study" columns in Table 3. Since they are based on an unbiased study these performance characteristics are accurate approximations to the true population characteristics.

Table 2

Illustrative Summaries of Distribution of 100 Men by PSA Level and Prostate
Cancer Status from an Unbiased Study (Assuming Prostate Cancer Prevention
Trial rates Representative of the General Population) and for a Biased Study, which
for the Same Group of 100 Men, Only Biopsied Those with PSA > 2.0 ng/mL

| PSA (ng/mL) | Men in unbiased study N = 100 | Positive biopsy in unbiased study N = 21 | Negative biopsy in unbiased study N = 79 | Men in biased study N = 34 | Positive biopsy in biased study N = 11 | Negative biopsy in biased study N=23 |
|---|---|---|---|---|---|---|
| > 4.0 | 11 | 5 | 6 | 11 | 5 | 6 |
| 2.1–4.0 | 23 | 6 | 17 | 23 | 6 | 17 |
| ≤ 2.0 | 66 | 10 | 56 | 0 | 0 | 0 |

Table 3

Sensitivity, Specificity, Positive Predictive Value (PPV) and Negative Predictive
Value (NPV) for PSA Cutoffs 2.0 and 4.0 ng/mL for an Unbiased Sample of 100
Men from the General Population (Unbiased Study) and a Biased Subsample
(Biased Study) from the Same 100 Men that Only Included Those with
PSA > 2.0 ng/mL

| Characteristic | PSA cutoff 2.0 ng/mL | | PSA cutoff 4.0 ng/mL | |
|---|---|---|---|---|
| | Unbiased study | Biased study | Unbiased study | Biased study |
| Sensitivity | 52.4% | 100.0% | 23.8% | 45.5% |
| Specificity | 70.9% | 0.0% | 92.4% | 73.9% |
| PPV | 32.4% | 32.4% | 45.5% | 45.5% |
| NPV | 84.8% | Not calculable | 88.8% | 73.9% |

To understand how selection of the population for study could yield biased estimates
of the true operating characteristics, consider the case where only men with PSA exceeding 2.0 ng/mL receive a biopsy by clinical indication (i.e., that digital rectal examination
is an unnecessary screening test among men with low PSA values, a concept supported
by Schroeder and colleagues (3)) and for simplicity that prostate biopsy is 100% sensitive and specific for prostate cancer. This yields the study results listed under the "Biased
study" columns of Table 3.

The last row of Table 2 (men with PSA ≤ 2.0 ng/mL) is not included at all in the
performance characteristic calculations because the cancer status for these men is not
verified by biopsy. The biased study thus obtains the performance characteristics for
PSA cutoffs 2.0 and 4.0 ng/mL in the "Biased study" columns of Table 3. For both PSA
cutoffs, 2.0 and 4.0 ng/mL, the study grossly overestimates their sensitivity relative to
the true population values and underestimates their specificities. The study obtains the
correct PPV for the two PSA cutoffs but the NPV of the cutoff 2.0 ng/mL is not estimable
and the NPV for the cutoff 4.0 ng/mL underestimates the true value. The problem that
this example demonstrates is how a lack of *verification* of presence or absence of disease, in this case, prostate cancer diagnosis with prostate biopsy, can directly bias the
performance characteristics of the test.

In 2004, when we published the first results of our analysis of the risk of prostate cancer among men with a PSA value less than or equal to 4.0 ng/mL, the concept above became better understood and the importance of *verification* of presence or absence of prostate cancer gained attention in the development and validation of prostate cancer biomarkers *(4)*. Nonetheless, current studies continue to evaluate prostate cancer biomarkers in the absence of verification. Indeed, the majority of current studies have this characteristic. Commonly, control subjects are included who have "low" PSA values and who are deemed "cancer-free" simply due to their PSA value. Study performance is then calculated, calling these controls "True Negatives" when indeed, we now know that some will have cancer. Additionally, as the vast majority of men have lower PSA values (about 50% of the population will have a PSA under 1 ng/mL and about 75% will have a PSA less than 2 ng/mL), the problem is exacerbated for applying study results to the general population.

### Spectrum Bias

A second, less well-characterized problem must also be considered as new prostate cancer screening tests are developed. By way of background, let us presume that there exists a gene that is overexpressed in the prostate and that a product of this gene, which we will call PCGP1 (Prostate Cancer Gene Product One), can be measured in the serum. Our initial investigations find that the gene is only rarely identified in normal epithelium while it is overexpressed many fold levels greater in prostate cancer cells.

We will now pause for a moment and consider the following. We do know that prostate cancer is ubiquitous in the general population if the prostate is completely examined. Autopsy series have found that prostate cancer will be found in 30% of men in their 60s and in 50% or more in men in their 70s *(5)*. Most of these tumors cannot be detected by biopsy as they are small but some larger tumors may be undetected with current biopsy strategies. We would then hypothesize that the PCGP1 measure would almost certainly have a range of values among men with prostate cancer and would most likely have higher levels in larger tumors and lower levels in smaller tumors.

Let us now assume that we have determined from preliminary investigations that we will use a threshold value of 100 µg/mL as a positive test for PCGP1. As PSA is a relatively useful surrogate for prostate cancer volume, if we assume an extraordinarily good performance of our new marker, we might find the results in Table 4 of PCGP1 if applied to our population of men.

Table 4
Hypothetical Distribution of a New Marker PCGP1 (%) Relative to the
Distribution of PSA and Prostate Cancer Status in the USA

| PSA | Men | Prostate cancer | Of cancer cases, PCGP1 levels | | No prostate cancer | Of non-cancer cases, PCGP1 levels | |
|---|---|---|---|---|---|---|---|
| | | | >100 | <100 | | >100 | <100 |
| 4.1–10 | 6 | 2 | 2 | 0 | 4 | 0 | 4 |
| 2.1–4.0 | 24 | 6 | 4 | 2 | 18 | 2 | 16 |
| 0–2.0 | 70 | 9 | 4 | 5 | 61 | 6 | 55 |

As can be seen, for the larger tumors the test does quite well, but as the size of the tumor (again, PSA is a good surrogate for this) falls, the sensitivity falls. Simultaneously, although few non-cancer cases are positive by PCGP1, there are still about 10% of non-cancer cases with a falsely positive signal with this marker.

Let us now explore what happens with this marker when it is undergoing developmental testing. One of the most common applications will be to examine how it performs against PSA in the population of men with a PSA between 4 and 10 ng/mL. One of the first tests of this marker to determine its performance characteristics will be in a group of men whose PSA is in this range and of whom all are biopsied. If an investigator performs his initial study in a group of men undergoing biopsy for a PSA above 4 ng/mL, he will find the PCGP1 assay sensitivity to be 100% and specificity to be 100%. In truth, actual sensitivity of the assay for the entire population is only 59% while specificity is 90%. In practice, there are no biomarkers that will have performance characteristics as good as our hypothetical marker PCGP1 and, as a result, the error could be much worse than these examples. As can be seen the conditions used to select patients for analysis have the potential to give falsely optimistic results of a biomarker that, when applied to a general population, will not be replicated.

## WHAT ARE THE ACTUAL PERFORMANCE CHARACTERISTICS OF PSA?

The reader is directed to the previous chapter by Canby-Hagino and Hernandez to understand how the performance of PSA has changed over the years and how ascertainment bias led to misunderstandings about its performance. The problems arose simply due to the fact that men with PSA values less than 4.0 ng/mL were not biopsied due to the perception that prostate cancer did not occur at these levels. When one recognizes that *the greatest risk factor for prostate cancer is a prostate biopsy*, it is not surprising that a PSA cutoff level of 4.0 ng/mL persisted for about two decades.

### *The First PCPT Analysis*

The first glimpse into the actual performance characteristics of the test was noted in our 2004 publication *(4)*. This study examined 2,950 men in the placebo group of the Prostate Cancer Prevention Trial who never had a PSA above 4.0 ng/mL over the course of their 7 years of participation in the study, never had an abnormal rectal examination, and had an end-of-study biopsy. As such, there was *full ascertainment* for cancer in all of these subjects. Table 5 displays the results of this study. The implications of this first analysis were the following:

1. There is no lower limit of PSA at which prostate cancer cannot be detected.
2. PSA is not a dichotomous marker (positive or negative) but reflects a range of risk of prostate cancer.
3. Prostate cancer is actually quite common at levels of PSA between 2 and 4 ng/mL.
4. The risk of high-grade prostate cancer can be meaningful at some levels of PSA below 4.0 ng/mL.

Table 5
Results of Prostate Cancer Prevention Trial End-of-Study
Biopsies in Men with PSA ≤ 4.0 ng/mL and a Normal Rectal
Examination all 7 Years of Study

| PSA range (ng/mL) | Percent with cancer | Percent with high-grade (Gleason grade ≥ 7) cancer |
|---|---|---|
| 0–0.5 | 6.6 | 0.8 |
| 0.6–1.0 | 10.1 | 1.0 |
| 1.1–2.0 | 17.0 | 2.0 |
| 2.1–3.0 | 23.9 | 4.6 |
| 3.1–4.0 | 26.9 | 6.7 |

5. Like all other clinical tests, setting a threshold value (or cutpoint) for PSA requires a consideration of the trade-offs in sensitivity and specificity for the test; higher threshold values optimize specificity (minimize the number of negative biopsies) while lower levels maximize sensitivity (number of cancers detected).

## The Second PCPT Analysis

The first analysis of the risk of prostate cancer at levels of PSA at or below 4.0 ng/mL was a stunning revelation to the urologic and general medical community, breaking the notion that PSA was either "normal" or "elevated." This analysis, however, was limited by a *spectrum bias*: it only included levels of PSA at or below 4.0 ng/mL. It was in the next year that we completed the formal analysis across a range of PSA values *(6)*. In this analysis, we examined all men in the placebo group of the PCPT who had a prostate biopsy. Due to the end of study biopsies, this meant that a full range of PSA values were available, not limited by an artificial cutoff. A total of 5,587 men, 65% of the entire placebo group, underwent a biopsy and of these, 1,225 ultimately were found to have prostate cancer.

Table 6 summarizes the overall findings of this analysis. With the wider range of PSAs in the analysis, it could now be seen that the until-then commonly used PSA value of

Table 6
Sensitivities and Specificities of PSA for Prostate Cancer and High-Grade
(Gleason Grade ≥ 8) Disease Reported by the Prostate Cancer Prevention Trial

| PSA cutoff for a positive test (ng/mL) | Cancer | | High-grade cancer (Gleason 8–10) | |
|---|---|---|---|---|
| | Sensitivity (%) | Specificity (%) | Sensitivity (%) | Specificity (%) |
| 1.1 | 83.4 | 38.9 | 94.7 | 35.9 |
| 2.6 | 40.5 | 81.1 | 78.9 | 75.1 |
| 4.1 | 20.5 | 93.8 | 50.9 | 89.1 |
| 6.1 | 4.6 | 98.5 | 26.3 | 97.5 |
| 10.1 | 0.9 | 99.7 | 5.3 | 99.5 |

4.0 ng/mL to prompt a prostate biopsy had obvious advantages but major disadvantages. The advantage was that the number of unnecessary biopsies was quite low – specificity was approximately 90%. Unfortunately, this value failed to diagnose 80% of prostate cancers and, despite the better detection of aggressive and often-lethal high-grade Gleason 8–10 cancer, missed half of these aggressive tumors. Unfortunately, to identify more prostate cancers, it becomes necessary to substantially lower PSA threshold values.

A major observation from this second analysis of the PCPT was that PSA has a superior performance for the detection of high-grade prostate cancer than for prostate cancer overall. As can be noted in Table 6, to achieve a 90% sensitivity for prostate cancer detection, a PSA cutoff below 1.1 ng/mL would be necessary. From our analysis, we found that a PSA cutoff of 1.5 ng/mL achieved a 89.5% sensitivity for Gleason 8–10 cancer detection (data not in the table). Using receiver operating characteristic curve analyses, we found that the C-statistic (also known as the Area under the Receiver Operating Characteristic Curve or AUC) for PSA for prostate cancer detection was 0.678. A C-statistic of 0.5 is identical to the flip of a coin while the perfect test has a value of 1.0. What an acceptable C-statistic is for cancer detection or risk assessment is uncertain but a recent prediction model for breast cancer, deemed possibly superior to the traditional Gail model, had values of 0.631 for premenopausal women and 0.624 for postmenopausal women (7). As such, the AUC for PSA is superior to methods for breast cancer prediction. Interestingly and fortunately, the C-statistic for detection of high-grade prostate cancer was substantially better; 0.782 and 0.827 for Gleason 7–10 and 8–10 cancer, respectively.

## CLINICAL IMPLICATIONS OF PSA PERFORMANCE CHARACTERISTICS

The performance characteristics may seem to be only numbers to the clinician who is interested in one issue: what to recommend to his/her patient? If the only information available is PSA (see the later chapter on the *PCPT Risk Calculator* for integration of other risk variables into clinical decision-making), the physician must then make a determination as to what is the goal of PSA interpretation. As we have noted above, some patients may summarize the reason for their visit as, "I'm very worried about my prostate cancer risk. If I have it, I want to know about it and to take steps to control it." What this patient has effectively stated is that *test sensitivity is the dominant issue*. The clinician can then help the patient decide how certain he wants to be that he does not have cancer. If 90% is the level of certainty a relatively low PSA level is required. The clinician can then state to the patient that there will be a high likelihood of a negative (or unnecessary) biopsy. With this discussion, the patient may then understand the reason for a higher PSA level.

There are other circumstances where a given patient may be more interested in his risk of aggressive prostate cancer and may actually be interested in minimizing the risk of an unnecessary (negative) prostate biopsy. This may occur in patients with comorbidities or with conditions in which a biopsy may pose them a greater risk. Examples may include patients who are anticoagulated (who would require discontinuation of their anticoagulant before and immediately after the biopsy) or who may require more complicated antibiotic prophylaxis (with, for example, a history of endocarditis). In these patients, *test specificity* will dominate decision-making and a higher PSA level will often be selected for recommending and accepting a prostate biopsy.

Clearly, there is no single level of PSA at which the term "normal" can be applied. The patient's expectations and other risk factors must be taken into account. Ideally, as well, the patient should be informed of the "downstream" effects of a biopsy that is negative or positive. For example, he should understand that if the biopsy is positive, treatments are available but that there are side effects of these treatments and, regardless of the grade and stage of disease, treatment is not always successful and cancer can recur. A recommended resource for the patient is the 2007 Prostate Cancer Guidelines from the American Urological Association *(8)*. On the other hand, if the biopsy is negative, it does not completely preclude the presence of cancer and that repeated biopsies may be recommended.

### *PSA Standardization*

Although the previous discussion shows the challenges faced by setting a single "range of normal" for PSA, the practical aspect of PSA today is that it is generally reported in that "normal/abnormal" fashion. The most commonly reported range of normal of 0–4.0 ng/mL was originally set using the Hybritech PSA test in 1994. More recently, the WHO IRP 96/670 PSA standard has been used by some PSA test manufacturers to recalibrate their PSA test. This calibration change is generally reported to lower PSA results by about 20% *(9)*. It is thus important for clinicians who use PSA alone as a measure of prostate cancer risk to understand which assay is being used and with which calibration method. Ideally, in the future, ranges of normal will be adjusted for these changes in calibration. It is also important for patients whose PSA values are being tracked closely for clinical decision-making purposes to consider using the same assay or assays that are highly correlated. Examples of patients for whom differences in assays may adversely affect patient care include those on surveillance or those with a rising PSA after therapy; in both, a change in the assay with up to 20% difference in results could lead to inappropriate treatment or, conversely, a delay in therapy.

## CONCLUSIONS

This chapter has illustrated a number of important points regarding both the performance characteristics of PSA and new diagnostic tests for prostate cancer. Prostate cancer poses challenges for both the developers of these tests as well as for clinicians who then offer these tests to the patient population.

Properly performed validation studies for prostate cancer detection tests will require extremely well-defined populations in whom full ascertainment is achieved. These types of studies are difficult as this requirement means that prostate biopsies must be performed in *all subjects*. Without this information, the true performance of the test in the general population will be unknown. Similarly the number of missed cancers in the unbiopsied patients simply will not be inferable and the benefit to the population will be uncertain. A parallel observation is that even with full ascertainment, the conclusions of tests of new biomarkers will only be applicable to the population studied. For example, if a test proves useful in a group of men aged 55–65 with a PSA above 2.5 ng/mL, the utility in all other groups may be better, the same, or worse than current methods.

Because of the extraordinary impact of prostate cancer screening on the general population, it is essential that clinicians and investigators understand these issues to maximize the benefit and minimize harm to the enormous group of men worldwide who are at risk of this disease.

## REFERENCES

1. Thompson, I. M., Ankerst, D.P., Chi, C., Goodman, P.J., Tangen, C.M., Lucia, M.S., Feng, Z., Parnes, H.L., Coltman, C.A., Jr. (2006) Assessing prostate cancer risk: Results from the Prostate Cancer Prevention Trial *J Natl Cancer Inst* **98**, 529–34.
2. Porter, M.P., Stanford, J.L., Lange, P.H. (2006) The distribution of serum prostate-specific antigen levels among American men: implications for prostate cancer prevalence and screening *Prostate* **66**,1044–51.
3. Schroeder, F.H., van der Maas, P., Beemsterboer, P., Kruger, A.B., Hoedemaeker, R., Rietbergen, J., Kranse, R. (1998) Evaluation of the digital rectal examination as a screening test for prostate cancer. Rotterdam section of the European Randomized Study of Screening for Prostate Cancer *J Natl Cancer Inst* **90**, 1817–23.
4. Thompson, I.M., Pauler, D.K., Goodman, P.J., Tangen, C.M., Lucia, M.S., Parnes, H.L., Minasian, L.M., Ford, L.G., Lippman, S.M., Crawford, E.D., Crowley, J.J., Coltman, C.A., Jr. (2004) Prevalence of prostate cancer among men with a prostate-specific antigen level < or = 4.0 ng per milliliter *New Engl J Med* **350**, 2239–46.
5. Delongchamps, N.B., Sing, A., Haas, G.P. (2006) The role of prevalence in the diagnosis of prostate cancer *Cancer Control* **13**, 158–68.
6. Thompson, I.M., Ankerst, D.P., Chi, C, Lucia, M.S., Goodman, P.J., Crowley, J.J., Parnes, H.L., Coltman, C.A. (2005) Operating characteristics of Prostate Specific Antigen in men with an initial PSA level of 3.0 ng/mL or lower *JAMA* **294**, 66–70.
7. Barlow, W.E., White, E., Ballard-Barbash, R., Vacek, P.M., Titus-Ernstoff, L., Carney, P.A., Tice, J.A., Buist, D.S., Geller, B.M., Rosenberg, R., Yankaskas, B.C., Kerlikowske, K. (2006) Prospective breast cancer risk prediction model for women undergoing screening mammography *J Natl Cancer Inst* **98**, 1204–14.
8. Thompson, I., Thrasher, J.B., Aus, G., Burnett, A.L., Canby-Hagino, E.D., Cookson, M.S., D'Amico, A.V., Dmochowski, R.R., Eton, D.T., Forman, J.D., Goldenberg, S.L., Hernandez, J., Higano, C.S., Kraus, S.R., Moul, J.W., Tangen, C.M. (2007) AUA Prostate Cancer Clinical Guideline Update Panel. Guideline for the management of clinically localized prostate cancer: 2007 update *J Urol* **177**, 2106–31.
9. Cook B. PSA Testing. Clinical Laboratory News. 34(6) June 2008. Found at http://www.aacc.org/publications/cln/2008/June/Pages/series_0608.aspx. Verified 6/29/2008.

# 7

# The Performance of PSA for Predicting Prostate Cancer After a Prior Negative Prostate Biopsy

*Catherine M. Tangen*

## Contents

## SUMMARY

Some have suggested that prostate-specific antigen (PSA) has no predictive value for prostate cancer after a first negative biopsy has been performed. Because of its required end-of-study biopsy, the Prostate Cancer Prevention Trial (PCPT) was an ideal place to compare the performance operating characteristics of PSA for prostate cancer between a first and subsequent prostate biopsies. This chapter reviews the results of the PCPT analysis and puts those results into context with other studies that have been published on this topic.

**Key Words:** Prostatic neoplasms, Prostate-specific antigen, Screening, Sensitivity, Specificity.

## BACKGROUND

There is considerable debate as to what level of PSA should prompt prostate biopsy or whether it should be combined with other factors related to prostate cancer to conduct risk assessment for the individual patient *(1–3)*. For the group of men with a negative biopsy, optimal management is uncertain. Should a biopsy be repeated? If a biopsy is to be repeated, how soon should this be done and under what circumstances?

From: *Current Clinical Urology: Prostate Cancer Screening*, Edited by: D. P. Ankerst et al.
DOI 10.1007/978-1-60327-281-0_7 © Humana Press, a part of Springer Science+Business Media, LLC 2009

A number of new biomarkers related to prostate cancer have been developed with the goal of addressing when to biopsy the man whose previous biopsy, often based on PSA, is negative. These biomarkers include percent-free PSA, human kallikrein 2, and prostate cancer gene 3 (PCA3) to name just a few *(1–3)*. An alternative approach, which was previously demonstrated in a study of 5,519 men on the placebo arm of the Prostate Cancer Prevention Trial (PCPT), all who underwent prostate biopsy and had several key established risk variables available, was to include whether or not the patient had a prior negative biopsy as a potential risk factor in constructing a multivariable risk tool for prostate cancer *(4)*. After accounting for the effects of PSA, digital rectal exam (DRE), and family history, a prior negative biopsy decreased the risk of finding prostate cancer on the subsequent biopsy (adjusted odds ratio 0.64; 95% confidence interval of 0.53, 0.78, $p < 0.001$) *(4)*.

Another approach for assessing the role of PSA in the setting of a repeat prostate biopsy is to estimate the receiver operating characteristic curve (ROC) and corresponding area under the curve (AUC or C-statistic) for the role of PSA in accurately predicting prostate cancer status. This was done by Thompson et al. using the PCPT placebo data *(5)*.

## METHODS FOR PCPT ANALYSIS

The Prostate Cancer Prevention Trial randomized 18,882 men 55 years and older with a normal DRE and a PSA $\leq 3.0$ ng/ml to either finasteride or placebo *(6)*. Men underwent annual DRE and PSA determination and, if either were abnormal (DRE suspicious for cancer; PSA $\geq 4.0$ ng/ml on placebo, adjusted PSA $\geq 4.0$ ng/ml on finasteride), prostate biopsy was recommended. After 7 years of study, participants without a prior cancer diagnosis were recommended to undergo prostate biopsy. To compare the performance of PSA for predicting outcomes of a first prostate biopsy to a second, we examined men from the placebo group of the study who had either only one biopsy or a first and second prostate biopsies (the first negative for prostate cancer) during the study, and additionally, a PSA and DRE within 1 year prior to each biopsy.

Among men with two biopsies, McNemar's test for paired observations was used to compare between the two biopsies: percent of biopsies performed for cause (PSA $\geq$ 4 ng/ml or abnormal DRE), percent of participants with abnormal DRE at the time of biopsy, and percent with elevated PSA (PSA $\geq 4.0$ ng/ml); the paired *t*-test was used to compare mean values of PSA. Differences in distribution of age, race, and family history of prostate cancer between men who had one and two prostate biopsies were compared using a chi-square test. Performance operating characteristics of PSA at the first and second biopsies were evaluated in terms of sensitivity (Sens), specificity (Spec), the ROC curve, C-statistic (area underneath the ROC curve = AUC), positive predictive value (PPV), and negative predictive value (NPV). For each possible PSA cutpoint, sensitivity was defined as the proportion of cancer cases with PSA greater than or equal to that cutpoint, specificity as the proportion of cancers less than the cutpoint, PPV as the proportion of cancers among all individuals with PSA greater than the cutpoint, and NPV as the proportion of non-cancers among men with PSA less than or equal to the cutpoint. The ROC was constructed as a plot of the false positive rate (1-Specificity) on the *x*-axis versus sensitivity on the *y*-axis and the C-statistic calculated as the area underneath this curve (AUC). A test of whether the C-statistic equals 0.5 (50% chance that PSA correctly predicts prostate cancer) was performed using the Wilcoxon rank sum test. All statistical tests and confidence intervals were performed at the two-sided 0.05-level of statistical significance.

## RESULTS FROM PCPT

This section summarizes the results from Thompson et al. *(5)*. Of the 9,457 men randomized to the placebo arm of the PCPT, 4,921 men had a first and only prostate biopsy during the study with DRE and PSA within 1 year prior to it. An additional 687 men had a negative first biopsy and underwent a second one during the study. Characteristics of these men and the clinical indications related to their biopsies can be found in Table 1. Men who had two biopsies tended to be older at study entry than those who had only one.

Among men with two biopsies, a statistically significantly greater number of the first biopsies (87.5%) were prompted by an elevated PSA or abnormal DRE than the second (47.0%) ($p < 0.0001$), but this result is largely artificial, driven by the design of the PCPT: many of the second biopsies would have fallen at the end of the 7 years of the study, where all men without a prior prostate cancer diagnosis were requested to undergo prostate biopsy. By the same reasoning, there is a higher proportion of elevated PSAs, and abnormal DREs at the time of first biopsy. Average PSA values did not statistically significantly differ between the first biopsy (3.1 ng/ml (standard deviation (SD)) = 2.5) and the second (3.0, SD = 2.7) ($p = 0.10$).

Figure 1 displays the ROC curve for PSA for the first and second biopsies using the PCPT placebo data. The C-statistic for the first biopsy was 0.650 (95% confidence interval 0.632, 0.668), the second biopsy had a slightly higher C-statistic and its 95% confidence interval overlapped with that from the first 0.664 (95% confidence interval

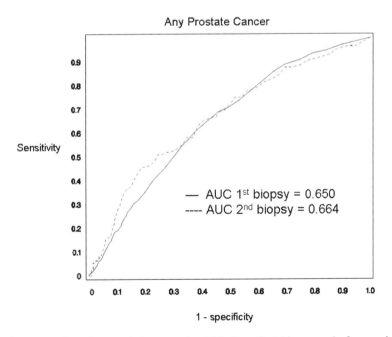

**Fig. 1.** Receiver operating characteristic curve for PSA for a first biopsy and after a prior negative biopsy in the Prostate Cancer Prevention Trial.

Table 1
Patient Characteristics of Those Undergoing One or Two Biopsies in the PCPT Analysis

| Characteristic | *Placebo group* | | |
| --- | --- | --- | --- |
| | Men who had only one biopsy (*n* = 4,921) | Men who had two biopsies (*n* = 687) | |
| Age at study entry, *n* (%) | | | |
| Less than 60 | 1,659 (33.7%) | 173 (25.2%) | |
| 60–64 | 1,537 (31.2%) | 226 (32.9%) | |
| 65–69 | 1,102 (22.4%) | 175 (25.5%) | |
| 70 or older | 623 (12.7%) | 113 (16.4%) | |
| | *p*-value <0.0001 | | |
| Family history of prostate cancer, *n* (%) | 824 (16.7%) | 111 (16.2%) | |
| | *p*-value = 0.70 | | |
| Race, *n* (%) | | | |
| White | 4,689 (95.3%) | 662 (96.4%) | |
| African American | 159 (3.2%) | 20 (2.9%) | |
| Other | 73 (1.5%) | 5 (0.7%) | |
| | *p*-value = 0.25 | | |
| | **Only biopsy** *n* = **4,921** | **First biopsy** (*n* = **687**) | **Second biopsy** (*n* = **687**) |
| PSA at time of biopsy (ng/ml) Median (25%, 75%) | 1.4 (0.8, 2.4) | 2.6 (1.1, 4.5) | 2.3 (1.0, 4.2) |
| For cause* at time of biopsy, *n* (%)** | 882 (17.9%) | 601 (87.5%) | 323 (47.0%) |
| DRE abnormal at time of biopsy, *n* (%)** | 451 (9.2%) | 351 (51.1%) | 151 (22.0%) |
| PSA elevated at time of biopsy (> 4.0 ng/ml), *n* (%)** | 472 (9.6%) | 269 (39.2%) | 189 (27.5%) |
| Months since prior biopsy Median (25%, 75%) | N/A | N/A | 32 (12, 56) |
| Prostate cancer detected | 1,074 (21.8%) | 0 (0%) | 112 (16.3%) |

*"For cause" indicates an abnormal DRE or elevated PSA. **$p$-Value<0.0001 for comparison between the first and second biopsies among men with two biopsies.

0.607, 0.721). Note a formal statistical comparison is not permitted since the second biopsy results are from a subset of the first biopsy results. A test of whether the C-statistic for PSA on the second biopsy equals 0.5 (PSA as a test is no better than a flip of a coin) provided a $p$-value less than 0.001 indicating that among men with a prior negative biopsy, PSA still has value as a diagnostic test.

Sensitivity and specificity for clinical cutoffs of PSA for first and second biopsies are shown in Table 2. For a PSA cutoff of 4.0 ng/ml, the sensitivity for an initial biopsy

Table 2

PSA Properties for Predicting Prostate Cancer by First and Second Biopsy Status in the PCPT

| First biopsy, 1,074 cancers, 4,534 non-cancers | | | | | Second biopsy, 112 cancers, 575 non-cancers | | | |
|------|------|------|------|------|------|------|------|------|
| PSA | Sens | Spec | PPV | NPV | Sens | Spec | PPV | NPV |
| 1.0 | 81.3 | 39.2 | 24.1 | 89.8 | 87.5 | 28.7 | 19.3 | 92.2 |
| 1.5 | 65.8 | 57.3 | 26.8 | 87.6 | 80.4 | 39.1 | 20.5 | 91.1 |
| 2.0 | 51.7 | 68.8 | 28.2 | 85.7 | 73.2 | 49.2 | 21.9 | 90.4 |
| 2.5 | 40.2 | 77.1 | 29.4 | 84.5 | 66.1 | 57.6 | 23.3 | 89.7 |
| 3.0 | 32.2 | 82.2 | 30.0 | 83.7 | 58.0 | 63.1 | 23.5 | 88.5 |
| 4.0 | 21.0 | 88.6 | 30.4 | 82.6 | 48.2 | 76.5 | 28.6 | 88.4 |
| 6.0 | 3.7 | 97.6 | 26.5 | 81.1 | 16.1 | 93.0 | 31.0 | 85.1 |
| 8.0 | 1.4 | 99.0 | 25.4 | 80.9 | 6.3 | 97.4 | 31.8 | 84.2 |
| 10.0 | 0.7 | 99.5 | 25.0 | 80.9 | 2.7 | 98.4 | 25.0 | 83.9 |

Sens = sensitivity, Spec = specificity, PPV = positive predictive value, NPV = negative predictive value.

is 21.0%, and the specificity is 88.6%. For the second biopsy, the increased cutoff of 5.0 ng/ml (data not shown) provides approximately the same specificity as 4.0 ng/ml did for the first biopsy and obtains sensitivity of 33.0%. At a cutoff of 2.5 ng/ml for a first biopsy, the specificity is 77.1% and sensitivity is 40.2%. A PSA of 4.0 ng/ml for the second biopsy yields the same specificity (approximately 76%) and a sensitivity of 48.2%. The ROC analysis reveals that the PSA cutoff needs to be elevated at the second biopsy in order to obtain the same false positive rate, and subsequent similar true positive rate, as at the first biopsy. A scan down the rows of Table 2 reveals that the PPV and NPV at all cutoffs of PSA are very similar at the first and second biopsies.

## RESULTS FROM OTHER STUDIES

Djavan et al. performed an analysis of 820 men to assess the ability of PSA to predict the outcome of repeat prostate biopsy (7). Those men had a total PSA of 4–10 ng/ml and were diagnosed with benign prostatic hyperplasia after their initial biopsy. Mean age was 68 years (standard deviation 8.5) and mean PSA was 6.4 (std dev = 1.8). Ten percent of men were diagnosed with prostate cancer on repeat biopsy. The AUC for PSA was 60.0, but no confidence interval or p-value was reported (7).

A recent study by Marks et al. reported that, after a previous prostate biopsy, PSA was of no utility in assessing a patient's risk for prostate cancer (8). Their study included 233 men with persistent levels of PSA 2.5 ng/ml or greater who had one or more negative prostate biopsies. The average age at biopsy was 64 years (median 64, range 45–83), the average prostate volume by transrectal ultrasonography was 49 cm$^3$ (median 43, range 13–225), and the population was 95% white, 4% black, and 1% Hispanic. Biopsies typically consisted of 12 cores from the peripheral zone. The AUC for PSA was 0.52 (95% confidence interval 0.44, 0.61). Since it was not significantly different from 0.5 the investigators concluded that PSA had little predictive utility in this setting, contradicting the results from the PCPT.

One explanation for the conflicting results between the PCPT and the study by Mark et al. could be that their study had spectrum bias at the second biopsy. Their study only included men with PSA levels persistently greater than or equal to 2.5 ng/ml. Truncation of PSA values in an ROC computation introduces bias to the estimates of sensitivity, specificity, and AUC, moving sensitivity upward and specificity and the AUC downward; see Chapter 6, this volume. On the other hand, in the PCPT analysis half of the second biopsies were not prompted by an elevated PSA or DRE due to the study design of an end-of-study biopsy so the data from that study more closely approximated the full spectrum of PSA values that are seen in a screening setting, and thereby minimizing the confounding effects of verification bias *(9–11)*.

Although the AUC for PSA reported by Djavan et al. (0.60) was similar to that from PCPT (AUC = 0.66), their study also suffered from PSA spectrum bias. Additionally, only men with BPH were included in the analysis, potentially limiting the generalizability of their results.

The ideal biomarker for prostate cancer is both dichotomous (abnormal or normal) and accurate (if abnormal, cancer is present; if normal, cancer is not present). Unfortunately, PSA is not dichotomous; instead, accuracy is dependent on the threshold level selected for biopsy. At lower levels of the test, sensitivity is maximized with lower levels of specificity. At higher levels, while specificity is improved, sensitivity is less with the potential risk of missing a cancer diagnosis. These relationships are difficult for the general public to understand and have led to conclusions that "The PSA Test Fails" when anecdotes are related of cancer at very low levels of PSA or a patient with a higher level of PSA with multiple biopsies showing no cancer *(12)*.

## CONCLUSION

Thompson et al. showed with the placebo arm of the PCPT that PSA does have predictive value in the setting of a repeat prostate biopsy *(5)*. The AUC was estimated at 0.66 and is significantly better than what would be expected by chance ($p < 0.001$). Those investigators also showed that in order to have the same PSA sensitivity from the first to the second biopsy, the PSA threshold should probably be increased. Despite their significant finding, the sensitivity and specificity for PSA in this setting are far from ideal, and ongoing research into new markers to use when deciding whether to conduct a repeat biopsy is greatly needed.

## REFERENCES

1. Groskopf J, Aubin SM, Deras IL, Blase A, Bodrug S, Clark C, Brentano S, Mathis J, Pham J, Meyer T, Cass M, Hodge P, Macairan ML, Marks LS, Rittenhouse H.(2006) APTIMA PCA3 molecular urine test: development of a method to aid in the diagnosis of prostate cancer. *Clin Chem.* **52**:1089–95.
2. Lee R, Localio AR, Armstrong K, Malkowicz SB, Schwartz JS.; Free PSA Study Group. (2006) A meta-analysis of the performance characteristics of the free prostate-specific antigen test. *Urology.* **67**:762–8.
3. Martin BJ, Cheli CD, Sterling K, Ward M, Pollard S, Lifsey D, Mercante D, Martin L, Rayford W. (2006) Prostate specific antigen isoforms and human glandular kallikrein 2 – which offers the best screening performance in a predominantly black population? *J Urol.* **175**:104–7.
4. Thompson IM, Ankerst DP, Chi C, Goodman PJ, Tangen CM, Lucia MS, Feng Z, Parnes HL, Coltman CA Jr. (2006) Assessing prostate cancer risk: results from the Prostate Cancer Prevention Trial. *J Natl Cancer Inst.* **98**:529–34.

5. Thompson IM, Tangen CM, Ankerst DP, Chi C, Lucia MS, Goodman PH, Parnes H, Coltman CA. (2008) The performance of PSA for predicting prostate cancer is maintained after a prior negative biopsy. *J Urol.* **180**:544–7.
6. Thompson IM, Goodman PJ, Tangen CM, Lucia MS, Miller GJ, Ford LG, Lieber MM, Cespedes RD, Atkins JN, Lippman SM, Carlin SM, Ryan A, Szczepanek CM, Crowley JJ, Coltman CA Jr. (2003) The influence of finasteride on the development of prostate cancer. *N Engl J Med.* **349**:215–24.
7. Djavan B, Zlotta A, Remzi M, Ghawidel K, Basharkhah A, Schulman CC, Marberger M. (2000) Optimal predictors of prostate cancer on repeat biopsy: A prospective study of 1, 051 men. *J Urol* **163**:1144–1149.
8. Marks LS, Fradet Yves, Deras IL, Blase A, Mathis J, Aubin SMJ, Cancio AT, Desaulniers M, Ellis WJ, Rittenhouse H, Groskopf J. (2007) PCA3 molecular urine assay for prostate cancer in men undergoing repeat biopsy. Urology **69**;532–35.
9. Nadler RB, Loeb S, Roehl KA, Antenor JA, Eggener S, Catalona WJ. (2005) Use of 2.6 ng/ml prostate specific antigen prompt for biopsy in men older than 60 years. *J Urol.* **174**:2154–7.
10. Keetch DW, Catalona WJ, Smith DS. (1994) Serial prostatic biopsies in men with persistently elevated serum prostate specific antigen values. *J Urol* **151**:1571–4.
11. Punglia RS, D'Amico AV, Catalona WJ, Roehl KA, Kuntz KM. (2003) Effect of verification bias on screening for prostate cancer by measurement of prostate-specific antigen. *N Engl J Med.* **349**:335–42.
12. Stamey TA, Caldwell M, McNeal JE, Nolley R, Hemenez M, Downs J. (2004) The prostate specific antigen era in the United States is over for prostate cancer: What happened in the last 20 years? *J Urol.* **172**:1297–301.

# 8

# Subfractions and Derivatives of Total Prostate-Specific Antigen in the Early Detection of Prostate Cancer

*Alexander Haese and Alan W. Partin*

## SUMMARY

Subfractions, derivatives, and isoforms of Prostate-specific antigen provide the urologist with additional valuable information in the management of prostate cancer patients. While some parameters, such a free PSA are well-established in some total PSA ranges, evidence cumulates that free PSA application can be extended toward lower total PSA concentrations. Likewise derivatives of PSA, in particular PSA velocity has gained significant influence in decision-making as to when a prostate biopsy should be performed, and – more recently – as a marker for disease progression after therapy and as a marker of outcome even before therapy. More challenging – due to their delicate nature, their need for extremely careful preanalytical preparation and complexity as molecules – are subfractions of free PSA, some of which are associated with benign and some with malignant disease. Constant development in the field of total PSA and its derivatives requires regular update. In this chapter, we will review the current utility of subfractions, derivatives, and isoforms of prostate-specific antigen.

**Key Words:** PSA, Free PSA, ProPSA, Isoform.

From: *Current Clinical Urology: Prostate Cancer Screening*, Edited by: D. P. Ankerst et al.
DOI 10.1007/978-1-60327-281-0_8 © Humana Press, a part of Springer Science+Business Media, LLC 2009

# INTRODUCTION

Prostate-specific antigen (PSA) as a tumor marker with exceptional organ specificity has outperformed any other urologic marker *(1)* This unique development was unforeseeable, when in 1971 Hara et al. extracted a protein from human seminal plasma and proposed that it serves as a forensic tool to identify rape victims *(2)*. This was followed by purification of PSA from prostate tissue *(3)*, and subsequent detection in human serum *(4)*. The development of immunoassays for detection of PSA in blood demonstrated the unique potential of PSA as a marker for prostate cancer *(5)*. Today, PSA is the main parameter for early detection, follow-up, and disease monitoring of clinically localized, advanced, and metastatic prostate cancer and, along with clinical stage and histologic grading, contributes to the prediction of pathologic stage and prognosis.

The global term "total immunoreactive PSA" or simply "PSA" neglects a heterogeneous blend of different, complexed, and free molecular forms of PSA. In serum, 65–95% of the total PSA is in a stable covalent complex with alpha-1-antichymotrypsin (PSA–ACT) and constitutes the vast majority ($\geq$98%) of the immunodetected PSA-complexes, whereas free PSA, accounting for 5–35% of the total PSA, is inert and unable to interact with the large excess of antiproteases in blood. The concentration of free noncomplexed PSA in blood contributes little disease-specific information for the early detection of prostate cancer in comparison to the information provided by total PSA levels. Therefore, the most widely used utility of free PSA measurements is to generate the ratio of free to total PSA (%fPSA). For reasons yet poorly understood, a higher ratio of free to total PSA occurs in patients without evidence of cancer than in those with prostate cancer *(6)*. By measuring both free and total PSA, the calculated %fPSA significantly enhances the efficacy of early detection of prostate cancer, in particular within the "diagnostic gray zone" area at total PSA-levels from 4 to 10 ng/ml *(7)*. However, in men with suspicion for prostate cancer, three men need to be biopsied to find one cancer. Therefore, there is a need to improve the diagnostic armamentarium to avoid costly, morbidity-associated and unnecessary biopsies.

Among the most interesting recent research developments for the improved detection in prostate cancer serum markers is the accumulating knowledge of different free PSA isoforms. Free PSA consists of several subfractions and there is now increasing evidence reported that selective measurements of at least some of the free PSA-subfractions may further enhance discrimination of benign from malignant prostatic diseases.

# FREE PSA IN THE EARLY DETECTION OF PROSTATE CANCER

The discovery of various different molecular forms of PSA in circulation in the early 1990s facilitated the development of immunoassays for PSA subforms with improved cancer specificity. This section illustrates the diagnostic value of free PSA for early detection of prostate cancer and describes its clinical implication to date.

## *PSA in Peripheral Blood, Free, and Complexed PSA*

Two major metabolic routes are speculated after PSA is released into blood circulation:

1. PSA that is proteolytically processed during passage through the secretory pathway eventually forms a minor proportion of 5–40% of total PSA in the blood. This subfraction lacks enzymatic activity, thus is unable to form complexes with the abundant amount of antiproteases in the circulation and remains as free (or "unbound") PSA. Free PSA is cleared from the blood by renal glomerular filtration with a half-life of 12–18 h *(8)*.

2. The majority of PSA (60–95%) that enters the peripheral blood is catalytically active, thus capable to form stable, covalent complexes with several of the major physiologic protease inhibitors, such as serine protease inhibitors ($\alpha_1$-antichymotrypsin [ACT], protein C inhibitor [PCI], $\alpha_1$-antitrypsin [API]) and another class of antiproteases, encompassing $\alpha_2$-macroglobulin (AMG) and pregnancy-zone protein (PZP) *(9)*. Active PSA reacts preferentially with AMG (about 20 times more promptly than in the formation of PSA–ACT complexes). However, PSA–AMG is rapidly metabolized by efficient hepatic clearance mechanisms with a half-life of only 6.7 min. This results in serum concentrations close to or below detection limits *(8)*. Moreover, PSA–AMG is not immunoreactive since all antigenic epitopes of PSA are encapsulated and thus hidden by the AMG molecule. Elimination of PSA–ACT complexes is comparatively slow with an estimated half time of 3 days, which corresponds to a decrease of PSA–ACT by approximately 1 ng/ml per day *(10)*. Consequently, PSA–ACT accumulates in blood and forms the major component of detectable PSA–antiprotease complexes (= complexed PSA), the minor component being PSA–API (0.5–5%).

For reasons yet poorly understood, a higher ratio of free to total PSA occurs in patients without than in those with prostate cancer *(6)*. This is consistent with the finding that the proportion of complexed PSA is higher in patients with prostate cancer than in those without *(6,11)*. The most valuable application of free PSA measurement is the identification of the unique, free PSA-specific antigenic epitope structures that are unavailable when PSA forms stable covalent complexes with antiproteases such as ACT *(8,9,12)*. This discovery forms the molecular basis for the generation of specific immunoassays that can accurately measure the free PSA fraction in circulation *(6)*. By analyzing both free and total PSA, the calculated percent of free PSA (%fPSA) improves the armamentarium for early prostate cancer detection *(6)*.

### Clinical Application of Free PSA (fPSA)

Currently, at least three fPSA assay systems are approved as adjuncts to PSA-based prostate cancer screening. Initial data from the Dutch ERSPC-section clearly demonstrated that lower %fPSA levels predict the risk of prostate cancer more accurately than a given level of total PSA alone. For example, when total PSA is between 4 and 10 ng/ml, the average probability of harboring a tumor is about 25% in patients with a normal DRE, but varies from only 8% to as high as 56% when the %fPSA is 40% and 5%, respectively (see Tables 1 and 2).

Numerous studies evaluated sensitivity and specificity of %fPSA for prostate cancer detection (Table 3). These studies demonstrated that by using %fPSA cut-offs between 14 and 28%, 19–64% of unnecessary biopsies could have been avoided while preserving a sensitivity for prostate cancer detection of 71–100% *(13–15)*. One of the largest multicenter trials evaluated a total of 773 men with normal DRE over the truncated range of total PSA between 4 and 10 ng/ml *(7)*. Each had a free and total PSA test using the Hybritech Tandem PSA and Tandem free PSA assay, and had a histologically confirmed

Table 1
Likelihood of a Positive Biopsy Finding in Initial
Biopsy in Men with an Unremarkable Digital Rectal
Examination Adjusted by Total PSA Concentration

| PSA (ng/ml) | Percent cancer on biopsy (%) |
|---|---|
| 0–2 | 1 |
| 2–4 | 15 |
| 4–10 | 25 |
| >10 | >50 |

Table 2
Likelihood of a Positive Biopsy Finding in Initial Biopsy in
Men with an Unremarkable Digital Rectal Examination
Adjusted by %fPSA Concentration

| PSA | %fPSA | Percent cancer on biopsy (%) |
|---|---|---|
| 4–10 ng/ml | 0–10 | 56 |
| | >10–15 | 28 |
| | >15–20 | 20 |
| | >20–25 | 16 |
| | >25 | 8 |

diagnosis by at least a sextant prostate biopsy. Applying a cut-off value for %fPSA below 25% would have provided detection of 95% of cancers. At the same time, it would have reduced the biopsy rate by 20% in the total PSA range of 4–10 ng/ml. On the basis of these results %fPSA has been established and Food and Drug Administration (FDA) approved for clinical use in the 4–10 ng/ml PSA range.

Subsequent investigations focused on the lower PSA range of 2–4 ng/ml PSA, found in up to 22% of all patients with significant, yet predominantly favorable prostate cancers. A %fPSA threshold of 27% in this PSA range provided detection of 90% of cancers while, at the same time sparing 18% of unnecessary biopsies (16). In addition, Haese and colleagues reported that an 18–20% %fPSA cut-off can be applied to detect prostate cancer in the 2–4 ng/ml range and only moderately increase the number of patients biopsied to detect one significant cancer (biopsy-to-cancer ratio of 3–4:1) (17). These findings support the use of %fPSA in this lower total PSA range as well.

Several reports are available that emphasize the role of %fPSA to predict outcome of a repeated prostate biopsy after an initial negative attempt in men suspected of having prostate cancer. In a multivariable analysis of 298 consecutive men who presented for subsequent biopsy, Fowler and colleagues showed that %fPSA was a significant predictor of outcome, whereas simple derivatives of total PSA (PSA density, PSA velocity) were not (18). Similar findings were reported by Djavan et al., who studied the role of PSA adjusted for the volume of the transition zone (PSA TZ-density) to detect prostate cancer among 820 men invited for secondary biopsy (19). Best diagnostic performance was obtained when a 30% cut-off for %fPSA was applied; the AUC (74.5%) exceeded that for PSA TZ-density (69.1%). In another study based on secondary analysis, the pivotal trial which led to FDA approval of free PSA diagnostic performance

Table 3
Overview on the Literature for the Ratio of Free to Total PSA for the Discrimination of Benign Vs. Malignant Prostatic Disease

| Author/year | Patients neg/PCa | DRE | tPSA range (ng/ml) | Cut-off % | Sensitivity % | Specificity |
|---|---|---|---|---|---|---|
| Christenson et al., 1993 | n/a | – | 4–20 ng/ml | 18% | 71 | 95 |
| Catalona et al., 1995 | 63/50 | – | 4–10 ng/ml | 20% | 90 | 38 |
|  | 26/48 | neg |  | 23% | 90 | 31 |
| Prestigiacomo et al., 1996 | 20/28 | – | 4–10 ng/ml | 23% | 95 | 64 |
|  |  |  |  | 14% | 95 | 56 |
| Catalona et al.* 1998 | 379/394 | neg | 4–10 ng/ml | 25% | 95 | 20 |
|  |  |  |  | 22% | 90 | 29 |
| Catalona et al., 1997 | 73/259 | neg | 2.6–4 ng/ml | 27% | 90 | 18 |

* = multi-institutional

of %fPSA and PSA density were equivalent *(16)*. A lowered PSA density cut-point of 0.09 ng/ml/cc was identical to a %free PSA threshold of 25% in maintaining 95% sensitivity and 80% specificity for cancer detection in repeated biopsy among 163 patients with a serum PSA level between 4 and 10 ng/ml. However, skilled transrectal ultrasonography, an uncomfortable and expensive procedure to accurately measure the prostate volume required for a PSA density calculation, can be avoided using %fPSA, which only needs a simple blood draw to analyze.

Percent-free PSA has also been shown useful to provide aspects of prognostic value, such as identification of those patients who will develop highly aggressive cancer in the future. In a study by Carter et al., measurement of free and total PSA was performed up to 10 years before diagnosis of prostate cancer with extraprostatic extension, lymph node, or bone metastases and compared to a group of patients who had prostate cancer with a more favorable pathology. They demonstrated a statistically significant difference in %fPSA between disease entities ($p=0.008$) 10 years prior to diagnosis. Total PSA failed to demonstrate this difference *(20)*.

Even though the diagnostic value of %fPSA has been confirmed in numerous clinical trials and is widely used in current clinical practice, its application requires careful considerations. Several recent studies evaluating novel prostate-related markers for early cancer detection were not able to reproduce the diagnostic performance of %fPSA initially reported in the studies of Catalona and colleagues *(21,22)*. These discrepancies may find an explanation in any, or in a combination of its properties:

1. Because free PSA increases with age and prostate volume, and decreases as the total PSA increases, demographic differences among populations studied can influence the results of free PSA trials *(23)*. In particular prostatic volume influences %fPSA in patients with prostate cancer *(24)*. In smaller prostates there is a statistically significant difference in %fPSA between patients with benign disease and prostate cancer. However, with increasing total prostate volume, differences in %fPSA between both cancer and no cancer diminish and at large volumes %fPSA concentrations may be indistinguishable. A similar result was found when prostates < 35cc vs. ≥ 35cc were compared: A cut-off of 14% for small prostates and a cut-off of 25% of %fPSA for larger prostates detected prostate cancer with 95% sensitivity *(25)*.
2. %fPSA-immunodetection is highly susceptible to preanalytical bias. The limited in vitro stability of free PSA, particularly in serum, warrants very careful handling of specimens including very rapid separation of serum/plasma from the blood cells and analysis of serum within 24 h of sample collection *(26)*. Prostatic manipulation (vigorous DRE), prostate biopsy, and urethral instrumentation have all been shown to increase total PSA concentrations primarily due to an increase in the free PSA component of total PSA *(27)*. Therefore any manipulation of the prostate gland should be avoided for at least 48–72 h prior to the collection of a sample for measurement of free PSA.
3. Probably the most significant problem in comparing diagnostic performance from study to study is that the results vary depending on the manufacturer of the assay. The clinical effect of significant inter-assay variation was clearly demonstrated by Nixon and associates. In their comparative study of three investigational assays for free PSA among 123 consecutively accrued patients, different %fPSA cut-points of 22%, 34%, and 34% were identified that would ensure a 95% sensitivity cancer detection, and the number of negative biopsies that would have been prevented were 38%, 19%, and 34%, respectively *(28)*.

In conclusion, %fPSA provides a valuable improvement in the specificity while main-taining high sensitivity for prostate cancer in men with a total PSA of 2–10 ng/ml. A reference value of %fPSA cannot be exactly recommended, since it is affected by multiple factors. Common ranges between 14% and 25% are applied *(6,7,14,15)*. Narrowing this range to an optimal, widely accepted cut-off value has not been pos-sible up till now. It is therefore the decision of physicians along with their patients to be either more aggressive to detect cancer at the risk of an unnecessary biopsy (e.g. trend to higher sensitivity) or more restrictive, less inclined to perform the biopsy that would ultimately reveal a benign result, at the risk of overlooking a cancer.

## PSA-DERIVATES IN THE DETECTION OF PROSTATE CANCER

PSA-derivates are permutations of total serum PSA used in an attempt to improve sensitivity and specificity of prostate cancer detection. These permutations are PSA den-sity, PSA velocity, and age-specific PSA ranges. Their meaning in the early detection of prostate cancer will be described in this section.

### *PSA Density*

The concept of PSA density was first described by Benson et al. *(29)*. The rationale behind PSA density is the observation of a positive relationship between serum PSA and prostatic volume. The background is, that the majority of prostatic enlargement is due to benign hyperplastic tissue of the transition zone. Normalization by prostate volume might enhance cancer specificity. PSA-D divides the serum PSA by prostatic volume. It was created to normalize a certain PSA for the volume of the respective prostate, assum-ing that a certain volume of prostate cancer would increase PSA to a greater extent than benign prostatic hyperplasia. However, two aspects limit the use of PSA-D. First, it depends on the examiner to estimate the prostatic volume correctly. Secondly, the ratio of stroma to epithelium varies considerably between individuals. Since only the epithe-lium produces PSA and the stroma cannot be estimated from transrectal ultrasound, this influences PSA density to an unforeseeable extent *(30,31)*. Therefore, results of PSA-D have been discordant. A cut-off of 0.15 for PSA density has been reported, and it was found that PSA-D enhanced prostate cancer detection when PSA was below 10 ng/ml *(32)*. Another study, however, found that about 50% of all prostate cancers would have been missed, when a cut-off of 0.15 was used *(33)*. Another could not find any statisti-cal significant difference between 107 men with positive or negative biopsy result when PSA-D was used *(34)*. Therefore, at present the role of PSA-D in the early detection of prostate cancer has not yet been proven to be useful when PSA is 4–10 ng/ml and DRE is unremarkable.

A modification of PSA-D, transition zone density (PSA-TZD) is the normalization of PSA to the transition zone volume *(19)*. It focuses on the assumption that, histologically, hyperplasia occurs almost exclusively in the transition zone. PSA from the peripheral zone and central zone is assigned to be a constant and less substantial source of PSA in the absence of cancer. In an initial study with a cut-off of 0.35 ng/ml/cc, the high-est positive predictive value for prostate cancer detection was found using PSA-TZD

(74%) (35). However, methodological problems of volume measurement and epithelial-to-stroma ratio affect PSA-TZ-density in the same way as simple PSA-D. Since other centers failed to reproduce the advantage of PSA-TZD, to date it cannot be considered to be a routine tool for prostate cancer detection.

### Age-Specific PSA Ranges in the Early Detection of Prostate Cancer

As outlined earlier the upper limit of normal PSA concentration is commonly assigned to 4 ng/ml. This, however, does not compensate for increasing prostate volume with increasing age. Hence, the principle of age-specific PSA ranges has been intro-duced (36) to improve sensitivity of prostate cancer detection in younger patients (e.g., age 50) while sparing unnecessary biopsies for insignificant cancers (improve specificity in older patients, e.g., age 70). Several studies have evaluated age-specific PSA ranges. In evaluation of nearly 4,600 men, age-specific PSA ranges detected 74 additional can-cers in those 60 years or younger. In 80% of all cancers detected in the younger men, pathologic work-up was favorable (Gleason score below 7, organ confined or capsular penetration, no lymph node metastases, or seminal vesicle invasion). The detection of prostate cancer increased by 18% in younger men while decreasing by 22% in older men (37). The comparison of age-specific PSA ranges to normal PSA cut-offs of 4 ng/ml in a screened population showed that the number of cancers detected increased by 8% using age-specific ranges in men below 59 years when DRE was unremarkable. Moreover, in men older than 60 years, 21% of biopsies could have been spared while missing only 4% of organ-confined cancers. It was concluded that age-specific PSA ranges improve sensitivity in younger populations (38). Other studies, however, concluded that the stan-dard PSA cut-off of 4 ng/ml was optimal for all age groups (39) and in addition, the most cost-effective tool (40) (Table 4).

Race-corrected age-specific PSA ranges take reports into account that describe higher PSA in black as compared to white or Asian men, even after controlling for age, Gleason grade, or clinical stage, which has been associated with a larger tumor volume in black compared to white men (1.3–2.5 times larger). It was reported that 40% of cancers in a black population would have been missed when traditional age-specific ranges would have been used (36,41,42).

Table 4
Age-Adjusted PSA Ccut-Off Value in Normal Men of Different Races, Suggested
by Studies from Oesterling et al. and Morgan et al.

| Author | N | Race | PSA-Cut-off (ng/ml) adjusted by Age (years) | | | |
|--------|---|------|-------|-------|-------|-------|
| | | | 40–49 | 50–59 | 60–69 | 70–79 |
| Oesterling et al., 1995 | 422 | White | 2.5 | 3.0 | 4.0 | 5.5 |
| Oesterling et al., 1995 | 286 | Asian | 2.0 | 3.0 | 4.0 | 5.0 |
| Morgan et al. 1996 | 1,673 | African-American | 2.0 | 4.0 | 4.5 | 5.5 |

# MOLECULAR ISOFORMS OF FREE PSA FOR EARLY DIAGNOSIS OF PROSTATE CANCER

Molecular studies have reported significant heterogeneity of free PSA in serum, seminal plasma, hyperplastic, and cancerous tissue. Isoforms of free PSA that have retained some or all of the pro-peptide sequence or that have developed internal cleavages have been identified and have demonstrated remarkable disease-related specificity. Based on this information, a panel of new serum markers has been developed and evaluated in various single and even some multi-institutional trials, however, these assays are not yet available for routine clinical use.

## *I: Biological Description of the Free Isoforms of PSA*

*Background:* Precise biochemical description of the free isoforms of free PSA in serum is an extraordinarily difficult task, which is to a large extent caused by the low serum concentrations in serum. Several studies tried to overcome the low concentrations by analyzing serum from patients with metastatic disease and exceedingly high total PSA concentrations *(43,44)*. Drawbacks of such procedures are that purification steps might eliminate or modify some of the free forms and that it is likely that a massive untreated tumor has a different pattern of free PSA than a cancer that is in a curable stage. Clinically relevant information for early detection of curable cancers, the main task for any tumor marker, may therefore be difficult to obtain. While the concentration of free PSA in seminal plasma is about one million times higher than in serum, making appropriate amounts for analysis more easily obtainable, analysis of free PSA isoforms therein can at most give an approximate reflection of its distribution in serum. This is because of the fundamentally different nature of free PSA in serum and seminal plasma. In seminal plasma about 60–70% of PSA is found as a catalytically active free form *(9,45)*, whereas less than 5% of PSA is in complex with antiproteases. The major antiprotease to which active single-chain PSA is covalently linked in a 1:1 molar ratio is PCI *(46)*. The lesser amount (30–40%) of catalytically inactive PSA in seminal fluid exists mainly as free, internally cleaved, two-chain or multichain forms of the protein *(9,47)*, reported to be the result from not only cleavages of C-terminal of mainly Lys145, but also cleavages of C-terminal of Lys182 *(47)*. In serum, in contrast to seminal plasma, a dominant amount (typically 65–95%) of PSA enters complex formation of covalent 1:1 molar complexes with ACT *(8,11)*. About 2% forms a complex with API *(48)*. A minority, 5–35%, of the immunodetectable PSA in blood, is found in free noncomplexed and catalytically inactive form, as it remains unreactive with the very large excess of antiproteases (ACT or AMG) in blood *(27)*. In vitro, PSA rapidly forms complexes with AMG *(49)*.

### CLASSIFICATION OF FREE PSA ISOFORMS

Classification of free PSA isoforms can be done by assessing the presence or absence of internal cleavages, in which case the respective forms are termed nicked (= with internal cleavages) or intact (= without internal cleavages). From the intact PSA isoforms a subgroup can be identified that comprises "underprocessed" isoforms, called precursor PSA or proPSA (Fig. 1 and Color Plate 1).

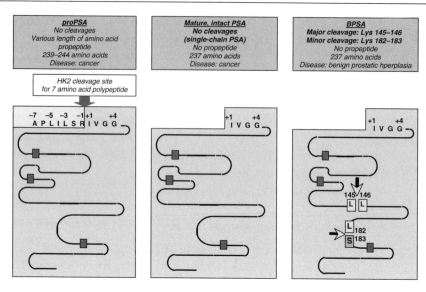

Fig. 1. Depiction of isoforms of free PSA. (*see* Color Plate 1)

*(1) Precursor or proPSA Isoforms*: Physiologically a 7-amino acid propeptide is cleaved from the inactive 244-amino acid proPSA at the N-terminal end of the polypeptide chain, resulting in the enzymatically active, intact free PSA. In vitro several serine proteases of prostatic origin are able to cleave the proPSA signal peptide, e.g., hK2 *(50)*, Prostase (hK4), or Prostin (hK15) *(51)*. The proPSA isoforms reported so far contain the native proleader peptide of 7-amino acids (–7proPSA) and truncated proleader peptides containing 1 (–1proPSA), 2 (–2proPSA), 4 (–4proPSA), or 5 (–5proPSA) amino acids *(43,52)*. These isoforms are precursors of the mature, enzymatically active free PSA. As a potential explanation for the existence of inactive free PSA in serum, precursor forms of free PSA are candidates, since they do not possess enzymatic activity. This inability precludes the common complex formation with antiproteases normally observed. A potential explanation of why these proPSA isoforms accumulate in prostatic tissue, and subsequently can be detected in patient serum, is the observation of an increased resistance of these forms toward activation, that is, the complete removal of an already partially cleaved propeptide. This has been shown for the –2proPSA isoform, but may also be the case for other truncated variants. The initial report describing a proPSA isoform was by Mikolajczyk et al. who in 1997 found a –4proPSA isoform that contributed about 25% of all free PSA in pooled prostate cancer serum. Subsequent studies by the same group demonstrated the presence of –2proPSA in tissue extracts of peripheral zone cancers. Moreover, the concentration of –2proPSA was higher in cancer than in benign tissue. Using immunohistochemical staining with specific MAbs against –2proPSA and –5/–7proPSA, Chan et al. *(53)* demonstrated the presence of both proPSA isoforms in needle biopsies of the prostate with benign and malignant differentiation. Mikolajczyk et al. detected –2proPSA in prostate cancer sera with moderately elevated tPSA, suggesting the presence and immunodetectability of this isoform at early cancer stages. Other models studying proPSA isoforms are LnCap-cell lines, which have been shown to generate predominantly –7proPSA and –5proPSA, plus mature, intact, but enzymatically inactive free PSA *(54,55)*. A clear issue in the detection of proPSA isoforms in

serum is their stability. However, likely, it is not known whether these isoforms interfere differently with proteolytic enzymes. Likewise, in the process of purification, these isoforms are potentially more susceptible to cleavages, which might be an explanation for the conflicting results of several studies.

(2) *Isoforms With Internal Cleavages:* Analogous to the proPSA isoforms, free PSA variants with internal cleavages offer a potential explanation for the nonreactivity of free PSA in serum. In studies presented so far, cleavage sites at Isoleucine 1, Histidine 54, Phenylalanine 57, Lysine 145 *(56)*, and Lysine 182 were reported, however, more than one cleavage site occurs, such as at Lysine 145 and Lysine 182. The structural and potentially conformational changes of these clipped isoforms disable complex formation with ACT, however, most of the epitopes responsible for antibody recognition are not affected. Enzymatic activity studies with different substrates demonstrated that PSA from seminal fluid and benign prostatic hyperplasia (BPH) nodules had similar specific trypsin-like activity. However, serum free PSA with an internal cleavage at Lys145 had much lower specific chymotrypsin-like activity than seminal fluid active free PSA with an internally intact amino acid backbone, which offers more chymotrypsin-like activity. N-Terminal sequence analysis showed that Lys145-nicked PSA was neither in the preproenzyme form (261 amino acids) nor in the zymogen proenzyme form (244 amino acids) of PSA, both of which are known precursors of mature PSA (237 amino acids) *(56)*. Because chymotrypsin-like activity of PSA is a prerequisite for complex formation, mostly with alpha-1-antichymotrypsin, Lys145-nicked PSA (and potentially other nicked variants of free PSA) should form much less PSA-antichymotrypsin complex in the presence of antichymotrypsin and, therefore, more will remain in the free, non-complexed form of PSA. Among the reported nicked PSA-forms, one variant with the singular cleavage site at Lysine 182 has been termed BPSA (= BPH-associated PSA) *(57–59)*, due to its elevated concentration in prostatic issue derived from the transition zone of symptomatic BPH-nodules. Clinical application of nicked PSA isoforms will be discussed later.

(3) *Intact PSA Isoforms:* As described earlier, intact free PSA isoforms are those that comprise free, mature PSA isoforms that for unknown reasons are enzymatically inactive, but are not characterized by a propeptide, or by internal cleavages. The reasons for their enzymatic inactivity are unclear, but they may harbor conformational or structural modifications. Noldus et al. *(44)* and Qian et al. *(60)*, using pooled serum of PCa patients with metastatic disease (tPSA >2,000 ng/ml), and Mikolajczyk et al., using pooled serum of PCa patients *(52)* with a total PSA concentration of 63 ng/ml described intact mature free PSA as a dominant isoform. These studies differed, however, since Noldus et al. found a free PSA isoform with a clip at Lys145–Lys146 *(44)*, whereas Mikolajczyk demonstrated that a –4proPSA isoform accounted for nearly 25% of all free PSA in serum *(52)*. Peter et al., using individual patient sera with tPSA-concentrations between 1,900 and 8,500 ng/ml, also demonstrated intact, mature free PSA in three of five samples in combination with truncated proPSA isoforms (–7), (–5), and (–4) *(43)*. Detection of intact, mature free PSA has also occurred in seminal plasma and LnCaP-cells.

(4) *Glycosylation Variants*: PSA is a glycoprotein. Eight percent of PSA consists of a carbohydrate side chain which is linked to asparagine on position 45 of the PSA amino acid chain *(61)*. This oligosaccharide unit accounts for the capability of PSA to interact with lectins. Research analyzing differences in the glycosylation pattern in benign and malignant prostatic disease, however, produced conflicting results. Initial reports that

concluded a significant difference *(62,63)* were not replicated in later analyses *(64)*. It is likely that methodological pitfalls in the analyses of different glycosylation patterns are responsible for such differences. Most notably, some authors have questioned the suitability of lectins for assessing differences in glycosylation variants *(65)*.

*(5) Truncated PSA Forms*: Truncated PSA forms lack amino acids at the N-terminal end of the amino acid backbone after complete removal of the propeptide. These isoforms have been detected in both spent medium of LnCap-cell lines *(66)* and in prostatic issue *(56)*. Deletion of N-terminal amino acids causes conformational changes, resulting in enzymatic inactivity. Whether these truncated PSA forms are expressed in prostate cancer or have a significant role among the free PSA forms remains an open question.

## II: Clinical Application of Free PSA Isoforms

From a clinical point of view the present literature associates some isoforms with malignant prostatic disease and others with benign prostatic enlargement.

Precursor forms of free PSA: Precursor forms of free PSA, commonly referred to as proPSA-isoforms, are among the most studied variants in terms of their clinical application. Initially a form with removal of only three amino acids, termed –4proPSA, was described in pooled cancer serum (see above) *(67)*. More recently a –2proPSA (removal of five amino acids) was detected in PCa extracts. When, subsequently, serum of PCa patients with a tPSA range of 6–24 ng/ml was analyzed for –2proPSA, it could be shown that 25–95% of free PSA consisted of –2proPSA as opposed to 6–19% in men with no evidence of the disease *(68)*. The use of proPSA detection was explored in the tPSA range 2.5–4 ng/ml range. By using the percentage of proPSA to free PSA (%proPSA) one study found that 75% of all cancers could have been detected while sparing 59% of unnecessary biopsies, whereas %fPSA would have spared only 33% of unnecessary biopsies *(69)*. Recent data by Catalona et al. showed an improved prostate cancer detection rate in men with a total PSA between 2 and 4 ng/ml, where the ratio of proPSA to fPSA (%proPSA) spared 19% of all unnecessary biopsies compared to 10% for the ratio of free to total PSA. In the total PSA range 4–10 ng/ml, at a sensitivity of 90%, %proPSA spared 31% of all unnecessary biopsies compared to 20% for the ratio of free to total PSA *(70)*. Partin et al. *(22)* analyzed total PSA, free PSA, BPSA, and all proPSA forms combined in the tPSA range 2–24 ng/ml and %fPSA ranges less than 15%. They found an area under curve (AUC) of 0.71 for proPSA/BPSA (compared to tPSA AUC = 0.51 and fPSA AUC = 0.54). At the proPSA/BPSA cut-off of 0.71, sensitivity was 90% and specificity 46%. Looking at prognostic features, Shariat et al. examined associations of serum levels of –7proPSA, –4proPSA, and –2proPSA with clinical and pathologic features of prostate cancer in 62 patients who underwent radical prostatectomy for clinically localized disease. They found total PSA, –7proPSA, and –2proPSA to be significantly higher in patients with extraprostatic extension than in those with organ-confined disease and showed a positive correlation with tumor volume at prostatectomy. Furthermore, the serum levels were higher in patients at high risk for recurrent cancer, compared to patients with favorable outcome prognosis. They concluded that proPSA forms measured in preoperative serum specimens are associated with advanced prostate cancer and identified patients at higher risk of recurrence after radical prostatectomy *(71)*. Comparably, Catalona et al. *(72)*, analyzing the total PSA range 2–4 ng/ml found that –2proPSA differed statistically significantly between aggressive ($\geq$Gleason grade 7, extraprostatic extension) and nonaggressive (Gleason grade $\leq$ 6, organ confined) PCa.

## INTACT PSA ISOFORMS

Construction of monoclonal antibodies with the ability to discriminate such single-chain free PSA forms (which represent the sum of latent and mature PSA formats) from multichain PSA forms with internal cleavage sites at Lys145–Lys146 made it possible to design an assay to discriminate multichain forms of fPSA, nicked PSA or "PSA-N," from intact single-chain fPSA, "PSA-I" *(73)*. It is, however, important to stress that this immunoassay also detects proPSA isoforms, since they also do not have internal cleavages. Analysis of plasma samples with tPSA levels greater than 3.0 ng/ml from a subset of a screening study population in Sweden showed that proportions of intact/free PSA were significantly higher in men with PCa than in those without *(74)*. A subsequent study of 178 men with no evidence of disease and 255 patients with biopsy-proven prostate cancer demonstrated that measurements of intact PSA enhanced discrimination of patients with negative systematic prostate biopsy from those with biopsy-proven PCa *(75)*.

## NICKED PSA ISOFORMS

The characteristic feature of BPSA is a cleavage at Lys182–Ser183, which categorizes it into the multichain free PSA isoforms. BPSA was initially described in nodular tissue samples of the transition zone of BPH *(58)*, subsequently in seminal plasma *(57)* and finally in serum *(76)* of men with benign prostatic disease. Tissue samples from prostates larger than 50 g due to BPH, benign prostates smaller than 25 g, and PCa demonstrated an almost exclusive BPSA expression in the transition zone compared to normal and in cancerous prostates *(58)*. Wang et al. characterized the immunoreactivity of BPSA by competition assays for different epitopes on the PSA-molecule and demonstrated a different immunoreactivity of the six antibodies used, implying that the development of MAbs for BPSA should allow the construction of an immunoassay for specific BPSA measurement *(77)*. From the same group, Linton et al. developed such an immunoassay and estimated 15–50% of free PSA in serum samples of men with benign disease to be BPSA whereas it was undetectable in normal control males *(76)*. It may be concluded that BPSA is an isoform that to some extent reflects BPH and may have potential to monitor it under surgical or medical treatment.

In summary, free PSA isoforms present a promising new tool for further and more accurate assessment of men with prostate cancer, including improved specificity in early detection as well as potential hints for pathological staging and prognosis. The general hypothesis of a different contribution of benign and malignant prostatic tissue to different free PSA isoforms in serum and a potentially disease-specific pattern is presently supported by the detection of isoforms that are more associated with BPH or PCa. Still a clear picture as to the nature and clinical utility of free PSA isoforms is lacking. Preanalytical sample work-up and analytical detection techniques are far from standardized, which makes comparison of different studies difficult. In an optimized setting, through multicenter based evaluations it may be possible to correctly assess their true potential for early detection of clinically significant PCa.

# REFERENCES

1. Polascik, T. J., Oesterling, J. E. and Partin, A. W. (1999) Prostate specific antigen: a decade of discovery – what we have learned and where we are going *J Urol* **162**, 2; 293–306.
2. Hara, M., Koyanagi, Y., Inoue, T. and Fukuyama, T. (1971) [Some physico-chemical characteristics of "gamma-seminoprotein", an antigenic component specific for human seminal plasma. Forensic immunological study of body fluids and secretion. VII] *Nippon Hoigaku Zasshi* **25**, 4; 322–4.
3. Wang, M. C., Valenzuela, L. A., Murphy, G. P. and Chu, T. M. (1979) Purification of a human prostate specific antigen *Invest Urol* **17**, 2; 159–63.
4. Papsidero, L. D., Wang, M. C., Valenzuela, L. A., Murphy, G. P. and Chu, T. M. (1980) A prostate antigen in sera of prostatic cancer patients *Cancer Res* **40**, 7; 2428–32.
5. Kuriyama, M., Wang, M. C., Lee, C. I., Papsidero, L. D., Killian, C. S., Inaji, H., et al. (1981) Use of human prostate-specific antigen in monitoring prostate cancer *Cancer Res* **41**, 10; 3874–6.
6. Christensson, A., Bjork, T., Nilsson, O., Dahlen, U., Matikainen, M. T., Cockett, A. T., et al. (1993) Serum prostate specific antigen complexed to alpha 1-antichymotrypsin as an indicator of prostate cancer *J Urol* **150**, 1; 100–5.
7. Catalona, W. J., Partin, A. W., Slawin, K. M., Brawer, M. K., Flanigan, R. C., Patel, A., et al. (1998) Use of the percentage of free prostate-specific antigen to enhance differentiation of prostate cancer from benign prostatic disease: a prospective multicenter clinical trial *JAMA* **279**, 19; 1542–7.
8. Lilja, H., Christensson, A., Dahlen, U., Matikainen, M. T., Nilsson, O., Pettersson, K., et al. (1991) Prostate-specific antigen in serum occurs predominantly in complex with alpha 1-antichymotrypsin *Clin Chem* **37**, 9; 1618–25.
9. Christensson, A., Laurell, C. B. and Lilja, H. (1990) Enzymatic activity of prostate-specific antigen and its reactions with extracellular serine proteinase inhibitors *Eur J Biochem* **194**, 3; 755–63.
10. Bjork, T., Ljungberg, B., Piironen, T., Abrahamsson, P. A., Pettersson, K., Cockett, A. T., et al. (1998) Rapid exponential elimination of free prostate-specific antigen contrasts the slow, capacity-limited elimination of PSA complexed to alpha 1-antichymotrypsin from serum *Urology* **51**, 1; 57–62.
11. Stenman, U. H., Leinonen, J., Alfthan, H., Rannikko, S., Tuhkanen, K. and Alfthan, O. (1991) A complex between prostate-specific antigen and alpha 1-antichymotrypsin is the major form of prostate-specific antigen in serum of patients with prostatic cancer: assay of the complex improves clinical sensitivity for cancer *Cancer Res* **51**, 1; 222–6.
12. Piironen, T., Villoutreix, B. O., Becker, C., Hollingsworth, K., Vihinen, M., Bridon, D., et al. (1998) Determination and analysis of antigenic epitopes of prostate specific antigen (PSA) and human glandular kallikrein 2 (hK2) using synthetic peptides and computer modeling *Protein Sci* **7**, 2; 259–69.
13. Luderer, A. A., Chen, Y. T., Soriano, T. F., Kramp, W. J., Carlson, G., Cuny, C., et al. (1995) Measurement of the proportion of free to total prostate-specific antigen improves diagnostic performance of prostate-specific antigen in the diagnostic gray zone of total prostate-specific antigen *Urology* **46**, 2; 187–94.
14. Prestigiacomo, A. F., Lilja, H., Pettersson, K., Wolfert, R. L. and Stamey, T. A. (1996) A comparison of the free fraction of serum prostate specific antigen in men with benign and cancerous prostates: the best case scenario *J Urol* **156**, 2 Pt 1; 350–4.
15. Bjork, T., Piironen, T., Pettersson, K., Lovgren, T., Stenman, U. H., Oesterling, J. E., et al. (1996) Comparison of analysis of the different prostate-specific antigen forms in serum for detection of clinically localized prostate cancer *Urology* **48**, 6; 882–8.
16. Catalona, W. J., Smith, D. S. and Ornstein, D. K. (1997) Prostate cancer detection in men with serum PSA concentrations of 2.6 to 4.0 ng/ml and benign prostate examination. Enhancement of specificity with free PSA measurements *JAMA* **277**, 18; 1452–5.
17. Haese, A., Dworschack, R. T. and Partin, A. W. (2002) Percent free prostate specific antigen in the total prostate specific antigen 2 to 4 ng./ml. range does not substantially increase the number of biopsies needed to detect clinically significant prostate cancer compared to the 4 to 10 ng./ml. range *J Urol* **168**, 2; 504–8
18. Fowler, J. E., Jr., Sanders, J., Bigler, S. A., Rigdon, J., Kilambi, N. K. and Land, S. A. (2000) Percent free prostate specific antigen and cancer detection in black and white men with total prostate specific antigen 2.5 to 9.9 ng./ml *J Urol* **163**, 5; 1467–70.
19. Djavan, B., Zlotta, A. R., Byttebier, G., Shariat, S., Omar, M., Schulman, C. C., et al. (1998) Prostate specific antigen density of the transition zone for early detection of prostate cancer *J Urol* **160**, 2; 411–8; discussion 18–9.

20. Carter, H. B., Partin, A. W., Luderer, A. A., Metter, E. J., Landis, P., Chan, D. W., et al. (1997) Percentage of free prostate-specific antigen in sera predicts aggressiveness of prostate cancer a decade before diagnosis *Urology* **49**, 3; 379–84.

21. Djavan, B., Remzi, M., Schulman, C. C., Marberger, M. and Zlotta, A. R. (2002) Repeat prostate biopsy: who, how and when?. a review *Eur Urol* **42**, 2; 93–103

22. Partin, A. W., Mangold, L. A., Sokoll, L. J., Chan, D. W., Mikolajczyk, S. D., Linton, H. J., et al. (2003) Clinical utility of proPSA and BPSA when percent free PSA is below 15% *J Urol* **169**, 4; 384 (A1436)

23. Woodrum, D., French, C. and Shamel, L. B. (1996) Stability of free prostate-specific antigen in serum samples under a variety of sample collection and sample storage conditions *Urology* **48**, 6A; 33–39

24. Haese, A., Graefen, M., Noldus, J., Hammerer, P., Huland, E. and Huland, H. (1997) Prostatic volume and ratio of free-to-total prostate specific antigen in patients with prostatic cancer or benign prostatic hyperplasia *J Urol* **158**, 6; 2188–92.

25. Partin, A. W., Catalona, W. J., Southwick, P. C., Subong, E. N., Gasior, G. H. and Chan, D. W. (1996) Analysis of percent free prostate-specific antigen (PSA) for prostate cancer detection: influence of total PSA, prostate volume, and age *Urology* **48**, 55–61

26. Piironen, T., Pettersson, K., Suonpaa, M., Stenman, U. H., Oesterling, J. E., Lovgren, T., et al. (1996) In vitro stability of free prostate-specific antigen (PSA) and prostate-specific antigen (PSA) complexed to alpha 1-antichymotrypsin in blood samples *Urology* **48**, 6A Suppl; 81–7.

27. Lilja, H., Haese, A., Bjork, T., Friedrich, M. G., Piironen, T., Pettersson, K., et al. (1999) Significance and metabolism of complexed and noncomplexed prostate specific antigen forms, and human glandular kallikrein 2 in clinically localized prostate cancer before and after radical prostatectomy *J Urol* **162**, 6; 2029–34; discussion 34–5.

28. Nixon, R. G., Wener, M. H. and Smith, K. M. B. (1997) Biolgical variation of prostate specific antigen levels in serum: an evaluation of day-to-day physiological fluctuations in a well-defined cohort of 24 patients *J Urol* **157**, 2183–90

29. Benson, M. C., Whang, I. S., Olsson, C. A., McMahon, D. J. and Cooner, W. H. (1992) The use of prostate specific antigen density to enhance the predictive value of intermediate levels of serum prostate specific antigen *J Urol* **147**, 3 Pt 2; 817–21.

30. Partin, A. W., Carter, H. B., Chan, D. W., Epstein, J. I., Oesterling, J. E., Rock, R. C., et al. (1990) Prostate specific antigen in the staging of localized prostate cancer: influence of tumor differentiation, tumor volume and benign hyperplasia *J Urol* **143**, 4; 747–52.

31. Stamey, T. A., Kabalin, J. N., McNeal, J. E., Johnstone, I. M., Freiha, F., Redwine, E. A., et al. (1989) Prostate specific antigen in the diagnosis and treatment of adenocarcinoma of the prostate. II. Radical prostatectomy treated patients *J Urol* **141**, 5; 1076–83.

32. Seaman, E., Whang, I. S., Olsson, C. A., Katz, A. E., Cooner, W. H. and Benson, M. (1993) PSA-Density (PSAD). Role in patient evaluation and management *Urol Clin North Am* **20**, 635

33. Catalona, W. J., Richie, J. P., de Kernion, J. B., Ahmann, F. R., Ratliff, T. L., Dalkin, B. L., et al. (1994) Comparison of prostate-specific antigen concentration versus prostate-specific antigen density in the early detection of prostate cancer: Receiver operator characteristic curves *J Urol* **152**, 2031

34. Brawer, M. K., Aramburu, E. A. G., Chen, G. L., Preston, S. D. and Ellis, W. J. (1993) The inability of prostate-specific antigen index to enhance the predictive value of prostate specific antigen in the diagnosis of prostatic carcinoma *J Urol* **150**, 369

35. Djavan, B., Marberger, M., Zlotta, A. R. and Schulman, C. C. (1998) PSA, f/tPSA, PSAD, PSA-TZ and PAS-velocity for prostate cancer prediction: A multivariate analysis *J Urol* **159**, 898(A)

36. Oesterling, J. E. (1996) Age-specific reference ranges for serum PSA *N Engl J Med* **335**, 5; 345–6.

37. Partin, A. W., Criley, S. R., Subong, E. N., Zincke, H., Walsh, P. C. and Oesterling, J. E. (1996) Standard versus age-specific prostate-specific antigen reference ranges among men with clinically localized prostate cancer: A pathological analysis *J Urol* **155**, 1336

38. Reissigl, A., Pointner, J., Horniger, W., Ennemoser, O., Strasser, H., Klocker, H., et al. (1995) Comparison of different prostate-specific antigen cutpoints for early detection of prostate cancer: Results of a large screening study *Urology* **46**, 662

39. Catalona, W. J., Richie, J. P., Ahmann, F. R., Hudson, M. A., Scardino, P. T., Flanigan, R. C., et al. (1994) Comparison of digital rectal examination and serum prostate specific antigen in the early detection of prostate cancer: results of a multicenter clinical trial of 6,630 men *J Urol* **151**, 5; 1283–90.

40. Littrup, P. J., Kane, R. A., Mettlin, C., Murphy, G. P., Lee, F., Toi, A., et al. (1994) Cost-effective prostate cancer detection. Reduction of low-yield biopsies *Cancer* **74**, 3146

41. Morgan, T. O., Jacobsen, S. J., McCarthy, W. F., Jacobson, D. J., McLeod, D. G. and Moul, J. W. (1996) Age-specific reference ranges for prostate-specific antigen in black men *N Engl J Med* **335**, 304

42. Oesterling, J. E., Kumamoto, Y., Tsukamoto, T., Girman, C. J., Guess, H., Masumori, N., et al. (1995) Serum prostate-specific antigen in a community based population of health Japanese men: lower values than for similarly aged white men *Br J Urol* **75**, 347

43. Peter, J., Unverzagt, C., Krogh, T. N., Vorm, O. and Hoesel, W. (2001) Identification of precursor forms of free prostate-specific antigen in serum of prostate cancer patients by immunosorption and mass spectrometry *Cancer Res* **61**, 957–62

44. Noldus, J., Chen, Z. X. and Stamey, T. A. (1997) Isolation and characterization of free form prostate-specific antigen (f-PSA) in sera of men with prostate cancer *J Urol* **158**, 1606–09

45. Lilja, H. (1985) A kallikrein-like serine protease in prostatic fluid cleaves the predominant seminal vesicle protein *J Clin Invest* **76**, 5; 1899–903.

46. Christensson, A. and Lilja, H. (1994) Complex formation between protein C inhibitor and prostate-specific antigen in vitro and in human semen *Eur J Biochem* **220**, 1; 45–53.

47. Leinonen, J., Zhang, W. M. and Stenman, U. H. (1996) Complex formation between PSA isoenzymes and protease inhibitors *J Urol* **155**, 3; 1099–103.

48. Zhang, W. M., Finne, P., Leinonen, J., Vesalainen, S., Nordling, S. and Stenman, U. H. (1999) Measurement of the complex between prostate-specific antigen and alpha1- protease inhibitor in serum *Clin Chem* **45**, 6 Pt 1; 814–21.

49. Zhang, W. M., Finne, P., Leinonen, J., Vesalainen, S., Nordling, S., Rannikko, S., et al. (1998) Characterization and immunological determination of the complex between prostate-specific antigen and alpha2-macroglobulin *Clin Chem* **44**, 12; 2471–9.

50. Lovgren, J., Rajakoski, K., Karp, M., Lundwall, a. and Lilja, H. (1997) Activation of the zymogen form of prostate-specific antigen by human glandular kallikrein 2 *Biochem Biophys Res Commun* **238**, 2; 549–55.

51. Takayama, T. K., Carter, C. A. and Deng, T. (2001) Activation of prostate-specific antigen precursor (pro-PSA) by prostin, a novel human prostatic serine protease identified by degenerate PCR *Biochemistry* **40**, 6; 1679–87.

52. Mikolajczyk, S. D., Grauer, L. S., Millar, L. S., Hill, T. M., Kumar, A., Rittenhouse, H. G., et al. (1997) A precursor form of PSA (pPSA) is a component of the free PSA in prostate cancer serum *Urology* **50**, 5; 710–4.

53. Chan, T. Y., Mikolajczyjk, S. D., Lecksell, K., Shue, M. J., Rittenhouse, H., Partin, A. W., et al. (2003) Immunohistochemical staining of prostate cancer with monoclonal antibodies to the precursor of prostate-specific antigen *Urology* **62**, 177–81

54. Vaisänen, V., Lovgren, J., Hellman, J., Piironen, T., Lilja, H. and Pettersson, K. (1999) Characterization and processing of prostate-specific antigen (hK3) and human glandular kallikrein 2 (hK2) secreted by LNCaP cells. *Prostate Cancer Prostatic Dis* 2; 91–97

55. Kumar, A., Mikolajczyjk, S. D., Hill, T. M., Millar, L. S. and Saedi, M. S. (2000) Different proportions of various prostate-specific antigen (PSA) and human kallikrein 2 (hK2) forms are present in noninduced and androgen induced LNCap cells *Prostate* **44**, 248–54

56. Chen, Z. X., Chen, H. and Stamey, T. (1997) Prostate Specific Antigen in Benign Prostatic Hyperplasia: Purification and Characterization *J Urol* **157**, 6; 2166–70

57. Mikolajczyk, S. D., Millar, L. S., Marker, K. M., Wang, T. J., Rittenhouse, H. G., Marks, L. S., et al. (2000) Seminal plasma contains "BPSA," a molecular form of prostate-specific antigen that is associated with benign prostatic hyperplasia *Prostate* **45**, 3; 271–6

58. Mikolajczyk, S. D., Millar, L. S., Wang, T. J., Rittenhouse, H. G., Wolfert, R. L., Marks, L. S., et al. (2000) "BPSA", a specific molecular form of free prostate-specific antigen is found predominantly in the transition zone of patients with nodular benign prostatic hyperplasia *Urology* **55**, 41–45

59. de Vries, S. H., Raaijmakers, R., Blijenberg, B. G., Mikolajczyk, S. D., Rittenhouse, H. G. and Schröder F. H. (2005) Additional use of [-2] precursor prostate-specific antigen and "benign" PSA at diagnosis in screen-detected prostate cancer *Urology* **65**, 5; 926–30.

60. Qian, Y., Sensibar, J., Zelner, D. J., Schaeffer, A. J., Finlay, J. A., Rittenhouse, H., et al. (1997) Two-dimensional gel electrophoresis detects prostate-specific antigen alpha-1-antichzmotrypsin complex in serum but not in prostatic fluid *Clin Chem* **43**, 352–59

61. Belanger, A., van Halbeck, H., Graves, H. C., Grandbois, K., Stamey, T., Huang, L., et al. (1995) Molecular mass and carbohydrate structure of prostate-specific antigen: Studies for establishment of an international PSA standard *Prostate* **27**, 187–97

62. Barak, M., Mecz, Y., Lurie, A. and Gruener (1989) Binding of serum prostate antigen to concanavalin A in patients with cancer or hyperplasia of the prostate *Oncology (Huntingt)* **46**, 375–77

63. Chan, D. and Gao, Y. M. (1991) Variants of prostate-specific antigen separated by concanavalin A *Clin Chem* **37**, 1133–34

64. van Dieijen-Visser, M. P., van Pelt, J. and Delaere, K. P. (1994) Pitfalls in the differentiation of N-glycosylation variants of prostate-specific antigen using concanavalin A *Eur J Clin Chem Clin Biochem* **32**, 473–78

65. Jung, K., Lein, M., Henke, H., Schnorr, D. and Loening, S. (1996) Isoforms of prostate-specific antigen in serum: A result of the glycosylation process in dysplastic prostatic cells? *Prostate* **29**, 65–66

66. Herrala, A., Kurkela, R., Vihinen, M., Kalkkinen, N. and Vihko, P. (1998) Androgen-sensitive human prostate cancer cells, LnCap, produce both N-terminally mature and truncated prostate-specific antigen isoforms *Eur J Biochem* **255**, 329–35

67. Mikolajczyk, S. D., Millar, L. S., Wang, T. J., Rittenhouse, H. G., Marks, L. S., Song, W., et al. (2000) A Precursor Form of Prostate-specific Antigen Is More Highly Elevated in Prostate Cancer Compared with Benign Transition Zone Prostate Tissue. *Cancer Res* **60**, 756–59

68. Mikolajczyk, S. D., Marker, K. M., Millar, L. S., Kumar, A., Saedi, M. S., Payne, J. K., et al. (2001) A truncated precursor form of prostate-specific antigen is a more specific serum marker of prostate cancer *Cancer Res* **61**, 18; 6958–63

69. Sokoll, L. J., Chan, D. W., Mikolajczyk, S. D., Rittenhouse, H. G., Evans, C. L., Linton, H. J., et al. (2003) Proenzyme PSA for the early detection of prostate cancer in the 2.5–4.0 ng/ml total PSA range: preliminary analysis *Urology* **61**, 2; 274–6

70. Catalona, W. J., Bartsch, G., Rittenhouse, H., Evans, C. L., Linton, H. J., Amirkhan, A., et al. (2003) Serum Pro Prostate-specific Antigen improves cancer detection compared to free and complexed prostate-specific antigen in men with prostate-specific antigen 2 to 4 ng/ml *J Urol* **170**, 2181–85

71. Shariat, S., Mikolajczyk, S. D., Singh, H., Rittenhouse, H. G., Canto, E., Fleissner, E. Y., et al. (2003) Preoperative serum levels of proPSA isoforms are associated with biologically aggressive prostate cancer *J Urol* **169**, 4 (A230); 60

72. Catalona, W. J., Mikolajczyk, S. D., Linton, H. J., Evans, C. L., Amikan, A., Rittenhouse, H. G., et al. (2003) ProPSA helps to detect more aggressive prostate cancer in the 2–4 ng/ml range *J Urol* **169**, 4 (A1127); 290

73. Nurmikko, P., Vaisanen, V., Piironen, T., Lindgren, S. and Lilja, H. (2000) Production and characterisation of novel anti-prostate-specific antigen (PSA) monoclonal antibodies that do not detect internally cleaved Lys145-Lys146 inactive PSA *Clin Chem* **46 (10)**, 1610–18

74. Nurmikko, P., Pettersson, K., Piironen, T., Hugosson, J. and Lilja, H. (2001) Discrimination of prostate cancer from benign disease by plasma measurement of intact, free prostate-specific antigen lacking an internal cleavage site at Lys145-Lys146 *Clin Chem* **47**, 8; 1415–23.

75. Steuber, T., Nurmikko, P., Haese, A., Pettersson, K., Graefen, M., Hammerer, P., et al. (2002) Discrimination of benign from malignant prostatic disease by selective measurements of single chain, intact free prostate specific antigen *J Urol* **168**, 5; 1917–22

76. Linton, H. J., Marks, L. S., Millar, L. S., Knott, C. L., Rittenhouse, H. G. and Mikolajczyk, S. D. (2003) Benign prostate-specific antigen (BPSA) in serum is increased in benign prostate disease *Clin Chem* **49**, 2; 253–9

77. Wang, T. J., Slawin, K. M., Rittenhouse, H. G., Millar, L. S. and Mikolajczyk, S. D. (2000) Benign prostatic hyperplasia-associated prostate-specific antigen (BPSA) shows unique immunoreactivity with anti-PSA monoclonal antibodies *Eur J Biochem* **267**, 13; 4040–5

# 9

# PSA Velocity at Presentation as a Predictor of Prostate Cancer Aggressiveness

*Jason A. Efstathiou and Anthony V. D'Amico*

## SUMMARY

Prostate-specific antigen (PSA) remains the best available marker for the detection of prostate cancer and for monitoring evidence of recurrence after treatment; yet, it has limitations both as a diagnostic and as a prognostic tool when considered on its own. Methods to improve the predictive and prognostic significance of PSA have led to innovations such as considering the rate of rise in serial PSA levels prior to diagnosis of prostate cancer. PSA velocity has significant advantages over a single-PSA measurement not only in differentiating between men with prostate cancer and those with benign disease, but also in predicting

From: *Current Clinical Urology: Prostate Cancer Screening*, Edited by: D. P. Ankerst et al.
DOI 10.1007/978-1-60327-281-0_9 © Humana Press, a part of Springer Science+Business Media, LLC 2009

the biological aggressiveness of prostate cancer at presentation. PSA velocity at presentation, and in particular an increase in the PSA level by more than 2 ng/ml during the year prior to diagnosis, is significantly associated with more advanced tumor stage, higher grade, and a shorter time to PSA failure, prostate cancer-specific and all-cause mortality following radical prostatectomy or radiation therapy in men with prostate cancer.

**Key Words:** Prostate-specific antigen, PSA velocity, Prostate cancer, Radical prostatectomy, Radiation therapy.

## INTRODUCTION

The introduction of serum prostate-specific antigen (PSA) as a biomarker for prostate cancer and its use in the United States beginning in 1989 led to a marked increase in prostate cancer detection. Since the advent of the PSA era, however, stage migration has occurred with diagnosis occurring at a younger age and at a lower-serum PSA level and Gleason score resulting in disease that is more likely to be confined to the prostate (1). Consequently, there has been an increase in the use of local only monotherapy, including radical prostatectomy (RP) and various forms of radiation therapy (RT), intended to cure these smaller volume and lower-grade cancers.

Treatments for localized prostate cancer impact quality of life (2–7), so the issues of over-diagnosis and over-treatment of clinically insignificant tumors remain (8). Specifically, some screen-detected cancers may have a low-lethal potential and thus may not necessarily require treatment (9,10). Whether population screening for prostate cancer using PSA measurement decreases mortality remains under study in the form of ongoing population-based randomized controlled screening trials in the United States and Europe (11,12).

In the interim, PSA remains the best available marker for the detection of prostate cancer and for monitoring evidence of recurrence after treatment (13); yet, it has limitations both as a diagnostic and as a prognostic tool when considered on its own. Specifically, due to serial annual PSA screening, levels greater than 10.0 ng/ml at diagnosis have become infrequent (14) and, as a result, the prognostic significance of any single value of PSA below 10.0 ng/ml while still present (15) is becoming more limited.

Methods to improve the prognostic significance of PSA and therefore guide management in the era of PSA screening have led to innovations such as considering the rate of rise in PSA levels prior to diagnosis of prostate cancer. This concept known as PSA velocity was introduced in 1992 by Carter et al. (16) using data compiled by the Baltimore Longitudinal Study on Aging after examining stored serum samples and comparing age-adjusted rates of PSA change among men with prostate cancer, benign prostatic hyperplasia (BPH), and controls. PSA velocity has significant advantages over a single-PSA measurement not only in differentiating between men with prostate cancer and those with benign disease (17,18), but also in predicting the biological aggressiveness of prostate cancer at presentation.

This chapter will review the evidence supporting the concepts that serial pre-diagnostic PSA values can be used to estimate the PSA velocity at presentation and that this parameter is significantly associated with tumor stage, grade, time to PSA failure, and time to prostate cancer-specific and all-cause mortality following RP or RT.

## ESTIMATING PROSTATE-SPECIFIC ANTIGEN VELOCITY

PSA velocity assesses the rate of PSA change over time. The clinical utility of PSA velocity is limited by the fact that serum PSA is not cancer-specific and is subject to intra-patient and inter-assay variabilities [19]. In the early studies by Carter et al. [20], PSA velocity was calculated using a linear regression analysis of PSA values during an interval of at least 18 months. Serum samples were not collected more frequently and thus shorter intervals could not be evaluated. Since then, numerous other methods of calculating PSA velocity have been used without any consensus and with the potential to produce markedly inconsistent results.

Connolly and colleagues [21] recently calculated PSA velocity in a large population-based database from Northern Ireland using three common methods and compared their test characteristics. These methods were as follows:

1. Linear regression analysis, using the equation: $p = at + b$
2. Arithmetic equation of change in PSA over time using the equation: $[1/(n-1)] \times (\Sigma_{i=2}^{n} p_i - p_{i-1}/t_i - t_{i-1})$
3. Rate of PSA change using first and last values only and the equation: $p_n - p_1/t_n - t_1$

Where $p$ = PSA value, $t$ = time at PSA test (year), $a$ = slope of regression line (equivalent to PSA velocity), $b$ = intercept at time zero, and $n$ = total number of PSA tests.

This study found that an individual PSA velocity result differs substantially depending on the method of calculation, suggesting that a uniform methodology should be employed. The authors concluded that linear regression analysis using all PSA values is less influenced by short-term PSA variability and should be the method of choice for calculating PSA velocity.

Studies by D'Amico and colleagues [22–25], looking at outcomes following therapy, have used a linear regression analysis to calculate PSA velocity in the year prior to diagnosis. This method includes the PSA measurement closest in time to diagnosis and all prior PSA values obtained within 12–18 months of diagnosis and separated by at least 6 months from the PSA value at diagnosis. A minimum of two and a maximum of three PSA values have been used in these studies. Such an approach seems reasonable since PSA velocity may be influenced by short-term PSA fluctuations if the component PSA measurements are too close together [26–28]. Similarly, PSA velocity increases over time in men diagnosed with prostate cancer [16] and using PSA values dating back several years may under-estimate the rate of change at the time of diagnosis [25] (see Fig. 1). The actual value at diagnosis more accurately reflects the clinical scenario and biological aggressiveness of the cancer at the time when important management decisions are occurring, while changes averaged over several years may also include changes in prostate size due to BPH [16]. In fact, a recent analysis by Nguyen et al. [25] demonstrated that PSA velocity estimated using pre-treatment PSA values obtained approximately 18 months prior to diagnosis as compared to all prior PSA values provides a stronger significant association (larger hazard ratios, smaller p-values) with the time to PSA recurrence, prostate cancer-specific mortality (PCSM), and all-cause mortality (ACM) following RT.

For everyday clinical use, arithmetic methods are attractive given their simplicity of calculation. Yu and colleagues [29] compared a variety of methods and showed

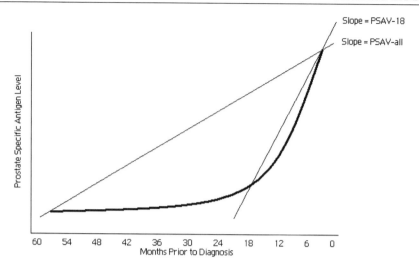

**Fig. 1.** Illustration of the impact of basing PSA velocity on values within 18 months of diagnosis vs. all prior PSA values *(25)*.

PSAV-18: PSA velocity determined based on linear regression of PSA values within 18 months prior to diagnosis

PSAV-all: PSA velocity determined based on linear regression of all PSA values available prior to diagnosis

This figure was published in Urology; 70(2), 288–93, Copyright Elsevier (2007).

that PSA velocity calculations using a simple arithmetic two-point calculation (PSA2-PSA1/Time2-Time1) and linear regression had a strong correlation ($r = 0.92$) when restricted to PSA values from 12 months before diagnosis of clinically localized prostate cancer. When PSA measurements beyond 1 year were included in the calculation, PSA velocity was significantly lower than in the 12 months before diagnosis potentially obscuring its prognostic value. None of the formulas involving three PSA values appeared to offer any additional benefit. Another recent report of 471 patients who underwent RP confirmed that a simple two-point method of calculating PSA velocity is sufficient and reliable and suggested that a minimum time interval of 12 months prior to radical prostatectomy is needed and that a PSA velocity cutoff of $\leq 2$ vs. $>2$ ng/ml/yr appears optimal *(30)*. These authors have suggested that simple arithmetic PSA velocity calculations may be used in daily clinical practice to help predict outcome following definitive therapy. Although the specific PSA velocity threshold level one chooses is arbitrary, a level of 2 ng/ml/yr seems reasonable for clinical usage *(22,23,30,31)*.

Establishing a consensus on how best to estimate PSA velocity is paramount to ensure that patients can be appropriately risk-stratified and that studies on the significance of PSA velocity can be directly compared. The optimal number of PSA tests, interval between PSA levels, and time interval before diagnosis by which PSA velocity most accurately reflects tumor biology remain to be determined.

## PRE-TREATMENT PSA VELOCITY AND ITS ASSOCIATION WITH TUMOR GRADE AND STAGE AT PRESENTATION

Evidence now exists that confirms that the pre-treatment PSA velocity is a significant predictor of higher-grade and more advanced-stage prostate cancer at diagnosis

*(16,22,31–39)*. Data collected from a cohort of over 1,400 men enrolled in the randomized Prostate, Lung, Colorectal, and Ovarian Cancer (PLCO) Screening Trial, who received $\geq 2$ PSA screens and were diagnosed with prostate cancer within 1 year of the last screen, showed that PSA velocity was independently associated with biopsy Gleason score *(32)*. After controlling for PSA and demographics, the odds of having a Gleason score of 7–10 were 1.3, 2.2, and 2.3 times higher for men with PSA velocity values from 0.5 to 1 ng/ml/yr, 1 to 2 ng/ml/yr, and >2 ng/ml/yr, respectively, compared with men who had PSA velocity values < 0.5 ng/ml/yr (*p* value for linear trend = 0.003).

In another report by D'Amico et al. of over 1,000 men who underwent RP, a high-PSA velocity was predictive of an elevated Gleason score (*p* = 0.03), advanced pathologic stage (*p* < 0.001), and lymph node metastases (*p* < 0.001) *(22)*. Specifically, among men who had PSA velocity levels <2 ng/ml/yr, 26% had pathologic Gleason scores of 7–10, and 25% had advanced pathologic stage disease. By comparison, among men who had PSA velocity levels > 2 ng/ml/yr, 31% had Gleason score of 7–10, and 30% had advanced-stage disease.

Additional studies have reported that pre-treatment PSA velocity is predictive of prostate cancer aggressiveness. In a group of 202 men who underwent RP, Patel et al. observed that those with PSA velocity levels of >2 ng/ml/yr were more likely to have pathologic T3 disease (*p* = 0.007), positive surgical margins (*p* = 0.01), and possess >10% grade 4/5 tumors (*p* = 0.04) than men with PSA velocity < 2 ng/ml/yr *(31)*. Similarly, in cohort of 358 men treated with RT, PSA velocity was significantly associated with the detection of Gleason score 4+3 or greater prostate cancer at biopsy (relative risk (RR) 1.06, 95% CI 1.02–1.10, *p* = 0.004) *(34)*. In a serial PSA screening program over a 10-year period that evaluated 353 men who eventually developed prostate cancer, PSA velocity was significantly associated with Gleason score and pathologic stage *(35)*.

Even in studies where statistical significance might not have been reached, a trend appeared to exist between an elevated PSA velocity and worse disease. Thiel et al. reported a lower-average PSA velocity in 43 patients with pathologically organ-confined disease (1.12 ng/ml/yr) than in 38 patients with more extensive disease (1.88 ng/ml/yr) following RP *(40)*. An analysis of over 1,200 men diagnosed with prostate cancer by prostate biopsy on the placebo arm of the Prostate Cancer Prevention Trial (PCPT) indicated that PSA velocity was strongly and significantly associated with increased risk of high-grade disease on univariable analysis (RR 8.93, 95% CI 5.71–13.97, *p* < 0.001), but not on multivariable analysis (*p* = 0.54) after controlling for other known prognostic factors such as PSA level *(41)*. Similarly, among a subset of 658 men who underwent RP on the PLCO Screening Trial, PSA velocity was significantly associated with advanced pathologic stage (18% vs. 32% for PSA velocity < 0.5 ng/ml/yr and >2 ng/ml/yr, respectively) on univariable, but not multivariable analyses *(32)*. The European Randomized Study of Screening for Prostate Cancer (ERSPC) Rotterdam also reported a modest univariable association between PSA velocity and tumor aggressiveness as measured by Gleason score and clinical stage *(42)*.

On balance, a higher-PSA velocity is associated with more advanced pathologic features at presentation and at RP. Whether this association has translated into an increased risk of recurrence and death from prostate cancer following treatment is the subject of the following sections.

## PRE-TREATMENT PSA VELOCITY AND ITS ASSOCIATION WITH TIME TO POST-OPERATIVE AND POST-RADIATION THERAPY PSA RECURRENCE

In addition to being associated with higher-grade and more advanced-stage prostate cancer at diagnosis, an increasing pre-treatment PSA velocity has also been shown to be associated with an increased risk of recurrence after RP or RT (Table 1) after adjusting for known prognostic factors.

### *PSA Velocity and Post-Operative PSA Recurrence*

As shown in Fig. 2, in the study by D'Amico et al. of over 1,000 men, an annual pre-operative PSA velocity > 2 ng/ml was associated with a significantly shorter time to PSA recurrence (multivariable RR 1.5, 95% CI 1.1–1.9, $p = 0.003$) after RP *(22)*. These results were confirmed by Patel et al. in a study of 202 men who underwent RP at Stanford *(31)*. Kaplan–Meier relapse-free survival estimates at 5 years were 89% vs. 73% for PSA velocity $\leq$ 2 ng/ml/yr and >2 ng/ml/yr, respectively ($p = 0.003$). In multivariable analyses that controlled for the known prognostic factors: clinical T stage, initial PSA level, biopsy Gleason score, percent of positive cores, and amount of tumor within positive cores, PSA velocity > 2 ng/ml/yr remained significant (RR 3.0, 95% CI 1.2–7.7, $p = 0.02$) for predicting relapse-free survival after RP. Thus, men with an annual pre-operative PSA velocity of >2 ng/ml had a 3-fold increase in their risk of relapse after prostatectomy. Additional analyses that have examined PSA velocity as a continuous variable and employed different PSA velocity cutoff levels remained significant.

Other surgical series have demonstrated similar findings. In a large cohort of over 2,200 patients with non-standardized PSA measurements who underwent RP at Mayo Clinic, PSA velocity (with a cutoff value of 3.4 ng/ml/yr) was predictive of biochemical progression (RR 1.30, 95% CI 1.06–1.58, $p = 0.011$) in a multivariable model that accounted for pre- and post-operative prognostic factors *(37)*. Similarly, in 102 men from a screening population in Austria who underwent RP, the median PSA velocity in the year before diagnosis in those who relapsed biochemically was 1.98 ng/ml/yr vs. 1.05 ng/ml/yr in those who had no evidence of disease within 5 years after surgery ($p <$ 0.05) *(38)*. In a study that used pre-operative PSA doubling time as its metric for PSA kinetics, results were analogous *(39)*.

One report found that neither pre-operative PSA velocity nor doubling time was a predictor of adverse pathologic findings or biochemical failure after RP *(43)*. However, the trend suggested an effect (PSA velocity was 1.37 ng/ml/yr vs. 0.94 ng/ml/yr for men with and without PSA recurrence, respectively, $p = 0.58$) and it is possible that the study's power to measure an association between PSA velocity and recurrence was limited by sample and event size, and relatively short follow-up.

### *PSA Velocity and Post-Radiation PSA Recurrence*

An association between an increasing pre-treatment PSA velocity and shorter time to PSA recurrence has been described in men undergoing RT. Specifically, D'Amico et al. *(23)* reported on a cohort of 358 men who underwent RT for localized prostate cancer and found that a PSA velocity > 2.0 ng/ml/yr was significantly associated with a shorter time to PSA failure (RR 1.8, 95% CI 1.3–2.6, $p = 0.001$) after adjusting for

## Table 1
### Summary of Studies Examining PSA Velocity and Adjusted Risk of PSA Recurrence, Prostate Cancer-Specific, and All-Cause Mortality Following RP or RT

| Study | Rx | No. of men | Median F/u (yrs) | Covariate | PSA recurrence | | | PCSM | | | ACM | | |
|---|---|---|---|---|---|---|---|---|---|---|---|---|---|
| | | | | | No. of events | RR* (95% CI) | p-Value | No. of events | RR* (95% CI) | p-Value | No. of Events | RR* (95% CI) | p-value |
| D'Amico [22] | RP | 1,095 | 5.1 | PSAv >2.0 ng/ml/yr | 366 | 1.5 (1.1–1.9) | 0.003 | 27 | 9.8 (2.8–34.3) | <0.001 | 84 | 1.9 (1.2–3.2) | 0.01 |
| Sengupta[37] | RP | 2290 | 7.1 | PSAv>3.4 ng/ml/yr | 583 | 1.5 (1.2–1.9) | 0.001 | 42 | 5.1 (1.9–13.2) | – | – | – | – |
| Patel[31] | RP | 202 | 4.0 | PSAv >2.0 ng/ml/yr | 31 | 3.0 (1.2–7.7) | 0.02 | – | – | – | – | – | – |
| D'Amico[23] | RT | 358 | 4.0 | PSAv >2.0 ng/ml/yr | 160 | 1.8 (1.3–2.6) | 0.001 | 30 | 12.0 (3.0–54.0) | 0.001 | 79 | 2.1 (1.3–3.6) | 0.005 |
| Palma[44] | RT | 473 | 7.6 | PSAv >2.0 ng/ml/yr | 188 | – | 0.09 | 24 | – | 0.55 | 78 | – | 0.99 |

* = the relative risks represent adjusted values from multivariable analyses controlling for known prognostic factors including PSA level, Gleason score, and tumor category
— = not available

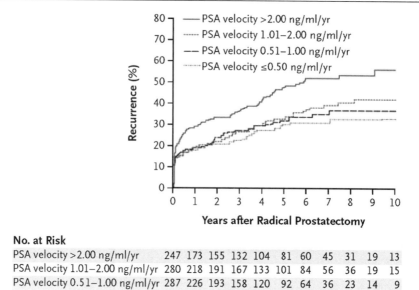

**Fig. 2.** Kaplan–Meier estimates of disease recurrence after radical prostatectomy, according to the quartile of PSA velocity during the year before diagnosis *(22)*.

the PSA level, Gleason score, and clinical tumor category at diagnosis. Notably, PSA velocity remained significant when analyzed as a continuous variable. There was also a significant interaction between PSA velocity and pre-treatment risk group for PSA recurrence. Specifically, the adjusted RRs for PSA failure were 1.4 (95% CI 1.2–1.6) and 1.03 (95% CI 1.02–1.05) for patients with low- and higher-risk disease, respectively. This suggests that for a given increase in PSA velocity the corresponding increment in the risk of PSA recurrence will be higher in a man with low-risk disease compared with higher-risk disease. Figure 3 illustrates a significant difference between the estimates of PSA recurrence when stratified by the pre-RT PSA velocity for men with low-risk disease, as well as for those with higher-risk disease. Among men presenting with low-risk disease, the 7-year estimates of PSA recurrence were 78% (95% CI 57–99%) vs. 54% (95% CI 40–69%) for those with a PSA velocity > 2 ng/ml/yr vs. $\leq$2 ng/ml/yr, respectively ($p = 0.005$); while among men presenting with higher-risk disease, the rates were 87% (95% CI 74–100%) vs. 60% (95% CI 46–74%) ($p < 0.001$).

A recent study of 473 patients treated with RT in British Columbia found that men with a PSA velocity > 2 ng/ml/yr had a shorter biochemical disease-free survival compared with men with a PSA velocity of $\leq$2 ng/ml/yr (median, 68 months vs. 97 months, $p = 0.0003$) *(44)*. On multivariable analysis, however, PSA velocity was no longer a significant predictor of PSA recurrence in the entire cohort ($p = 0.09$). Yet, in patients with high-risk disease, PSA velocity predicted biochemical failure on univariable ($p = 0.0002$) and multivariable ($p = 0.02$) analyses. However, significant differences existed in this study compared to the prior study by D'Amico and colleagues. Specifically, the median PSA velocity in this report was substantially lower (0.3 ng/ml/yr) than in other surgical and RT series, including the D'Amico RT study (1.5 ng/ml/yr), perhaps due to

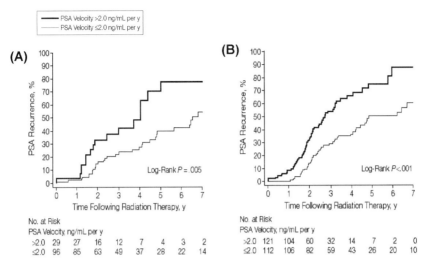

**Fig. 3.** Kaplan–Meier estimates of PSA recurrence stratified by the pre-treatment PSA velocity for men with (**A**) low-risk disease and (**B**) higher-risk disease *(23)*.

the method of calculation. In addition, the patients were of higher-risk, RT doses were lower, and an alternative definition of biochemical relapse was employed.

In summary, the pre-treatment PSA velocity appears to be predictive of biochemical progression following both RP *(22,31,37,38)* and RT *(23)*. However, not all men who experience a PSA recurrence will die of prostate cancer *(45)* because of the competing causes of mortality that can occur during the protracted clinical course that prostate cancer is known to have. Therefore, whether an increasing PSA velocity is associated with a shorter cancer-specific and overall survival is the subject of the next section.

## PRE-TREATMENT PSA VELOCITY AND ITS ASSOCIATION WITH TIME TO POST-OPERATIVE AND POST-RADIATION THERAPY PROSTATE CANCER-SPECIFIC AND ALL-CAUSE MORTALITY

While studies evaluating the prognostic significance of the PSA velocity assessed during the year prior to diagnosis now exist, one study evaluated whether an association existed between the diagnosis of lethal prostate cancer and PSA velocity more than a decade prior to diagnosis. Specifically, in a recent analysis of the Baltimore Longitudinal Study of Aging, PSA velocity measured 10–15 years before diagnosis identified men who developed non-fatal prostate cancer from men who developed fatal prostate cancer 25 years later *(33)*. Survival was 92% (95% CI 84–96%) among men with a PSA velocity $\leq 0.35$ ng/ml/yr and 54% (95% CI 15–82%) among men with PSA velocity $> 0.35$ ng/ml/yr ($p < 0.001$), translating into a higher-relative risk of prostate cancer death (RR 4.7, 95% CI 1.3–16.5, $p = 0.02$).

A PSA doubling time (DT) < 3 months in the setting of initial biochemical failure after primary RP or RT appears to be a surrogate endpoint for prostate cancer-specific mortality (PCSM) *(45)*. A pre-treatment PSA velocity > 2 ng/ml/yr has since been associated with a PSA DT of <3 months and as a result may be able to identify men at risk for clinically significant as compared to insignificant PSA relapse following RP or RT *(46)*. Given this association, it is not surprising that recent evidence shows a significant association between an increasing pre-treatment PSA velocity and a shorter time to cancer-specific and all-cause mortality following RP and RT as detailed below and as illustrated in Table 1.

### Prostate Cancer-Specific and All-Cause Mortality Following Radical Prostatectomy

In the study by D'Amico and colleagues based on an analysis of 1,095 men in a prospective PSA-based screening study, and as illustrated in Figs. 4 and 5, a >2 ng/ml increase in PSA level during the year prior to diagnosis was found in multivariable analyses to be significantly associated with a nearly 10-fold higher rate of death from prostate cancer (RR 9.8, 95% CI 2.8–34.3, $p < 0.001$) and nearly 2-fold higher rate of death from any cause (RR 1.9, 95% CI 1.2–3.2, $p = 0.01$) following RP *(22)*. Sengupta et al. confirmed an increase in cancer-specific mortality after RP in men with a PSA velocity > 3.4 ng/ml/yr using uncorrected PSA measurements derived from multiple sources *(37)*. In analyses that adjusted for clinical and pathological features, the risk of death from prostate cancer was 5-fold higher (RR 5.07, 95% CI 1.94–13.24). These authors did not comment on all-cause mortality (ACM).

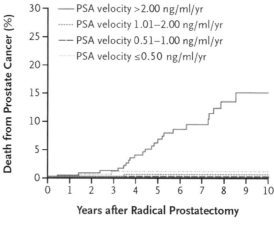

**No. at Risk**

| | | | | | | | | | | |
|---|---|---|---|---|---|---|---|---|---|---|
| PSA velocity >2.00 ng/ml/yr | 262 | 257 | 248 | 226 | 187 | 157 | 123 | 92 | 60 | 36 | 22 |
| PSA velocity 1.01–2.00 ng/ml/yr | 288 | 275 | 248 | 229 | 194 | 158 | 131 | 91 | 58 | 36 | 20 |
| PSA velocity 0.51–1.00 ng/ml/yr | 289 | 281 | 260 | 227 | 176 | 131 | 94 | 55 | 36 | 18 | 11 |
| PSA velocity ≤0.50 ng/ml/yr | 256 | 236 | 200 | 163 | 139 | 108 | 81 | 61 | 34 | 20 | 9 |

**Fig. 4.** Cumulative incidence estimates of death from prostate cancer after radical prostatectomy, according to the quartile of PSA velocity during the year before diagnosis *(22)*. Copyright © 2004 Massachusetts Medical Society. All rights reserved.

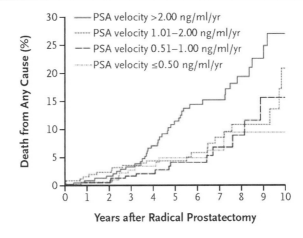

**No. at Risk**

| | | | | | | | | | | | |
|---|---|---|---|---|---|---|---|---|---|---|---|
| PSA velocity >2.00 ng/ml/yr | 262 | 257 | 248 | 226 | 187 | 157 | 123 | 92 | 60 | 36 | 22 |
| PSA velocity 1.01–2.00 ng/ml/yr | 288 | 275 | 248 | 229 | 194 | 158 | 131 | 91 | 58 | 36 | 20 |
| PSA velocity 0.51–1.00 ng/ml/yr | 289 | 281 | 260 | 227 | 176 | 131 | 94 | 55 | 36 | 18 | 11 |
| PSA velocity ≤0.50 ng/ml/yr | 256 | 236 | 200 | 163 | 139 | 108 | 81 | 61 | 34 | 20 | 9 |

**Fig. 5.** Kaplan–Meier estimates of death from any cause after radical prostatectomy, according to the quartile of PSA velocity during the year before diagnosis *(22)*.

## *Prostate Cancer-Specific and All-Cause Mortality Following Radiation Therapy*

In a study of RT managed patients *(23)*, similar to the reports of surgically managed patients *(22,37)*, the vast majority (28/30) of the observed prostate cancer deaths occurred in men whose PSA velocity exceeded 2 ng/ml/yr during the year prior to diagnosis. This translated into a 12-fold higher risk of experiencing PCSM (adjusted RR 12.0, 95% CI 3.0–54.0, $p = 0.001$) and 2-fold shorter time to ACM (adjusted RR 2.1, 95% CI 1.3–3.6, $p = 0.005$) following RT. An increasing PSA velocity remained significantly associated ($p < 0.001$) with a shorter time to both cancer-specific and ACM when analyzed as a continuous variable.

The prognostic importance of a PSA velocity > 2 ng/ml/yr in men with otherwise low-risk disease is shown in Fig. 6. Specifically, men presenting with low-risk disease and a PSA velocity > 2 ng/ml/yr had a 7-year estimate of PCSM of 19% (95% CI 2–39%) compared with 0% for men whose PSA velocity was ≤2 ng/ml/yr *(23)*. These respective values for ACM were 53% (95% CI 23–81%) vs. 14% (95% CI 5–24%) (Fig. 7). The corresponding values of PCSM for men with higher-risk disease were 24% (95% CI 12–37%) and 4% (95% CI 0–11%), respectively; and for ACM, 44% (95% CI 29–59%) vs. 31% (95% CI 16–46%). The adjusted RRs of PCSM were 2.4 (95% CI 1.6–3.5) and 1.08 (95% CI 1.05–1.10) for men with low- and higher-risk diseases, respectively; and these respective values for ACM were 1.5 (95% CI 1.2–1.8) and 1.04 (95% CI 1.02–1.06).

In the study by Palma et al. *(44)*, PSA velocity did not predict survival outcomes ($p = 0.55$ for PCSM and $p = 0.99$ for ACM). However, as previously noted, there were

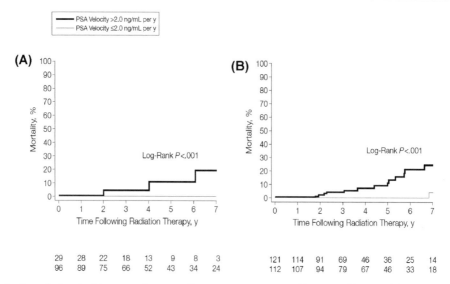

**Fig. 6.** Cumulative incidence estimates of prostate cancer-specific mortality stratified by the pre-treatment PSA velocity for men with (**A**) low-risk disease and (**B**) higher-risk disease *(23)*.
Copyright © 2005 American Medical Association. All rights reserved.

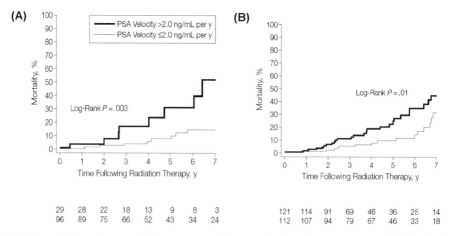

**Fig. 7.** Kaplan–Meier estimates of all-cause mortality stratified by the pre-treatment PSA velocity for men with (**A**) low-risk disease and (**B**) higher-risk disease *(23)*.
Copyright © 2005 American Medical Association. All rights reserved.

significant differences in the study reported by Palma et al., specifically a significantly lower-median PSA velocity compared to other studies.

### *Pre-Treatment PSA Velocity as the Single Higher-Risk Factor and its Association with Post-Operative and Post-Radiation Therapy Prostate Cancer-Specific Mortality*

Understanding the impact that the value of the PSA velocity and specifically a value > 2 ng/ml/yr has on the risk of PCSM following RP or RT compared to other known high-risk factors is important when counseling men facing prostate cancer management. A recent study *(47)* of 948 men who underwent RP or RT and had at least one high-risk factor (PSA velocity >2 ng/ml/yr, biopsy Gleason score ≥7, PSA level ≥10, clinical category ≥ T2b) addressed this question in men with clinically localized prostate cancer. As shown in Fig. 8, the solitary presence of a PSA velocity > 2 ng/ml/yr was associated with an increased risk of PCSM following RP (RR 7.3, 95% CI 1.0–59, $p = 0.05$) or RT (RR 12.1, 95% CI 1.4–105, $p = 0.02$) when compared to men who had any other single high-risk factor. Specifically, of all prostate cancer deaths in men with a single high-risk factor, 88% and 80% of these events were in men with a PSA velocity > 2 ng/ml/yr treated with RP or RT, respectively. Therefore, a pre-treatment PSA velocity > 2 ng/ml/yr alone may identify men with aggressive prostate cancer and in whom more aggressive therapy, including systemic treatment, is needed.

### *Prostate Cancer-Specific and All-Cause Mortality Following Androgen Suppression and Radiation Therapy in Men with PSA Velocity > 2 ng/ml/yr*

As shown in Figs. 4–8, despite RP or RT and despite apparent low-risk disease, it appears that an increase in PSA >2 ng/ml during the year prior to diagnosis incurs a higher-risk for cancer death and death from any cause, even when compared to other high-risk factors. This has led to consideration of more aggressive treatment in men with low-risk disease based on the PSA level, biopsy Gleason score, and T-category but with a pre-diagnostic PSA velocity >2 ng/ml/yr. Specifically, considering higher-RT doses, treatment of pelvic lymph nodes and addition of androgen suppression therapy (AST) as is commonly performed in men with high-risk prostate cancer have been suggested *(23)*. A recent non-randomized study of 241 men with PSA velocity >2 ng/ml/yr compared outcomes in those who received RT alone vs. RT with 6 months of AST *(24)*. Although the group receiving RT and AST as compared to RT alone had longer median follow-up and more advanced, higher-grade disease, they had significantly reduced risks of PSA recurrence (adjusted RR 0.22, 95% CI 0.14–0.35, $p<0.001$), PCSM (RR 0.23, 95% CI 0.09–0.64, $p = 0.005$), and ACM (RR 0.30, 95% CI 0.16–0.58, $p<0.001$) after adjusting for known prognostic factors (Fig. 9).

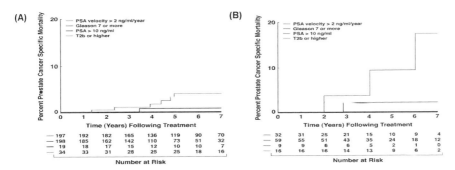

**Fig. 8.** Cumulative incidence estimates of prostate cancer-specific mortality following (**A**) radical prostatectomy and (**B**) radiation therapy stratified by the type of high-risk factor in men with a single high-risk factor *(47)*.

PSA velocity >2 ng/ml/yr as compared to all others, $p = 0.03$ for RP and $p = 0.005$ for RT

Reprinted with permission from John Wiley & Sons, Inc.

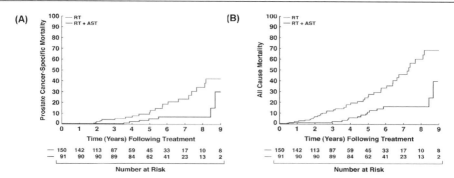

**Fig. 9.** Cumulative incidence estimates of (**A**) prostate cancer-specific mortality ($p = 0.007$) and Kaplan–Meier estimates of (**B**) all-cause mortality ($p<0.001$) after RT or RT and AST in men with pre-treatment PSA velocity $>2$ ng/ml/yr *(24)*.
Reprinted with permission from the American Society of Clinical Oncology.

Thus, in the setting of a newly diagnosed patient with a rapid pre-treatment increase in PSA, a hormone sensitive disease state may still exist and consideration of combined therapy appears warranted, although validation from a prospective randomized trial is needed. The addition of docetaxel chemotherapy to RT and AST or RP and AST in high-risk patients, including those with a PSA velocity of $>2$ ng/ml/yr, is the subject of ongoing randomized trials.

## PSA VELOCITY AND ITS ASSOCIATION WITH TIME TO PROSTATE CANCER-SPECIFIC AND ALL-CAUSE MORTALITY FOLLOWING THERAPY FOR NON-METASTATIC AND METASTATIC HORMONE REFRACTORY PROSTATE CANCER

With regard to biological aggressiveness, heterogeneity exists within each stage of prostate cancer from diagnosis to end-stage hormone refractory and metastatic disease. PSA kinetics have been studied to determine if they can aid in distinguishing men with non-metastatic hormone refractory prostate cancer destined to progress to a positive bone scan and cancer death rapidly from those who progress more slowly. Specifically, in a multi-institutional cohort of 919 men initially treated with RP or RT followed by salvage AST for PSA failure and who subsequently developed PSA defined recurrence while on hormonal therapy but maintained a negative bone scan, a PSA velocity $>1.5$ ng/ml/yr was significantly associated with time to PCSM and ACM ($p < 0.0001$) *(48)*. In these men the risk of PCSM was more than 200 times higher than in men with PSA defined recurrence in whom PSA velocity was $\leq1.5$ ng/ml/yr (adjusted RR 239, 95% CI 10–5,549, $p = 0.0006$). Further study to assess the impact of chemotherapy on time to bone metastases and mortality in such patients with a rapid PSA velocity are warranted.

Given time, men with metastatic prostate cancer develop androgen independence and ultimately die from their disease unless an intervening competing co-morbidity intercedes. An increasing PSA velocity was also significantly associated with shorter survival ($p = 0.005$) in a cohort of 213 men with metastatic, hormone refractory prostate cancer who were treated with cytotoxic, cytostatic, or combination therapy on three prospective, randomized phase II studies *(49)*. The adjusted RR for ACM was 1.8 (95% CI 1.3–2.5, $p = 0.0004$) for men who had a PSA velocity >0 ng/ml per month compared with men who had a PSA velocity ≤0 ng/ml per month after controlling for treatment and known prognostic factors. Estimates of survival 2 years after randomization for these men were 16% (95% CI 7–25%) and 44% (95% CI 35–53%), respectively. Similar results were obtained in the multi-institutional Southwest Oncology Group Study 99–16 *(50)* and in the TAX327 Study *(51)*, two randomized trials comparing cytotoxic chemotherapy regimens in patients with metastatic, hormone refractory prostate cancer. Significant associations were found between the PSA velocity *(50)*, as well as a PSA decline of 30% *(50,51)*, measured during the first 2–3 months of chemotherapy and the time to death. These studies indicate that PSA velocity and PSA decline may serve as surrogate markers for ACM following cytotoxic chemotherapy. These findings support the use of PSA velocity as an intermediate endpoint for death when assessing the clinical efficacy of novel agents in men with metastatic disease. Such an earlier endpoint can expedite drug discovery.

## SUMMARY AND CONCLUSIONS

As detailed in this chapter, the PSA velocity at presentation, and in particular an increase in the PSA level by more than 2 ng/ml during the year prior to diagnosis, is significantly associated with more advanced tumor stage, higher grade, and a shorter time to PSA failure, prostate cancer-specific, and ACM following RP or RT in men with clinically localized prostate cancer. Although prospective validation is ongoing, and a consensus on how best to estimate PSA velocity is planned, the inclusion of pretreatment PSA velocity in risk stratification is justified. As a distinct measure of the biological aggressiveness of prostate cancer, a PSA velocity >2 ng/ml/yr should have a role in patient selection for randomized trials evaluating the use of novel neoadjuvant and/or adjuvant systemic therapies in conjunction with current standards of care for men with clinically localized, high-risk and locally advanced prostate cancer. PSA kinetics during hormonal and cytotoxic chemotherapy has prognostic importance in men with advanced prostate cancer and is under study for use as a surrogate endpoint for survival in men with metastatic, hormone refractory prostate cancer.

## REFERENCES

1. Catalona, W.J., et al., Detection of organ-confined prostate cancer is increased through prostate-specific antigen-based screening. *JAMA*, 1993. 270(8): 948–54.
2. Essink-Bot, M.L., et al., Short-term effects of population-based screening for prostate cancer on health-related quality of life. *J Natl Cancer Inst*, 1998. 90(12): 925–31.
3. Begg, C.B., et al., Variations in morbidity after radical prostatectomy. *N Engl J Med*, 2002. 346(15): 1138–44.
4. Potosky, A.L., et al., Prostate cancer practice patterns and quality of life: the Prostate Cancer Outcomes Study. *J Natl Cancer Inst*, 1999. 91(20): 1719–24.
5. Talcott, J.A., et al., Time course and predictors of symptoms after primary prostate cancer therapy. *J Clin Oncol*, 2003. 21(21): 3979–86.
6. Clark, J.A., et al., Patients' perceptions of quality of life after treatment for early prostate cancer. *J Clin Oncol*, 2003. 21(20): 3777–84.
7. Stanford, J.L., et al., Urinary and sexual function after radical prostatectomy for clinically localized prostate cancer: the Prostate Cancer Outcomes Study. *JAMA*, 2000. 283(3): 354–60.

8. Draisma, G., et al., Lead times and overdetection due to prostate-specific antigen screening: estimates from the European Randomized Study of Screening for Prostate Cancer. *J Natl Cancer Inst*, 2003. 95(12): 868–78.

9. Stephenson, R.A., Prostate cancer trends in the era of prostate-specific antigen. An update of incidence, mortality, and clinical factors from the SEER database. *Urol Clin North Am*, 2002. 29(1): 173–81.

10. Thompson, I.M., et al., Prevalence of prostate cancer among men with a prostate-specific antigen level < or =4.0 ng per milliliter. *N Engl J Med*, 2004. 350(22): 2239–46.

11. Andriole, G.L., et al., Prostate Cancer Screening in the Prostate, Lung, Colorectal and Ovarian (PLCO) Cancer Screening Trial: findings from the initial screening round of a randomized trial. *J Natl Cancer Inst*, 2005. 97(6): 433–8.

12. de Koning, H.J., et al., Prostate cancer mortality reduction by screening: power and time frame with complete enrollment in the European Randomised Screening for Prostate Cancer (ERSPC) trial. *Int J Cancer*, 2002. 98(2): 268–73.

13. Stamey, T.A., et al., Prostate-specific antigen as a serum marker for adenocarcinoma of the prostate. *N Engl J Med*, 1987. 317(15): 909–16.

14. Cooperberg, M.R., et al., Time trends in clinical risk stratification for prostate cancer: implications for outcomes (data from CaPSURE). *J Urol*, 2003. 170(6 Pt 2): S21–5; discussion S26–7.

15. Makarov, D.V., et al., Pathological outcomes and biochemical progression in men with T1c prostate cancer undergoing radical prostatectomy with prostate specific antigen 2.6 to 4.0 vs 4.1 to 6.0 ng/ml. *J Urol*, 2006. 176(2): 554–8.

16. Carter, H.B., et al., Longitudinal evaluation of prostate-specific antigen levels in men with and without prostate disease. *JAMA*, 1992. 267(16): 2215–20.

17. Smith, D.S. and W.J. Catalona, Rate of change in serum prostate specific antigen levels as a method for prostate cancer detection. *J Urol*, 1994. 152(4): 1163–7.

18. Carter, H.B., et al., Prostate-specific antigen variability in men without prostate cancer: effect of sampling interval on prostate-specific antigen velocity. *Urology*, 1995. 45(4): 591–6.

19. Link, R.E., et al., Variation in prostate specific antigen results from 2 different assay platforms: clinical impact on 2304 patients undergoing prostate cancer screening. *J Urol*, 2004. 171(6 Pt 1): 2234–8.

20. Carter, H.B. and J.D. Pearson, PSA velocity for the diagnosis of early prostate cancer. A new concept. *Urol Clin North Am*, 1993. 20(4): 665–70.

21. Connolly, D., et al., Methods of calculating prostate-specific antigen velocity. *Eur Urol*, 2007. 52(4): 1044–50.

22. D'Amico, A.V., et al., Preoperative PSA velocity and the risk of death from prostate cancer after radical prostatectomy. *N Engl J Med*, 2004. 351(2): 125–35.

23. D'Amico, A.V., et al., Pretreatment PSA velocity and risk of death from prostate cancer following external beam radiation therapy. *JAMA*, 2005. 294(4): 440–7.

24. D'Amico, A.V., et al., Six-month androgen suppression plus radiation therapy compared with radiation therapy alone for men with prostate cancer and a rapidly increasing pretreatment prostate-specific antigen level. *J Clin Oncol*, 2006. 24(25): 4190–5.

25. Nguyen, P.L., et al., Effect of definition of preradiotherapy prostate-specific antigen velocity on its association with prostate cancer-specific mortality and all-cause mortality. *Urology*, 2007. 70(2): 288–93.

26. Roehrborn, C.G., G.J. Pickens, and T. Carmody, 3rd, Variability of repeated serum prostate-specific antigen (PSA) measurements within less than 90 days in a well-defined patient population. *Urology*, 1996. 47(1): 59–66.

27. Riehmann, M., et al., Analysis of variation in prostate-specific antigen values. *Urology*, 1993. 42(4): 390–7.

28. Prestigiacomo, A.F. and T.A. Stamey, Physiological variation of serum prostate specific antigen in the 4.0 to 10.0 ng./ml. range in male volunteers. *J Urol*, 1996. 155(6): 1977–80.

29. Yu, X., et al., Comparison of methods for calculating prostate specific antigen velocity. *J Urol*, 2006. 176(6 Pt 1): 2427–31; discussion 2431.

30. King, C.R., et al., Optimal timing, cutoff, and method of calculation of preoperative prostate-specific antigen velocity to predict relapse after prostatectomy: a report from SEARCH. *Urology*, 2007. 69(4): 732–7.

31. Patel, D.A., et al., Preoperative PSA velocity is an independent prognostic factor for relapse after radical prostatectomy. *J Clin Oncol*, 2005. 23(25): 6157–62.

32. Pinsky, P.F., et al., Prostate-specific antigen velocity and prostate cancer Gleason grade and stage. *Cancer*, 2007. 109(8): 1689–95.

33. Carter, H.B., et al., Detection of life-threatening prostate cancer with prostate-specific antigen velocity during a window of curability. *J Natl Cancer Inst*, 2006. 98(21): 1521–7.
34. Krejcarek, S.C., et al., Prediagnostic prostate-specific antigen velocity and probability of detecting high-grade prostate cancer. *Urology*, 2007. 69(3): 515–9.
35. Berger, A.P., et al., Longitudinal PSA changes in men with and without prostate cancer: assessment of prostate cancer risk. *Prostate*, 2005. 64(3): 240–5.
36. Goluboff, E.T., et al., Pretreatment prostate specific antigen doubling times: use in patients before radical prostatectomy. *J Urol*, 1997. 158(5): 1876–8; discussion 1878–9.
37. Sengupta, S., et al., Preoperative prostate specific antigen doubling time and velocity are strong and independent predictors of outcomes following radical prostatectomy. *J Urol*, 2005. 174(6): 2191–6.
38. Berger, A.P., et al., Relapse after radical prostatectomy correlates with preoperative PSA velocity and tumor volume: results from a screening population. *Urology*, 2006. 68(5): 1067–71.
39. Egawa, S., et al., Use of pretreatment prostate-specific antigen doubling time to predict outcome after radical prostatectomy. *Prostate Cancer Prostatic Dis*, 2000. 3(4): 269–274.
40. Thiel, R., et al., Role of prostate-specific antigen velocity in prediction of final pathologic stage in men with localized prostate cancer. *Urology*, 1997. 49(5): 716–20.
41. Thompson, I.M., et al., Assessing prostate cancer risk: results from the Prostate Cancer Prevention Trial. *J Natl Cancer Inst*, 2006. 98(8): 529–34.
42. Schroder, F.H., et al., Does PSA velocity predict prostate cancer in pre-screened populations? *Eur Urol*, 2006. 49(3): 460–5; discussion 465.
43. Freedland, S.J., F. Dorey, and W.J. Aronson, Preoperative PSA velocity and doubling time do not predict adverse pathologic features or biochemical recurrence after radical prostatectomy. *Urology*, 2001. 57(3): 476–80.
44. Palma, D., et al., Pretreatment PSA velocity as a predictor of disease outcome following radical radiation therapy. *Int J Radiat Oncol Biol Phys*, 2007. 67(5): 1425–9.
45. D'Amico, A.V., et al., Surrogate end point for prostate cancer-specific mortality after radical prostatectomy or radiation therapy. *J Natl Cancer Inst*, 2003. 95(18): 1376–83.
46. D'Amico, A.V., et al., Identifying patients at risk for significant versus clinically insignificant postoperative prostate-specific antigen failure. *J Clin Oncol*, 2005. 23(22): 4975–9.
47. D'Amico, A.V., et al., Prostate cancer-specific mortality after radical prostatectomy or external beam radiation therapy in men with 1 or more high-risk factors. *Cancer*, 2007. 110(1): 56–61.
48. D'Amico, A.V., et al., Surrogate end point for prostate cancer specific mortality in patients with nonmetastatic hormone refractory prostate cancer. *J Urol*, 2005. 173(5): 1572–6.
49. Rozhansky, F., et al., Prostate-specific antigen velocity and survival for patients with hormone-refractory metastatic prostate carcinoma. *Cancer*, 2006. 106(1): 63–7.
50. Petrylak, D.P., et al., Evaluation of prostate-specific antigen declines for surrogacy in patients treated on SWOG 99-16. *J Natl Cancer Inst*, 2006. 98(8): 516–21.
51. Armstrong, A.J., et al., Prostate-specific antigen and pain surrogacy analysis in metastatic hormone-refractory prostate cancer. *J Clin Oncol*, 2007. 25(25): 3965–70.

# III RISK ASSESSMENT FOR PROSTATE CANCER

# 10  Nomograms for Prostate Cancer

*Shahrokh F. Shariat and Michael W. Kattan*

## CONTENTS

## SUMMARY

Accurate estimates of risk are essential for physicians if they are to recommend a specific management to patients with prostate cancer. In addition their incorporation into clinical trial design ensures homogeneous high-risk patient groups for whom new cancer therapeutics are to be investigated. Using MEDLINE we performed a literature search on articles on prostate cancer predictive tools published during the period from January 1966 to July 2007. We recorded input variables, prediction form, number of patients used to develop the prediction tool, the outcome being predicted, prediction tool-specific features, predictive accuracy, and whether validation was performed. The literature search generated 109 published prediction tools from which only 68 had undergone validation. In this chapter we describe the criteria for evaluation (predictive accuracy, calibration, generalizability, head-to-head comparison, and level of complexity) and limitations of current predictive tools. Our review indicates that an increasing number of predictive tools addresses important endpoints such as disease recurrence, metastasis, and survival. For choosing among prediction tools, our recommendation is nomograms, which provide superior individualized risk estimation. Nevertheless, many more predictive tools, comparisons between them, and improvements to existing tools are needed.

From: *Current Clinical Urology: Prostate Cancer Screening*, Edited by: D. P. Ankerst et al.
DOI 10.1007/978-1-60327-281-0_10 © Humana Press, a part of Springer Science+Business Media, LLC 2009

**Key Words:** Prostate Cancer, Nomogram, Prediction, Artificial neural networks, Classification and regression trees.

## INTRODUCTION

Approximately 680,000 men are diagnosed with prostate cancer worldwide each year *(1)*. In the Unites States, this cancer is the most common solid malignancy and the second leading cause of cancer death in men *(2)*. The incidence of this disease will increase with more extensive use of serum prostate-specific antigen (PSA) testing. Although the survival benefits of PSA screening remain the subject of prospective studies in Western nations, the consequent rate of metastatic prostate cancer began to decrease from 18% in 1991 to 5% in 2007 *(2)*. This shift to earlier disease stage at diagnosis allows curative definitive local treatment.

While there are no randomized controlled trial data showing survival benefit for radiotherapy versus extirpative surgery, it is unlikely that consensus will be reached that any particular form of therapy is best for all patients. Owing to patient preferences regarding the potential adverse effects of treatment or observation, the treatment decision will always be a personal one. Patients differ in how much they value health-related quality of life aspects such as potency and continence, and in how much they fear cancer progression and the knowledge that they have prostate cancer; therefore, trading one adverse effect for another might be of great importance to one patient but inconsequential to another. Because of these differences in preference, the prostate cancer treatment decision will always need to be tailored to the individual patient. When comparing treatment alternatives, both quantity and quality of life should be considered. Quality of life, in the form of preferences regarding different adverse effects, must be considered. Therefore accurate estimates of the likelihood of treatment success, complications, and long-term morbidity are essential for patient counseling and informed decision-making. Toward this, properly informing the patient of the likelihood of treatment success and morbidity will improve his satisfaction after treatment. Lack of patient involvement has been identified as a major risk factor for regret of treatment choice *(3)*. Patients who make their own decisions when given adequate information should be less likely to regret their treatment choice than those whose physicians made the decision for them, particularly when complications arise *(4)*. Therefore, accurate estimates of risk are essential for physicians if they are to recommend a specific treatment and the rational application of neo-adjuvant/adjuvant treatment strategies for patients at risk of disease progression after definitive local therapy. Accurate risk estimates are also required for clinical trial design, to ensure homogeneous high-risk patient groups for whom new cancer therapeutics will be investigated.

## TRADITIONAL RISK ESTIMATION

Traditionally, physician judgment has formed the basis for risk estimation, patient counseling, and decision-making. However, humans have difficulty with predicting outcomes due to the biases that exist at all stages of the prediction process *(5–8)*. Clinicians do not recall all cases equally; certain cases can stand out and exert an unsuitably large influence when predicting future outcomes. Clinicians tend to be inconsistent when processing their memory and tend to resort to heuristics ("rules of thumb") when processing becomes difficult *(9)*. When it is time to make a prediction, they tend to predict the preferred outcome rather than the outcome with the highest probability *(7)*. In addition, clinicians find it difficult to learn from mistakes during the feedback process. Moreover, it is difficult to integrate the multitude of predictive variables that have been shown to be of importance in clinical judgment *(10,11)*. Finally, clinicians have difficulty weighing the relative importance of each of these factors when formulating predictions of outcome. Therefore, to obtain more accurate predictions, researchers have developed predictive tools based on statistical models *(12)*. In general, these predictive models have been shown to perform as well as or better than clinical judgment when predicting probabilities of outcome *(11)*. That said, physician input is obviously essential and crucial for the measurement of variables that are used in the prediction process and for the entire decision-making process.

Overall average is another commonly used method to predict outcomes. With this method, all patients have the same probability; there is no individualization. This approach is at least empirical and objective, but cannot discriminate low-risk from high-risk patients.

## EVALUATING PREDICTIVE TOOLS

Decision aids consist of the "Kattan-type" nomograms *(13,14)*, risk-groupings *(15–18)*, artificial neural networks (ANNs) that were pioneered by Snow et al. *(19)*, probability tables such as the most widely known and applied "Partin staging tables" *(20,21)*, and classification and regression tree (CART) analyses *(22,23)*. Several considerations apply when designing and judging predictive models.

*Predictive accuracy.* Accuracy represents the most important consideration. Predictive accuracy should be ideally confirmed in an external cohort, which represents the best method of validation. Alternatively, statistical methods such as bootstrapping may be used to internally validate the nomogram *(9,24–28)*. It is important to emphasize that predictive accuracy reflects two features at a time: discrimination and calibration. Conversely, the receiver operating characteristic (ROC) area under the curve (AUC) is only discriminatory. Usually, the discriminatory ability of predictive accuracy is derived from the ROC-AUC and expressed as a percentage. Discriminatory ability of predictive accuracy estimates ranges from 50 to 100%, where 50% is equivalent to a flip of a coin and 100% represents perfect prediction. No model is perfect and generally accepted accuracy ranges are 70–80%. Increases in predictive accuracy are not only of statistical significance but, more importantly, clinically meaningful. For example, an increase in predictive accuracy of 4% translates into 4 out of 100 patients having a more accurate prediction than the previous model. This figure then needs to be extrapolated to the disease prevalence and subsequently to the number of diagnostic and/or therapeutic procedures. Thus, from health, economic, and individual standpoints, a relatively small increase in predictive accuracy translates into a clinically important number of patients who deserve to be provided with accurate predictions.

*Calibration.* As indicated above, predictive accuracy indicates the overall ability of the model to predict the outcome of interest, but does not inform the user of its performance in specific patient subgroups. Some models may be ideally suited to predict in high-risk patients, but may predict poorly in low-risk patients. Other models may predict well throughout the range of predictions. Validation offers the possibility to graphically display and investigate a model's calibration that represents an equally important consideration. Calibration plots are used to graphically assess the model's performance characteristics at different risk levels (24,26–29).

*Generalizability.* General applicability of the model is important, as patient characteristics can vary. For example, the characteristics of prostate cancer might not be the same in Europe as in the USA (30). The performance of a predictive instrument can decline from the development set to an external validation set, in part because of change in the predictiveness of risk factors. Nomogram development depends heavily on its development cohort. Thus, prior to using a tool, the clinician should ensure that the nomogram is applicable to his patient (24,26–29).

Generalizability can be separated into two components: internal validity (reproducibility) and external validity (transportability) (27,31–33). A model has internal validity if it maintains its accuracy when applied to patients from the same underlying population as those in the sample used for the development. It has external validity if it maintains its accuracy when applied to patients from populations intrinsically different from the development sample, with respect to location, time period, or methods used for data collection. A model may lose accuracy when implemented in new settings if risk factors receive too little or too much weight. The internal validity of a model can be tested with split-sample, cross-validation, or bootstrapping methods (27), but external validity can be checked only by testing the model on new patients in new settings.

Several studies have shown that ethnicity may influence prostate cancer prevalence and/or disease characteristics. In consequence, studies need to provide proof of its generalizability in the same patients from different ethnicity (34–41) and geographical location (42–44).

*Level of complexity.* The level of complexity represents an important consideration. Excessively complex models are clearly impractical in busy clinical practice. Similarly, models that require computational infrastructure might pose problems with their applicability. For example, ANNs can accurately predict several outcomes, but the use of ANNs might be restricted due to lack of access to ANN code or lack of computer infrastructure. Look-up tables, such as the Partin tables, risk-grouping models, decision-trees based on CART models, and Kattan-type nomograms represent user-friendly, paper-based alternatives, which bypass these problems.

*Head-to-head comparison.* Finally, when judging a new tool, one should examine its predictive accuracy, validity, and performance characteristics relative to established models, with the intent of determining whether the new model offers advantages relative to available alternatives (25,27,28,45–49). In addition, for some outcomes, more than one model might be available, which makes model comparison necessary for selection of the best model. Furthermore, because the predictive accuracy will change at least to some degree with each new assessment, a direct comparison of alternatives greatly facilitates decision-making. Therefore, head-to-head comparison of different models applied to a common dataset is necessary to show which of the available models may be superior. With this approach, the alternatives are compared directly, without having to judge the concordance index in isolation or against a possibly arbitrary threshold.

## LIMITATIONS OF CURRENT PREDICTIVE TOOLS

All predictive tools have some limitations

*Development cohorts.* As mentioned above, predictive tools depend on their development cohorts. Most currently available tools are based on either single center of excellence series and/or represent data of high-volume surgeons/pathologists from highly specialized tertiary care centers. The outcomes of these datasets might differ considerably from those of patients treated at community health centers, since the quality and availability of treatments vary with the location and level of experience of the treating physician *(50–53)*. Therefore, before application, models should be validated in different patient populations.

*Retrospective statistical methodology.* Despite prospective data collection, modeling itself represents a retrospective statistical methodological approach with all its inherent limitations.

*Study selection criteria.* Specific model criteria such as inclusion and exclusion criteria restrict the use of the model to patients with similar characteristics and intervention. For example, since patients who received neo-adjuvant hormonal therapy have been excluded from most models, the models cannot be applied to patients treated with neo-adjuvant hormonal therapy. Another example is that models developed in patients treated with external beam radiotherapy cannot applied to patients treated with brachytherapy, intensity-modulated radiotherapy, or any other methodology.

*Change over time of the predictive value of model ingredients.* Tools that were developed in a different era may not provide equally accurate predictions in contemporary patients. Definitions of variables or methods of data collection may change. For example, pre-treatment total PSA, the primary parameter in most predictive tools has been observed to provide less reliable predictive information about prostate cancer as the proportion of men with more advanced prostate cancers and with higher total PSA levels, at presentation, continues to decrease *(54)*. Moreover, it has recently been shown that the correlation between total PSA and cancer has weakened over the last 20 years *(55–57)* and that the total PSA is mostly a significant marker for benign prostatic hyperplasia (BPH)-related prostate volume, growth, and outcomes *(58–60)*. Thus, there is a need for novel biomarkers that detect prostate cancer and, more importantly, distinguish indolent from biologically aggressive disease *(61)*.

Another example of a change in practice patterns affecting the applicability of predictive models is the modification of prostate biopsy technique over the last 20 years. Today, extended biopsy schemes are standard of care for prostate cancer detection and staging *(62)*. Therefore, models that are based on systematic sextant biopsy information may not be optimal anymore and should be updated. These two examples support that models need to be constantly updated and improved with novel predictors.

*Adjustment for competing risks.* Because of the protracted course of prostate cancer and competing causes of mortality in this patient population, *(63)* there is a need for competing-risk modeling to better inform the clinician counseling a patient. There is growing evidence to suggest that the anticipated survival benefit derived from the diagnosis and treatment for prostate cancer is non-uniform. Indeed, prostate cancer is now recognized as a heterogeneous disease with variable natural histories. For this reason, it is plausible that a proportion of newly diagnosed prostate cancers represent an indolent form of cancer, which may not merit treatment. Given the low-metastatic potential of prostate cancer and the slow growth rate observed for many PSA screen-detected tumors, it is also conceivable that age-related competing-cause mortality might dampen the benefits of treatment for some older patients with prostate cancer. Because the morbidity and mortality of prostate cancer treatment are non-trivial, clinicians must be able to better risk-stratify prostate cancer patients such that those who stand to gain the most from the intervention receive it. To date, the only modeling tool that allows adjustment for competing risks is the Kattan-type nomogram *(64,65)*.

*Restricted predictive accuracy.* None of the prediction models developed to date are perfect. This is mainly due to the lack of consideration of all predictive risk factors and the inability to assemble all known prognostic factors optimally. Prostate cancers with the same histopathologic features have a heterogeneous biologic behavior. Therefore, there is a need for novel biomarkers and imaging tools that are associated with the biologic behavior of prostate cancer to enhance the predictive accuracy of current tools *(47,66,67)*.

## "KATTAN-TYPE" NOMOGRAMS

Various distinct statistical methodologies have broadly been described as "nomograms." However, the statistical definition of a nomogram is a functional graphic representation of a mathematical formula or algorithm that incorporates several predictors modeled as continuous variables to predict a particular endpoint based on traditional statistical methods such as multivariable logistic regression or Cox proportional hazards analysis *(9,14)*. Nomograms consist of sets of axes; each variable is represented by a scale, with each value of that variable corresponding to a specific number of points according to its prognostic significance. For example, the nomogram in Fig. 1 *(14)* assigns to each PSA level a unique point value that represents its prognostic significance. In a final pair of axes, the total point value from all the variables is converted to the probability of reaching the endpoint. By using scales, nomograms calculate the continuous probability of a particular outcome.

One of the strengths of nomograms is that they are typically based on models that capture non-linear relationships, such as restricted cubic splines *(32)*. Unmodified regression models require variables to assume linear relationships, which are not ideal because it assumes that incremental changes represent the same significance across the spectrum of values. For example, a rise in PSA level from 1 to 5 ng/mL would represent the same impact as a rise from 101 to 105 ng/mL. The application of non-linear methods such as cubic splines imparts flexibility to the nomogram by allowing continuous variables to maintain non-linear relationships.

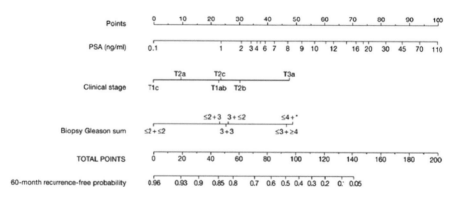

**Fig. 1.** Pre-operative nomogram based on 983 patients treated at the Methodist Hospital (Houston, TX, USA) for predicting the 5-year probability of freedom from PSA recurrence after definitive therapy with radical prostatectomy. Reprinted with permission from Kattan et al. *(14)*.

Nomograms are designed to extract the maximum amount of useful information from data. For example, the primary and secondary Gleason grades are used as independent variables, rather than the Gleason sum alone. Indeed, several combinations of primary/secondary Gleason grades can result in the same Gleason sum (e.g., 3+4=7 vs 4+3=7) *(68)* despite a different impact on prognosis.

The discrimination of nomograms should be measured using the concordance index (or *c*-index) rather than the receiver–operator characteristic curve area. While the area under the curve requires binary outcomes (e.g., cure/fail), the *c*-index functions in the presence of case censoring and is more appropriate for analyzing time-to-event data *(69)*. The concordance index is the probability that, given two randomly drawn patients, the patient who relapses first had a higher probability of disease recurrence. Note that this calculation assumes that the patient with the shorter follow-up relapses. If both patients relapse at the same time or a patient who does not relapse has a shorter follow-up than the other patient in the pair that does relapse, the probability does not apply to that pair of patients. With this measure, a *c*-index of 0.5 represents no discriminating ability and a value of 1.0 represents perfect discrimination. Nomograms have been adapted for use on personal digital assistants and personal computers to facilitate their use in the clinic or for research purposes. A suite of nomograms is available in the public domain for online use and free downloading (http://www.nomograms.org and www.nomogram.org).

## COMPARISON OF NOMOGRAMS WITH OTHER PREDICTION TOOLS

As more than one model is available for prediction of most outcomes, model comparison is necessary for selection of the best model. We review and compare the different predictive methodologies that have been used in the prostate cancer literature (Table 1).

### *Nomogram Versus Risk Grouping*

Physicians often use risk groups to determine the risk of an event. This approach consists of grouping patients with similar characteristics to discriminate between those at low-risk versus those at high-risk for a specific event. While risk-grouping is a logical approach, grouping patients is an inefficient use of the data and tends to reduce the predictive accuracy of a prognostic model. It assumes that all patients within a risk group are equal. However, risk groups comprise heterogeneous groups of patients. For example, some patients might barely qualify for a high-risk group, while others might have every known adverse prognostic factor. A commonly used risk-grouping tool is that developed by D'Amico et al. for prediction of biochemical recurrence in patients treated with radical prostatectomy, external-beam radiotherapy, or brachytherapy by placing patients into mutually exclusive risk groups based on clinical stage, biopsy Gleason sum, and pre-treatment PSA level *(15–18,70–74)*. When predicting the outcome for a subset of patients, the relative importance of prognostic variables in another patient group is ignored. In addition, risk-grouping requires the conversion of continuous to categorical variables, which limits information about the actual value.

Various studies have documented the superior performance of nomograms compared to risk-grouping *(25,45–47,49,75–77)*. This might stem from the fact that risk groups

Table 1
Techniques for the Development of a Clinical Prediction Model or Rule

| Technique | Advantages/strengths | Disadvantages/limitations |
| --- | --- | --- |
| Univariate analysis | Simple statistic methods<br>Easy clinical application | Reduced accuracy |
| Multivariable analysis (e.g., logistic regression) | Improved accuracy | More involved statistical methods |
| | Relative ease of clinical application | May miss complex variable relationships |
| Neural network | Improved accuracy | Difficult clinical application and dissemination |
| | Incorporation of complex variable relationships | Less intuitive |
| | | Unknown effect of any single variable |
| Nomogram | Improved accuracy<br>Ease of clinical application | Advanced statistics |
| CART analysis | Improved accuracy<br>Ease of clinical application<br>Intuitive partitioning | Advanced statistics |

consist of patients with similar (albeit not identical) characteristics, resulting in heterogeneity within a risk group that reduces the predictive accuracy (47,78,79). In contrast to risk groups, a nomogram makes a tailored predicted probability based on the characteristics of each patient. The heterogeneity inherent in risk groups is illustrated in Fig. 2, (14,73,80) where the 5-year recurrence-free probability after radical prostatectomy was calculated using a continuous, multivariable preoperative nomogram among patients classified as low-, medium- and high-risk, using the criteria of D'Amico et al. (73). While low-risk patients uniformly had a high likelihood of being free of biochemical recurrence by the nomogram, a substantial proportion of intermediate- and even high-risk patients had a calculated 5-year recurrence-free probability of ≥90%. A considerable overlap in the nomogram predictions is also evident among intermediate- and high-risk patients.

A risk group is composed of a mixture of patients and is only useful for gauging the prognosis for that group of patients. A patient does not care about the outcome of his (heterogeneous) group; he cares about his prognosis. By incorporating all relevant continuous predictive factors for individual patients, nomograms provide more accurate predictions than models based on risk-grouping (7,81). While nomograms are more complex than risk groups, this added complexity results in a better predictive accuracy for both the patient and physician. As mentioned above, nomograms have been adapted for use on personal digital assistants and personal computers to facilitate their use in the clinic or for research purposes.

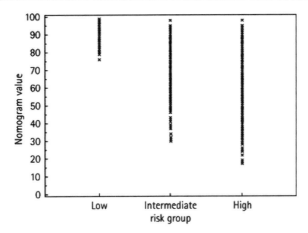

**Fig. 2.** Pre-operative nomogram predicting the 5-year recurrence-free probability after radical prosta-tectomy *(93)* for patients classified as low-, intermediate- or high-risk by D'Amico et al. *(73)*. Reprinted with permission from Mitchell et al. *(80)*.

Finally, the method of counting risk factors/variables should also be avoided because this assumes that each variable exerts an equal prognostic weight on the outcome, which is unlikely to represent the true relationship between variables and prognosis *(82–84)*.

### Nomogram Versus Look-Up Table

The superior predictive accuracy of continuous, multivariable nomograms versus look-up tables is illustrated by comparing the ability of the "Partin tables" *(20,21,85)* to predict the pathologic features of prostate cancer with a suite of nomograms. The "Partin tables" combined serum PSA level (four categories), clinical stage (seven categories), and biopsy Gleason sum (five categories) to predict the pathologic stage of prostate cancer that is assigned as one of four mutually exclusive groups, i.e., organ-confined, established extracapsular extension, seminal vesicle invasion, and lymph node involve-ment. These tables underestimate the probability of established extracapsular extension as a substantial proportion of patients with lymph node metastases and seminal vesicle invasion will also have established extracapsular extension. Therefore, several studies found that nomograms incorporating PSA level, clinical stage, and Gleason sum mod-eled as continuous variables had a superior predictive accuracy compared to the "Partin tables" for predicting organ-confined disease, seminal vesicle invasion, and lymph node invasion *(25,46,86–90)*.

Another example of the superiority of nomograms over look-up tables has been demonstrated by Chun et al. *(49,91)*. They showed that a logistic regression-based nomogram that included pre-operative PSA, clinical stage, primary and secondary biopsy Gleason grades had an accuracy of 80.4% for prediction of the probability of Gleason sum upgrading between biopsy and radical prostatectomy. In contrast, a pre-viously published look-up table *(92)* based on pre-operative PSA, clinical stage, and prostate gland volume had an accuracy of only 52.3% ($P < 0.001$). In addition, the nomogram had virtually ideal performance whereas the look-up table had important departures from ideal prediction. Taken together, these findings support that nomograms are more accurate than look-up tables and perform better throughout the range of predicted probabilities.

## Nomogram Versus Tree Analysis

Classification and Regression Trees (CART) are another type of predictive model that use non-parametric techniques to evaluate data, account for complex relationships, and present the results in a clinically useful form. In this type of analysis, there is a progressive splitting of the population into subgroups that are based on the independent predictive variables. The variables that are chosen, the discriminatory values of the variables, and the order in which the splitting occurs are all produced by the underlying mathematic algorithm to maximize predictive accuracy. A simplified example of a CART-recursive partitioning based on Cox proportional hazards regression analyses is shown in Fig. 3 (93). In this analysis, the clinician simply follows the paths of the tree that describe the characteristics of the patient being evaluated and arrives at the prediction of the outcome of interest for that particular patient.

Tree analysis is relatively easy to use for the clinician. First, in contrast to many logistic regression models, there are no complicated equations to remember or use. The structure of the tree is one that is appealing intuitively and congruent with methods of decision-making that a physician already uses on many occasions. For example, in trying to understand the best diagnostic test or treatment for a given patient, clinicians

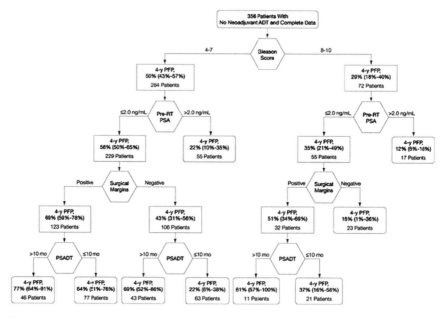

Stephenson, A. J. et al. JAMA 2004;291:1325–1332.

**Fig. 3.** Four-year actuarial progression-free probability after salvage radiotherapy. Progression-free probability (PFP) stratified by Gleason sum, pre-radiotherapy prostate-specific antigen (PSA) level, surgical margins, and PSA doubling time (PSADT). Patients receiving neo-adjuvant androgen deprivation therapy (ADT) were excluded from this analysis. All values in parentheses are 95% confidence intervals. RT indicates radiotherapy. Reprinted with permission from Stephenson et al. (93).

will use specific patient characteristics to determine progressively which modalities are most appropriate or which outcomes are most likely. CART not only uses this type of logic but also provides a formal structure and quantitative outcome assessment that can optimize the actual clinical decision.

Thus CART offer greater model-fitting flexibility than traditional statistical methods *(94)*, and theoretically might lead to enhanced predictive accuracy if datasets contain highly predictive non-linear or interactive effects. However, there are several issues to consider when deciding whether to use CART analysis. It is often important to estimate the overall impact of a single independent variable on the outcome of interest. This is especially true in studies with specific hypotheses about the effects of an independent variable or group of variables on the outcome. Because CART analysis is intended to identify distinct population subgroups, its hierarchical nature does not allow the estimation of net effects of a single variable *(95)*. Regression techniques, however, are largely used to estimate the "average" effect of an independent variable on the probability of having a dependent variable, while accounting for other factors. Thus, CART analysis would not be used as a substitute for proven regression techniques in this type of situation. Moreover, CART analysis can become very complex and difficult to interpret. Trees can grow into multiple levels and thereby result in splits that are not particularly important.

Several studies have shown that traditional statistical methods perform better than CART analysis. For example, using three real-world datasets, Kattan found that a Cox proportional hazards regression model provided superior predictive accuracy than four tree-based methods *(25)*. Similarly, Chun et al. compared a CART analysis *(23)* with a nomogram *(96,97)* for prediction of the side of extracapsular extension *(49)*. The nomogram yielded a predictive accuracy of 84% versus 70% for the CART model. Moreover, the nomogram calibration plot was virtually ideal whereas the CART calibration plot had appreciable divergence from ideal prediction. Thus the nomogram was statistically significantly more accurate than the CART model and performed better throughout the range of predicted probabilities.

### *Nomogram Versus Artificial Neural Networks (ANN)*

In the last 10 years a new class of techniques known as ANN has been proposed as a supplement or alternative to standard statistical techniques. For the purpose of predicting medical outcomes, an ANN can be considered a computer intensive classification method. It is a computational method that uses multifactorial analysis. It contains layers of richly interconnected computing nodes, for which weights are adjusted when data are presented to the network during a "training" process. Successful training can result in ANNs that predict output values or recognize patterns in multifactorial data *(98)*. Theoretically, an ANN should have considerable advantages over standard statistical approaches. Neural networks automatically allow (1) arbitrary non-linear relations between the independent and dependent variables, and (2) all possible interactions between the independent variables. Standard statistical approaches (e.g., logistic or Cox regression) require additional modeling to allow this flexibility. In addition, ANNs do not require explicit distributional assumptions (such as normality). These and other proposed advantages have generated considerable interest in the use of neural network techniques for the classification of medical outcomes.

However, ANNs are not without drawbacks. The primary disadvantage of an ANN is its black box quality, that is, without extra effort, it is difficult if not impossible to gain insight into a problem based on an ANN model. Regression techniques, for example, allow the user to sequentially eliminate possible explanatory variables that do not contribute to the fit of the model. Similarly, based on the underlying statistical theory, regression techniques allow hypothesis testing regarding both the univariate and multivariate associations between each explanatory variable and the outcome of interest. Furthermore, it yields other insights into the prediction model, such as hazard ratios and tests of significance for the predictors. These features are not available for the ANN. Moreover, regression analysis offers the added advantage of reproducibility and interpretability through the generation of hazard ratios and tests of significance for the predictors *(25)*. The same result is achieved each time it is run on a particular dataset, which is not necessarily true for machine learning techniques because they use random processes for sampling and/or coefficient estimation. In addition, regression analyses are common in many statistical software packages and are relatively fast to perform.

Based on a review of 28 studies comparing ANN and regression modeling, Sargent concluded that ANN should not replace standard statistical approaches as the method of choice for the classification of medical data *(99)*. In the eight largest studies (sample size > 5000), regression and ANN tied in seven cases, with regression winning in the remaining cases. In the more moderate-size datasets, ANN tended to be equivalent or outperform regression though it is unclear whether this is an artifact due to publication bias. The author pointed out that the regression methods are clearly superior to the ANN with respect to inferences based on the output. Inference and interpretation are frequently key desired outcomes of a modeling exercise. In addition to insight into the disease process, regression models provide explicit information regarding the relative importance of each independent variable. This information can be valuable in planning subsequent interventions, in eliminating possibly unnecessary tests and procedures (such as blood or tissue studies that are shown not to relate to the outcome of interest), and in determining which are the most critical data to store in a database.

Similarly, in a review of the literature, Schwarzer et al. concluded that machine learning methods often have failed to perform better than traditional statistical methods outlining numerous design flaws in the studies that show the superiority of neural networks *(100)*. For example, on numerous occasions the neural network was provided with additional data not available to the statistical method. Or many different neural networks were compared with a single statistical model, possibly contributing to a chance finding. In some cases the wrong statistical model was used as the benchmark.

Terrin et al. performed a simulation study that compared the external validity of logistic regression analyses, CART, and ANN on data simulated from a specified population and on data from perturbed forms of the population not representative of the original distribution *(101)*. They found that logistic regression models had the best performance followed by ANNs, and then CARTs. Similarly, using three real-world datasets, Kattan found that Cox proportional hazards regression models provided comparable or superior predictive accuracy than two neural networks *(25)*. Likewise, Chun et al. compared an ANN *(102)* with a nomogram *(103)* for predicting initial biopsy outcome in a cohort of 3,980 patients subjected to at least an 8-core initial biopsy *(48)*. The nomogram (70.6%) was 3.6% ($p<0.001$) more accurate than the ANN (67.0%). The nomogram calibration plot gave virtually ideal predictions. Conversely, the ANN had important departures from ideal predictions, which were manifested by underestimation throughout the range of predicted probabilities. These examples of direct comparison between nomograms and ANNs on the same dataset support that nomograms are statistically significantly more accurate and better calibrated than ANNs.

## CURRENTLY AVAILABLE PREDICTION TOOLS

The above discussion is meant to provide guidelines in the process of decision aid selection. It may be postulated that greater emphasis will be placed on standardized predictions, which will further promote the development of new predictive tools and/or the improvement/update of existing tools. Herein, we provide an overview of recent prostate cancer predictive tools organized by clinical states (Fig. 4). These tools address various prostate cancer outcomes such as prediction of initial and repeat biopsy outcomes in men considered at risk of prostate cancer (Tables 2 and 3, respectively), prediction of general and specific pathologic features at radical prostatectomy (Tables 4 and 5, respectively), prediction of biochemical recurrence after radical prostatectomy and radiotherapy (Tables 6 and 7, respectively), prediction of metastasis and survival (Table 8), prediction of life expectancy (Table 9), and finally prediction of pathologic features and biochemical recurrence based on new imaging tools or novel biomarkers (Table 10).

We recorded predictor variables, the outcome of interest, the number of patients utilized to develop the tools, tool-specific features, predictive accuracy estimates, and whether internal and/or external validation has been performed. Not all tools used the same analysis for calculation of the predictive accuracy (area under the curve, $c$-index, etc.) making the accuracy columns not entirely comparable.

Given the superiority of nomograms over other prediction methodologies in prostate cancer to date, we focused on the nomograms in the discussion.

### *Prediction of Biopsy Outcome*

Tables 2 and 3 show the multitude of predictive models for prediction of prostate cancer on the initial or repeat biopsy, respectively. Several authors explored the application of predictive models for estimation of risk of prostate cancer on initial needle biopsy. A nomogram developed by Eastham et al. for prediction of the probability of prostate cancer on initial biopsy in men with suspicious digital rectal

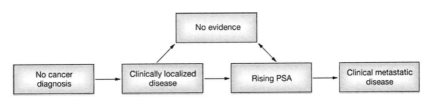

**Fig. 4.** Prostate cancer clinical states.

Table 2

Prostate Biopsy Nomograms for Prediction of Prostate Cancer Presence in the Initial biopsy Setting

| Year of publication | Reference | Prediction form | No of patients | Variables | Mean # of cores | Cancer detection (%) | Accuracy (%) | Validation |
|---|---|---|---|---|---|---|---|---|
| 1998 | Babaian et al. (145) | Risk group | 151 | Age, creatinine phosphokinase isoenzyme activity, prostatic acid phosphatase, PSA | 6 | 24 | 74 | Not performed |
| 1999 | Eastham et al. (36) | Probability nomogram development | 700 | Age, race, DRE, PSA (0–4 ng/mL) | 6 | 9 | 75 | Internal |
| 1999 | Virtanen et al. (146) | Neural network | 212 | Percent-free PSA, DRE, heredity | Not available | 25 | 81 | Internal |
| 2000 | Finne et al. (147) | Neural network | 656 | Percent-free PSA, PSA, DRE, TRUS | Not available | 23 | Not available | Not performed |
| 2001 | Horninger et al. (148) | Neural network | 3,474 | Age, PSA, percent-free PSA, DRE, TRUS, PSA density, PSA density of transition zone, transition zone volume | Not available | Not available | Not available | Not performed |
| 2003 | Kalra et al. (149) | Neural network | 348 | Age, ethnicity, heredity, IPSS, DRE, PSA, complexed PSA | 6 | Not available | 83 | Internal |

| | | | | | | | | |
|---|---|---|---|---|---|---|---|---|
| 2003 | Garzotto et al. (37) | Probability nomogram development | 1,239 | Age, race, family history, referral indications, prior vasectomy, DRE, PSA ($\leq$10 ng/mL), PSA density, TRUS findings | 6.7 (range 6–13) | 24 | 73 | Internal |
| 2004 | Finne et al. (150) | Neural network | 1,775 | DRE, percent-free PSA, TRUS, PSA | Not available | 22 | 76 | Internal |
| 2005 | Karakiewicz et al. (103) | Probability nomogram development | 6,469 | Age, DRE, PSA, percent-free PSA | 6 | 35–42 (multiple institutions) | 77 | Internal and external |
| 2005 | Porter et al. (151) | Neural network | 3,814 | Age, PSA, gland volume, PSA density, DRE, TRUS | 6 | 27–42 (multiple institutions) | 72–75 | Internal and external |
| 2006 | Suzuki et al. (35) | Probability nomogram development | 834 | Age, PSA, percent-free PSA, prostate volume, DRE | $\geq$6 | 29 | 82 | Internal |
| 2007 | Chun et al. (104) | Probability nomogram validation (103) and development | 2,900 | Age, DRE, PSA, percent-free PSA, sampling density* | 11 (range 10–20) | 41 | 77 | Internal and external |

DRE = digital rectal examination; PSA = prostate-specific antigen; TRUS = transrectal ultrasound prostate; HGPIN = high-grade prostatic intraepithelial neoplasia; ASAP = atypical small acinar proliferation of prostate; IPSS = international prostate symptom score *Sampling density = ratio of TRUS-derived total gland volume by the number of cores at biopsy

**Table 3**
**Prostate Biopsy Nomograms for Prediction of Prostate Cancer Presence in Other than the Initial biopsy Setting**

| Year of publication | Reference | Prediction form | Design | No of patients | Variables | Median no. of previous biopsy sessions | Mean no. of cores | Cancer detection (%) | Accuracy (%) | Validation |
|---|---|---|---|---|---|---|---|---|---|---|
| Repeat biopsy | | | | | | | | | | |
| 2000 | O'Dowd et al. (*106*) | Probability nomogram development | Repeat biopsy | 813 | Age, initial biopsy diagnosis, PSA, percent-free PSA | Not available | Not available | 29 | 70 | Not performed |
| 2003 | Lopez-Corona et al. (*107*) | Probability nomogram development | Repeat biopsy | 343 | Age, DRE, number of previous negative biopsies, HGPIN history, ASAP history, PSA, PSA slope, family history, months from initial negative biopsy | 2.9 (2–12) | 9.2 (6–22) | 20 | 70 | Internal |
| 2003 | Remzi et al. (*152*) | Neural network | Repeat biopsy | 820 | PSA, percent-free PSA, TRUS, PSA density, PSA density of the transition zone, transition zone volume | Not available | 8 | 10 | 83 | Not performed |

| Year | Author | Model | Biopsy type | N | Variables | | | | | Validation |
|---|---|---|---|---|---|---|---|---|---|---|
| 2005 | Yanke et al. (108) | Probability nomogram validation (107) | Repeat biopsy | 230 (356 biopsies) | Age, DRE, number of previous negative biopsies, HGPIN history, ASAP history, PSA, PSA slope, family history, months from initial negative biopsy, months from previous negative biopsy | 2.6 (2–7) | 17.9 (12–54) | 34 | 71 | Internal |
| 2007 | Chun et al. (105) | Probability nomogram development | Repeat biopsy | 2,393 | Age, DRE, PSA, percent-free PSA, number of previous negative biopsies, sampling density* | 1.5 (1–7) | 11 (10–24) | 30 | 76 | Internal and external |
| **Saturation biopsy** | | | | | | | | | | |
| 2006 | Walz et al. (153) | Probability nomogram development | Repeat saturation biopsy | 161 | Age, PSA, percent-free PSA, prostate and BPH volume, PSA doubling time, PSA density of the transition zone, number of previous biopsy sessions, number of cores at saturation biopsy | 2.5 (2–5) | 24.5 (20–32) | 41 | 75 | Internal |
| **Mixed – initial and repeat biopsy** | | | | | | | | | | |
| 1994 | Snow et al. (19) | Neural network | Initial and repeat biopsy | 1,787 | Age, change on PSA, DRE, PSA, TRUS | Not available | 6 | 34 | 87 | Not performed |
| 1998 | Carlson et al. (154) | Probability table | Initial and repeat biopsy | 3,773 | Age, PSA, Percent-free PSA | Not available | 6 | 33 | Not available | Internal |

(continued)

**Table 3**
**continued**

| | | | | | | | | | | |
|---|---|---|---|---|---|---|---|---|---|---|
| 2002 | Djavan et al. (155) | Neural network | Initial and repeat biopsy | 272 | PSA density of the transition zone, percent-free PSA, PSA density, TRUS (PSA 2.5–4.0 ng/mL) | Not available | 8 | 24 | 88 | |
| | | | | 974 | PSA density of the transition zone, percent-free PSA, PSA velocity, transition zone volume, PSA, PSA density (PSA 4.0–10.0 ng/mL) | 8 Not available | Not available | 35 | 91 | |
| 2002 | Stephan et al. (102) | Neural network | Initial and repeat biopsy | 1,188 | Age, DRE, PSA, percent-free PSA, TRUS | Not available | Not available | 61 | 86 | Not per-formed |
| 2002 | Porter et al. (38) | Neural network | Initial and repeat biopsy | 319 | Age, PSA, gland volume, TRUS, DRE, previous negative biopsy, African-American race | Not available | 9.7 (6–10) | 39 | 76 | Not per-formed |
| 2004 | Matsui et al. (156) | Neural network | Initial and repeat biopsy | 228 | PSA density, DRE, age, TRUS | Not available | 10–12 | 26 | 73 | Not per-formed |
| 2006 | Benecchi (157) | Neural network | Initial and repeat biopsy | 1,030 | Age, PSA, percent-free PSA | Not available | 6–12 | 19 | 80 | Not per-formed |
| 2006 | Yanke et al. (34) | Probability nomogram development | Initial and repeat biopsy | 8,851 | Age, race, PSA, DRE, number of cores | Not available | 6–13 | 27–38 | 75 | Internal |

DRE = digital rectal examination; PSA = prostate-specific antigen; TRUS = transrectal ultrasound prostate; HGPIN = high-grade prostatic intraepithelial neoplasia; ASAP = atypical small acinar proliferation of prostate. *Sampling density = ratio of TRUS-derived total gland volume by the number of cores at biopsy.

**Table 4**
**Prediction of Pathologic Stage in Men Treated with Radical Prostatectomy for Clinically Localized Prostate Cancer**

| Year of publication | Reference | Prediction form | Outcome | No of patients | Variables | Accuracy (%) | Validation |
|---|---|---|---|---|---|---|---|
| 1993 | Partin et al. (85) | Probability table | Pathologic stage | 703 | Biopsy Gleason sum, clinical stage, PSA | Not available | External (158) and updated (21,111) |
| 1995 | Narayan et al. (159) | Probability graph | Pathologic stage | 813 | Biopsy-based stage, biopsy Gleason sum, PSA | Not available | Not performed |
| 1997 | Partin et al. (20) | Probability table | Pathologic stage | 4,133 | Biopsy Gleason sum, clinical stage, PSA | 72 | Internal and external (160) |

**Table 5**
Prediction of Specific Pathologic Features in Men Treated with Radical Prostatectomy for Clinically Localized Prostate Cancer

| Year of publication | Reference | Prediction form | Outcome | No of patients | Variables | Accuracy (%) | Validation |
|---|---|---|---|---|---|---|---|
| 1994 | Epstein et al. (161) | Risk group | Clinically indolent cancer defined as pathologically organ-confined, tumor volume ≤0.2 cc, Gleason sum < 7) | 157 | Biopsy Gleason sum, millimeter core with cancer, PSA density, no adverse pathologic findings on needle biopsy | Not available | External (162) |
| 1996 | Goto et al. (163) | Risk group | Clinically indolent cancer defined as pathologically organ-confined, tumor volume ≤0.5 cc, Gleason sum < 7) | 569 | PSA density, maximal millimeter cancer in any core | Not available | Not performed |

| Year | Author | | | N | Variables | | Validation |
|---|---|---|---|---|---|---|---|
| 2003 | Kattan et al. (87) | Probability nomogram development | Clinically indolent cancer defined as pathologically organ-confined, tumor volume ≤0.5 cc, no Gleason grade 4 or 5 | 409 | PSA, primary and secondary biopsy Gleason sum | 64 | Internal |
| | | | | | PSA, primary and secondary biopsy Gleason sum, percent positive cores, TRUS volume | 74 | Internal |
| | | | | | PSA, clinical stage, primary and secondary biopsy Gleason sum, TRUS volume, millimeter core with cancer, millimeter core without cancer | 79 | Internal |

(continued)

## Table 5
### continued

| 2007 | Steyerberg et al. (29) | Nomogram validation (87) | Clinically indolent cancer defined as pathologically organ-confined, tumor volume $\leq$0.5 cc, no Gleason grade 4 or 5 | 247 | PSA, primary and secondary biopsy Gleason sum | 61 | – |
|------|------------------------|--------------------------|----------------------|-----|------|----|---|
| | | | | | PSA, primary and secondary biopsy Gleason sum, percent positive cores, TRUS volume | 72 | – |
| | | | | | PSA, clinical stage, primary and secondary biopsy Gleason sum, TRUS volume, millimeter core with cancer, millimeter core without cancer | 76 | – |

| Year | Author | Method | Endpoint | N | Predictors | Accuracy | Validation |
|---|---|---|---|---|---|---|---|
| 2006 | Chun et al. (91) | Probability nomogram development | Gleason upgrading between biopsy and radical prostatectomy | 2,982 | PSA, clinical stage, primary and secondary biopsy Gleason sum | 80 | Internal |
| 2006 | Chun et al. (164) | Probability nomogram development | Significant Gleason upgrading between biopsy and radical prostatectomy | 4,789 | PSA, clinical stage, biopsy Gleason sum | 76 | Internal |
| 2006 | Steuber et al. (118) | Probability nomogram development | Tumor location: transition versus peripheral zone | 945 | PSA, biopsy Gleason sum, positive biopsy cores at mid-prostate only, number of positive biopsy cores at base, cumulative percent biopsy tumor volume | 77 | Internal |
| 1995 | Peller et al. (165) | Probability table | Tumor volume | 102 | Biopsy Gleason sum, number of positive sextant cores, PSA | Not available | Not performed |

Table 5
continued

| Year | Author | Method | Outcome | N | Predictors | Accuracy | Validation |
|---|---|---|---|---|---|---|---|
| 1993 | Ackerman et al. (166) | Probability formula | Surgical margin positivity | 107 | Number of positive sextant cores, PSA density | 70 | Not performed |
| 1998 | Rabbani et al. (167) | Probability graph | Surgical margin positivity | 242 | Androgen deprivation, number of ipsilateral positive cores, PSA | Not available | Not perfromed |
| 1996 | Bostwick et al. (168) | Probability graph | Extracapsular extension | 314 | Biopsy Gleason sum, percent cancer in biopsy cores, PSA | 78 | Not performed |
| 1999 | Gilliland et al. (169) | Probability graph | Extracapsular extension | 3,826 | Age, biopsy Gleason sum, PSA | 63 | Not performed |
| 2000 | Gamito et al. (39) | Neural network | Extracapsular extension | 4,133 | Age, race, PSA, PSA velocity, Gleason sum, clinical stage | 30–76 | External |
| 2004 | Ohori et al. (96) | Probability nomogram development | Side-specific extracapsular extension | 763 | PSA, clinical stage, side-specific biopsy Gleason sum, side-specific percent positive cores, side-specific percent of cancer in cores | 81 | External (97) |

| | | | | | | | |
|---|---|---|---|---|---|---|---|
| 2006 | Steuber et al. (97) | Probability nomogram development | Side-specific extracapsular extension | 1,118 | PSA, clinical stage, biopsy Gleason sum, percent positive cores, percent of cancer in positive cores | 84 | Internal |
| 1996 | Badalament et al. (170) | Probability formula | Organ-confined disease | 192 | Biopsy Gleason sum, involvement of greater than 5% of base with or without apex biopsy, nuclear grade, PSA, total percent tumor involvement | 86 | Not performed |
| 1996 | Bostwick et al. (168) | Probability graph | Seminal vesicle invasion | 314 | Biopsy Gleason sum, percent cancer in cores, PSA | 76 | Not performed |
| 1996 | Pisansky et al. (171) | Probability graph | Seminal vesicle invasion | 2,953 | Biopsy Gleason primary grade, clinical stage, PSA | 80 | Internal |

(continued)

**Table 5**
**continued**

| Year | Author | Method | Outcome | N | Predictors | | Validation |
|------|--------|--------|---------|---|------------|---|------------|
| 2003 | Koh et al. (88) | Probability nomogram development | Seminal vesicle invasion | 763 | PSA, clinical stage, primary and secondary Gleason sum, and percent of cancer at the base | 88 | Internal |
| 2007 | Baccala et al. (172) | Probability nomogram development | Seminal vesicle invasion | 6,740 | Age, PSA, Biopsy Gleason sum, clinical stage | 80 | Internal |
| 2007 | Gallina et al. (90) | Probability nomogram development | Seminal vesicle invasion | 896 | PSA, clinical stage, biopsy Gleason sum, percent positive biopsy cores | 79 | Internal and external |
| 1993 | Ackerman et al. (166) | Probability formula | Lymph node invasion assessed with limited pelvic lymphadenectomy | 107 | Number of positive sextant cores, PSA | 94 | Not performed |
| 1994 | Bluestein et al. (173) | Probability graph | Lymph node invasion assessed with limited pelvic lymphadenectomy | 816 | Biopsy Gleason sum, clinical stage, PSA | 82 | Internal |

| 1994 | Roach et al. (174) | Probability graph | Lymph node invasion assessed with limited pelvic lymphadenectomy | 212 | Biopsy Gleason sum, PSA | Not available | Not performed |
| 2001 | Batuello et al. (175) | Neural network | Lymph node invasion assessed with limited pelvic lymphadenectomy | 6,454 | Biopsy Gleason sum, clinical stage, PSA | 77–81 | Internal and external |
| 2003 | Cagiannos et al. (86) | Probability nomogram development | Lymph node invasion assessed with limited pelvic lymphadenectomy | 5,510 | PSA, clinical stage, biopsy Gleason sum | 76 | Internal |
| | | | | | PSA, clinical stage, biopsy Gleason sum, institution | 78 | Internal |

(continued)

**Table 5**
**continued**

| | | | | | |
|---|---|---|---|---|---|
| 2006, 2007 | Briganti et al. (89, 114,176) | Probability nomogram development | Lymph node invasion assessed with extended pelvic lym-phadenectomy (≥10 nodes) | 602 (114) | PSA, clinical stage, biopsy Gleason sum | 76 | Internal |
| | | | | 781 (89) | PSA, clinical stage, biopsy Gleason sum, number of lymph nodes | 79 | Internal |
| | | | | 278 (176) | PSA, clinical stage, biopsy Gleason sum, percentage positive biopsy cores | 83 | Internal |

PSA = prostate-specific antigen; TRUS = transrectal ultrasound.

**Table 6**
**Pre- and Post-operative Prediction of Biochemical Recurrence in Men Treated with Radical Prostatectomy**

| Year of publication | Reference | Prediction form | Pre-versus post-operative | Biochemical recurrence (years) | No of patients | Variables | Accuracy (%) | Validation |
|---|---|---|---|---|---|---|---|---|
| 1994 | Snow et al. (19) | Neural network | Pre-operative | Not available | 240 | Age, PSA, clinical stage, biopsy Gleason grade, potency | 90 | Not performed |
| 1998 | Kattan et al. (14) | Probability nomogram development | Pre-operative | 5 | 983 | Biopsy primary and secondary Gleason grade, clinical stage, PSA | 74 | Internal and external (43,44, 177,178) |
| 1999 | Graefen et al. (179) | Probability graph | Pre-operative | 3.5 | 315 | Biopsy Gleason sum, number of positive cores, PSA | Not available | Not performed |
| 1999 | D'Amico et al. (17) | Probability table | Pre-operative | 2 | 892 | Biopsy Gleason sum, clinical stage, PSA | Not available | Not performed |
| 2000 | D'Amico et al. (18) | Probability graph | Pre-operative | 2 | 977 | Biopsy Gleason sum, endorectal coil magnetic resonance imaging T-stage, PSA, percent positive biopsy cores | Not available | Not performed |

(continued)

Table 6
continued

| | | | | | | | | |
|---|---|---|---|---|---|---|---|---|
| 1998 and 2002 | D'Amico et al. (15,16) | Probability graph | Pre-operative | 4 | 823 | Biopsy Gleason sum, clinical stage, PSA, percent positive biopsy cores | 80 | Internal and external (44,80) |
| 2001 | Tewari et al. (180) | Neural network | Pre-operative | 3.5 | 1,400 | Age, race, PSA, clinical staging, biopsy Gleason sum | 83 | Not performed |
| 2005 | Cooperberg et al. (84) | Probability graph | Pre-operative | 3 and 5 | 1,439 | Age, PSA, biopsy Gleason sum, clinical stage, percent positive biopsy | 66 | Internal and external (83) |
| 2006 | Stephenson et al. (120) | Probability nomogram development | Pre-operative | 10 | 1,978 and 1,545 | PSA, clinical stage, biopsy Gleason sum, year of surgery, number of positive and negative cores | 76–79 | Internal and external |
| 1998 | Bauer et al. (181) | Probability formula | Post-operative | 5 | 378 | Race, PSA, Gleason sum, organ-confined status | Not available | External (182) |

| Year | Author | Method | Timing | Time | Predictors | Accuracy | Validation |
|---|---|---|---|---|---|---|---|
| 1998 | D'Amico et al. (15) | Probability graph | Post-operative | 2 | Pathologic stage, PSA, Gleason sum, surgical margin status | Not available | Not performed |
| 1999 | Graefen et al. (179) | Probability graph | Post-operative | 3.5 | Pathologic stage, volume Gleason grade 4/5 | Not available | Not performed |
| 1999 | Potter et al. (183) | Neural network | Post-operative | 5 | Gleason sum, extraprostatic extension, surgical margin status, age, DNA ploidy, and quantitative nuclear grade | 94 | Internal |
| 1999 | Kattan et al. (13) | Probability nomogram development | Post-operative | 5 | PSA, Gleason sum, extracapsular extension, seminal vesicle invasion, lymph node invasion, surgical margin status | 88 | Internal and external (42,123, 184) |

(continued)

Table 6
continued

| | | | | | | | | |
|---|---|---|---|---|---|---|---|---|
| 2000 | Stamey et al. (185) | Probability formula | Post-operative | Unknown | 326 | PSA, percent Gleason grade 4/5, volume largest cancer, vascular invasion, prostate weight, percent intraductal cancer, lymph node invasion | Not available | Not performed |
| 2005 | McAleer et al. (186) | Probability graph | Post-operative | 7 | 2,417 | Gleason grade, stage, margin status, dichotomized PSA (cut point 10 ng/mL). | Not available | Not performed |
| 2005 | Stephenson et al. (119) | Probability nomogram development | Post-operative | 10 | 1,881, 1,782, and 1,357 | PSA, Gleason sum, extracapsular extension, seminal vesicle invasion, lymph node invasion, surgical margin status | 78–86 | Internal and external |

PSA = prostate-specific antigen; DNA = deoxyribonucleic acid

**Table 7**

**Pre-Treatment Prediction of Biochemical Recurrence in Men Treated with Radiotherapy**

| Year of publication | Reference | Prediction form | Treatment | Outcome | No of patients | Variables | Accuracy (%) | Validation |
|---|---|---|---|---|---|---|---|---|
| 1996 | Duchesne et al. (187) | Risk group | External beam radiotherapy | Biochemical recurrence (5) | 85 | PSA, biopsy Gleason sum | Not available | Not performed |
| 1997 | Pisansky et al. (188) | Risk group | External beam radiotherapy | Biochemical recurrence (5) | 500 | Biopsy Gleason sum, clinical stage, PSA | Not available | Not performed |
| 1997 | Zagars et al. (189) | Probability graph | External beam radiotherapy | Biochemical recurrence (6) | 938 | PSA, biopsy Gleason sum, clinical stage | Not available | Not performed |
| 1999 | D'Amico et al. (17) | Probability table | External beam radiotherapy | Biochemical recurrence (2) | 762 | Biopsy Gleason sum, clinical stage, PSA | Not available | Not performed |
| 1999 | Shipley et al. (190) | Probability table | External beam radiotherapy | Biochemical recurrence (5) | 1,607 | Biopsy Gleason sum, clinical stage, PSA | Not available | Not performed |
| 2000 | Kattan et al. (127) | Probability nomogram development | External beam radiotherapy | Biochemical recurrence (5) | 1,042 and 1,030 | PSA, biopsy Gleason sum, clinical stage, neo-adjuvant androgen deprivation therapy, radiation dose delivered | 73 | Internal and external (191) |

(continued)

Table 7
continued

| Year | Study | Type | Treatment | Endpoint (years) | N | Predictors | Accuracy | Validation |
|---|---|---|---|---|---|---|---|---|
| 1998 and 2002 | D'Amico et al. (72,73) | Probability graph | External beam radiotherapy | Biochemical recurrence (5) | 766 | Biopsy Gleason sum, clinical stage, PSA, treatment modality | Not available | Internal |
| 1998 | D'Amico et al. (73) | Probability graph | Brachytherapy | Biochemical recurrence (5) | 218 | Biopsy Gleason sum, clinical stage, PSA, neo-adjuvant therapy | Not available | Not performed |
| 1998 | Ragde et al. (192) | Risk group | Brachytherapy | Biochemical recurrence (10) | 98 | Age, biopsy Gleason sum, clinical stage, PSA, 45 Gy external beam radiotherapy | 76 | Internal |
| 2001 | Kattan et al. (128) | Probability nomogram development | Brachytherapy | Biochemical recurrence (5) | 920 (development cohort) and 1,827 (first external validation cohort) and 765 (second external validation cohort) | Biopsy Gleason sum, clinical stage, PSA, co-administration of external beam radiotherapy | Internal not available 61 (external) 64 (external) | External |

PSA = prostate-specific antigen

**Table 8**
**Prediction of Metastasis and Survival**

| Year of publication | Reference | Prediction form | Patient population | Outcome (years) | No of patients | Variables | Accuracy (%) | Validation |
|---|---|---|---|---|---|---|---|---|
| 2007 | Stephenson et al. (193) | Probability nomogram Development | Salvage radiotherapy for biochemical recurrence after radical prostatectomy | Biochemical recurrence after radiotherapy (7 years after biochemical recurrence) | 1,540 | Prostatectomy PSA, Gleason sum, seminal vesicle invasion, extracapsular extension, surgical margin status, lymph node metastasis, persistently elevated PSA after radical prostatectomy, pre-radiotherapy PSA, PSA doubling time, neo-adjuvant androgen deprivation therapy, radiation dose | 69 | Internal |
| 1994 | Partin et al. (194) | Probability graph | Radical prostatectomy | Local versus distant recurrence | 1,058 | PSA velocity, Gleason sum, pathologic stage | Not available | Not performed |

(continued)

Table 8
continued

| Year | Study | Purpose | Cohort | Outcome (years) | n | Predictors | Concordance index | Validation |
|---|---|---|---|---|---|---|---|---|
| 1999 | Pound et al. (124) | Probability table | Biochemical recurrence after radical prostatectomy | Metastasis (7 years after biochemical recurrence) | 315 | PSA doubling time, Gleason sum, time to biochemical recurrence | 56 | Not performed |
| 2003 | Kattan et al. (79) | Probability nomogram development | External beam radiotherapy | Metastasis (5) | 1,677 and 1,626 | PSA, clinical stage, biopsy Gleason sum | Internal not available External 81 | External |
| 1oo5 | Slovin et al. (133) | Probability nomogram development | Biochemical recurrence after radical prostatectomy or radiotherapy | Metastasis (1–2) | 148 | Baseline PSA, PSA doubling time, Pathologic T stage, Gleason sum | 69 | Not performed |
| 1005 | Dotan et al. (132) | Probability nomogram development | Biochemical recurrence after radical prostatectomy | Positive bone scan | 239 | Pre-treatment PSA, surgical margin status, seminal vesicle invasion, Gleason sum, trigger PSA, extracapsular extension, PSA slope, PSA velocity | 93 | Internal |

| Year | Author | Model type | Treatment | Endpoint | N | Predictors | Validation | Validation type |
|---|---|---|---|---|---|---|---|---|
| 2002, 2003 | D'Amico et al. (70,71) | Probability graph | External beam radiotherapy | Prostate cancer-specific mortality (10) | 381 / 94 | Biopsy Gleason sum, clinical stage, PSA, percent positive biopsy / Time to PSA failure, post-treatment PSA doubling time, timing of salvage hormonal therapy. | Not available | Internal |
| 2003 | D'Amico et al. (74) | Probability graph | Radical prostatectomy | Prostate cancer-specific mortality (8) | 4,946 | Biopsy Gleason sum, clinical stage, PSA | Not available | Internal |
| 2003 | D'Amico et al. (74) | Probability graph | External beam radiotherapy | Prostate cancer-specific mortality (8) | 2,370 | Biopsy Gleason sum, clinical stage, PSA | Not available | Internal |
| 2005 | Freedland et al. (125) | Probability table | Biochemical recurrence after radical prostatectomy | Prostate cancer-specific mortality (10 years after biochemical recurrence) | 379 | PSA doubling time, Gleason sum, time from surgery to biochemical recurrence | 59 | Not performed |

(continued)

**Table 8**
**continued**

| 2005 | Zhou et al. (195) | Probability graph | External beam radiotherapy | Prostate cancer-specific mortality (5) | 661 | PSA doubling time, biopsy Gleason sum | Not available | Internal |
| 2005 | Zhou et al. (195) | Probability graph | Biochemical recurrence after radical prostatectomy | Prostate cancer-specific mortality (5) | 498 | PSA doubling time | Not available | Internal |
| 2006 | Svatek et al. (196) | Probability nomogram development | Androgen-independent prostate cancer | Prostate cancer-specific mortality (1–5) | 129 | PSA at initiation of androgen deprivation therapy, PSA doubling time, nadir (SA on androgen deprivation therapy, time from androgen deprivation therapy to androgen independent prostate cancer) | 81 | Internal |

| Year | Author | Purpose | Population | Outcome (years) | N | Variables | Accuracy (%) | Validation |
|---|---|---|---|---|---|---|---|---|
| 2007 | Porter et al. (136) | Probability nomogram development | Men on androgen deprivation therapy after radical prostatectomy | Prostate cancer-specific mortality (2–5) | 66 | Pathologic T stage, Gleason sum, surgical margin status, age at androgen deprivation therapy, recurrence type | 66 | Internal |
| 2002 | Smaletz et al. (134) | Probability nomogram development | Men with progressive metastatic prostate cancer after castration | Overall survival (1–2) | 409 and 433 | Age, Karnofsky performance index, hemoglobin, PSA, lactic dehydrogenase, alkaline phosphatase, albumin | 71 | Internal and external |
| 2003 | Halabi et al. (135) | Probability nomogram development | Metastatic hormone-refractory prostate cancer | Overall survival (1–2) | 1,101 | Lactate dehydrogenase, PSA, alkaline phosphatase, Gleason sum, Eastern Cooperative Oncology Group performance status, hemoglobin, presence of visceral disease | 68 | Internal and external |

PSA = prostate-specific antigen

**Table 9**
**Prediction of Life Expectancy in Men with Prostate Cancer**

| Year of publication | Reference | Prediction form | Patient population | Outcome (years) | No of patients | Variables | Accuracy (%) | Validation |
|---|---|---|---|---|---|---|---|---|
| 1996 | Albertson et al. (197) | Probability formula | Clinically localized prostate cancer | Overall survival (10 years) | 451 | Age, Gleason sum and index of coexistent disease category | 71 | Not performed |
| 2004 | Tewari et al. (40) | Probability graph | Clinically localized prostate cancer | Overall survival (10 years) | 6,149 | Age, race, comorbidity, PSA, Gleason sum, treatment type | 63 | Not performed |

| 2006 | Cowen et al. (137) | Probability nomogram development | Clinically localized prostate cancer | Life expectancy (5–15 years) | 506 | Age, Charlson comorbidity index, presence of angina, systolic blood pressure, body mass index, smoking, marital status, PSA < Gleason sum, clinical stage, treatment type (radical prostatectomy versus radiotherapy versus other) | 73 | Internal |
| 2007 | Walz et al. (198) | Probability nomogram development | Clinically localized prostate cancer | Life expectancy (10 years) | 9,131 treated with either radical prostatectomy (n = 5,955) or external beam radiotherapy (n = 3,176) | Age, Charlson comorbidity index, treatment type (radical prostatectomy versus external beam radiotherapy) | 84.3 | Internal |

Table 10

Prediction of Specific Pathologic Features or Biochemical Recurrence in Men Treated with Radical Prostatectomy for Clinically Localized Prostate Cancer Based on Novel Variables

| Year of publication | Reference | Prediction form | Pre-versus post-operative | Novel variable | Outcome | No of patients | Variables | Accuracy (%) | Validation |
|---|---|---|---|---|---|---|---|---|---|
| 2006 | Wang et al. (67) | Probability nomogram development | Pre-operative | Magnetic resonance imaging and magnetic resonance spectro-scopic imaging | Lymph node invasion | 411 | MRI variables and Partin probability table (20) | 89 | Internal |
| 2007 | Wang et al. (66) | Probability nomogram Development | Pre-operative | Magnetic resonance imaging and magnetic resonance spectro-scopic imaging | Seminal vesicle invasion | 573 | MRI variables and pre-operative Kattan probability nomogram (14) | 87 | Internal |

| Year | Author | Type | Timing | Markers | Endpoint | N | Predictors | Score | Validation |
|---|---|---|---|---|---|---|---|---|---|
| 2007 | Shukla-Dave et al. (144) | Probability nomogram development | Pre-operative | Magnetic resonance imaging and magnetic resonance spectroscopic imaging | Insignificant cancer (organ-confined cancer of $\leq$ 0.5 cm³ with no poorly differentiated elements) | 220 | Pretreatment PSA, clinical stage, biopsy cores positive, pre-treatment MRI volume of prostate, and overall MRI/MRSI score | 85 | Internal |
| 2003 | Kattan et al. (47) | Probability nomogram development | Pre-operative | Plasma levels of transforming growth factor β1 and interleukin 6 soluble receptor | Biochemical recurrence | 714 | Preoperative plasma transforming growth factor β1 and interleukin 6 soluble receptor and pre-operative Kattan probability nomogram (14) | 83 | Internal and external (199) |

(continued)

**Table 10**
**continued**

| | | | | | | |
|---|---|---|---|---|---|---|
| 2005 | Stephenson et al. (*139*) | Probability nomogram development | Post-operative | Gene expression based on oligonucleotide microarrays | Biochemical recurrence | 79 | Gene expression signatures and post-operative Kattan probability nomogram (*13*) | 89 | Internal |
| 2007 | Shariat et al. (*200*) | Probability nomogram Development | Pre-operative | Plasma levels of plasminogen activator inhibitor 1 | Biochemical recurrence | 429 | Preoperative plasma plasminogen activator inhibitor 1 and pre-operative Kattan probability nomogram (*14*) | 79 | Internal |

MRI = magnetic resonance imaging.

examination and serum PSA <4.0 ng/mL yielded a $c$-index of 0.75 *(36)*. Despite good accuracy this nomogram suffers from limited generalizability. It was tested and validated in men with suspicious digital rectal examination and serum PSA <4.0 ng/mL. Therefore, the nomogram cannot be applied to men with unremarkable digital rectal examination findings and does not apply to PSA greater than 4.0 ng/mL (Tables 2 and 3).

Recently Garzotto et al. developed a nomogram predicting prostate cancer on needle biopsy using routinely available clinical and transrectal ultrasound variables which yielded a $c$-index of 0.73 *(37)*. Despite adequate predictive accuracy this model has an important limitation: the use of ultrasound-based input is highly impractical since men who undergo transrectal ultrasound are also likely to undergo ultrasound-guided needle biopsy and the predictions of this nomogram are only applicable after transrectal ultrasound since transrectal ultrasound variables are necessary for risk estimation. Predictions based on input that does not require ultrasound findings are more practical and may be interpreted before planned ultrasound-guided biopsy.

Karakiewicz et al. developed two nomograms for prediction of the probability of having prostate cancer *(103)*. In the first, the development dataset comprised 4,193 men from the University of Montreal, Montreal, Quebec, Canada, and the validation dataset comprised 1,762 men from the University of Hamburg, Hamburg, Germany. The nomogram was based on patient age, digital rectal examination, and serum PSA. Data from the men from Hamburg were subsequently used to develop a second nomogram in which percent-free PSA was added as a predictor and external validation was performed using 514 men from Montreal. Prostate cancer was detected in 37% of patients from Montreal and 42% of patients from Hamburg. External validation of the nomograms with and without percent-free PSA yielded $c$-indices of 0.77 and 0.69, respectively.

Unfortunately, many existing predictive models are based on sextant biopsy regimens limiting their transportability to current biopsy strategies. There has been a constant modification of prostate biopsy technique over the last 20 years. The poor sensitivity and specificity of ultrasound-guided biopsies sampling two or three cores from abnormal lesions for detecting cancer led to the creation of a systematic sextant random biopsy at the end of 1980s. Because prostate cancer is commonly found on the lateral edge of the peripheral zone, this method was later developed into an extended biopsy scheme in which more laterally directed cores were added. Today, extended biopsy schemes are standard of care for prostate cancer detection and staging *(62)*. Therefore, models that are based on systematic sextant biopsy information are not optimal anymore and need to be updated. Chun et al. recently demonstrated that nomograms developed in the sextant biopsy era may not be able to predict the probability of prostate cancer on needle biopsy in the extended biopsy era, equally accurate as they used to in the sextant biopsy era *(104,105)*. Therefore, they updated their previous nomogram *(103)* in three cohorts totaling 2,900 men. Moreover, they complemented the variables with sampling density (i.e., ratio of gland volume to the number of planned biopsy cores) to predict presence of prostate cancer on the initial 10 or more core biopsy. The contemporary external validation of the previously validated sextant nomogram *(103)* demonstrated a $c$-index of 0.70 accuracy. Internal validation of the new nomogram demonstrated a $c$-index of 0.77 and external cohorts demonstrated $c$-indices between 0.73 and 0.76.

Accurate prediction of repeat biopsy would be helpful to spare men who do not have prostate cancer a negative repeat biopsy and to identify patients who need a re-biopsy to detect prostate cancer. O'Dowd et al. used age, previous histological findings, percent-free PSA, and total PSA to predict biopsy result from 813 men at second prostate biopsy

*(106)*. Their multivariate logistic regression model yielded a *c*-index of 0.70 accuracy, but it was neither internally nor externally validated.

Lopez-Corona et al. developed a nomogram that predicts the probability of a positive repeat biopsy following one or more negative biopsies *(107)*. The input variables of the nomogram are patient age, result of digital rectal examination, cumulative number of negative cores previously taken from the patient, histories of high-grade prostatic intraepithelial neoplasia and/or atypical small acinar proliferations, PSA, PSA slope, and family history of prostate cancer. The nomogram was developed and internally validated using a sample of 343 men evaluated at the Memorial Sloan-Kettering Cancer Center and was externally validated using 230 patients from the Brooklyn Veterans Administration Medical Center *(108)*. The nomogram yielded a *c*-index of 0.71. Moreover, the nomogram was found to be more accurate than any of the common heuristics presently reported in the literature. However, the complexity of the nomogram makes it impractical in the clinical setting.

Therefore, Chun et al. developed and validated a nomogram for prediction of repeat biopsy outcome based on systematic 10 or more cores *(105)*. The model comprised patient age, digital rectal examination, PSA, percent-free PSA, number of previous negative biopsy sessions, and sampling density (i.e., ratio between prostate volume assessed at initial biopsy and the planned number of cores at repeat biopsy). Using three different cohorts of men, they reported *c*-indices of 0.68–0.78 after external validation.

### *Prediction of Pathologic Features*

Several multivariate statistical models have been proposed to estimate pathologic stage at radical prostatectomy with the intent of facilitating intraoperative decision-making. Of these methods the "Partin tables" represent the most widely used tool. This look-up table categorizes clinical stage, pre-treatment PSA, and prostate biopsy Gleason grade to predict pathologic stage at radical prostatectomy (Table 4) *(20)*. After its introduction in 1997, the validity of the "Partin tables" was confirmed *(109,110)* and the tables have been continuously updated to remain contemporaneous *(21,111)* (Tables 4 and 5).

In 2001, Graefen et al. enhanced the specificity of this approach by generating regression tree analysis capable of predicting the probability of extracapsular extension in a side-specific manner (Table 5) *(23)*. This model allows the identification of candidates for non-nerve sparing versus unilateral versus bilateral nerve sparing prostatectomy. As mentioned above, look-up tables and CART analyses have limitations that can be overcome with logistic regression nomogram modeling.

Therefore, Ohori et al. developed three nomograms to predict the presence of extracapsular extension specific to either side of the prostate in 2004 (Table 5) *(96)*. They modeled data from 763 patients to develop three different nomograms. The most basic model relies on pre-operative PSA, side-specific clinical stage, and side-specific biopsy Gleason grade. The intermediate model uses these variables plus the side-specific percent of positive cores. The enhanced model uses the ingredients from the intermediate model plus side-specific percent of cancer. The *c*-indices of these three models were 0.79, 0.80, and 0.81, respectively. These models predict the side-specific probability of extracapsular extension which is more helpful in surgical planning than knowledge of the overall probability of extracapsular extension. Another advantage of these models compared to the "Partin tables" *(20,21,111)* is that they predict the probability of extracapsular extension without regard to whether the seminal vesicles or lymph nodes are involved. "Partin tables" predict the probability of extracapsular extension assuming negative seminal vesicles and lymph nodes. Steuber et al. validated these nomograms (*c*-index of 0.83 for the base nomogram and 0.84 for the full nomogram) *(97)* and demonstrated that these models were more accurate than the CART analysis of Graefen et al. by 13% *(23)*.

Using the same cohort as Ohori et al. *(96)*, Koh et al. derived a nomogram to predict the probability of seminal vesicle invasion *(88)*. The predictors in this nomogram are pre-operative PSA, clinical stage, primary and secondary biopsy Gleason grade, and percent of cancer at the base of the prostate. The *c*-index of this nomogram was 0.88. Similar to the extracapsular extension nomogram, the seminal vesicle invasion nomogram differs from the "Partin tables" in that it does not make any assumption about the status of the lymph nodes.

Recently, Gallina et al. developed a new nomogram for prediction of seminal vesicle invasion in a contemporary series of European patients *(90)*. They then compared head-to-head the performance of their model to that of Koh et al.'s nomogram *(88)* and the "Partin tables" *(20,21,111)*. Gallina et al.'s nomogram was more accurate and better calibrated than Koh et al.'s nomogram *(88)* and the "Partin tables" *(20,21,111)*.

Cagiannos et al. pooled the data from 5,510 patients from six institutions to construct a nomogram for predicting lymph node status *(86)*. The predictors were pre-operative PSA, biopsy Gleason sum, and clinical stage. This nomogram had a *c*-index of 0.76, which was higher than that of the "Partin tables" (0.74) when applied to the same population. Adding institution as a predictor improved the *c*-index to 0.78. This nomogram might help with the surgical decision of whether to avoid performing lymph node dissections, which are associated with the cost and possible morbidity. While this nomogram is a useful tool, it was developed in a population of men who underwent a limited or standard lymphadenectomy. Lymph node invasion prevalence is, however, directly related to the extent of pelvic lymph node dissection *(112,113)*. Thus, extended lymph node dissection might be necessary to detect clinically occult lymph node metastases that would not otherwise be detected by a more limited lymph node dissection.

Therefore, Briganti et al. developed a nomogram predicting the probability of lymph node invasion among patients undergoing radical prostatectomy and an extended pelvic lymphadenectomy *(114)*. In addition, the authors considered landing zones of positive lymph nodes and developed, based on the assumption of being able to spare extended lymph node dissection in low-risk patients, a second highly accurate nomogram to predict presence of extra-obturator lymph node involvement *(115)*.

PSA screening leads to the early detection of cancers, of which some are so small, low-grade and non-invasive that they may be assumed to pose little risk to the patient (indolent cancer) *(116)*. Kattan et al. developed nomograms that predict the probability of harboring indolent prostate cancer (pathologically organ-confined cancer, 0.5 cc or less in volume and without poorly differentiated elements) *(87)*. The authors developed three models: the first included pre-operative PSA and primary and secondary biopsy Gleason grade; the second model added ultrasound volume and percent of positive cores as predictors to the predictors of the first model; and the third model further added millimeters of cancerous and non-cancerous tissues found in biopsy cores. The *c*-indices for these three models were 0.64, 0.74, and 0.79, respectively. The models might help in deciding when aggressive therapy can be delayed or avoided. Steyerberg et al. evaluated transportability of these nomograms to the screening setting *(29)*, where overdiagnosis and overtreatment are of key concern *(117)*. They found that the proportion of patients with indolent cancer was higher in the setting of a screening trial *(29)* than in the non-screened setting in which the models were created (49% vs 20%). They concluded that models predicting indolent prostate cancer in the clinical setting provide probabilities that are too low for cancers identified in a screening setting. Therefore, they developed an updated model that predicts the probability of indolent disease in patients with screen-detected prostate cancer.

Beyond pathologic features, nomograms predicting Gleason upgrading between biopsy and radical prostatectomy *(91)* and of tumor location *(118)* have been developed. For example, Chun et al. developed and internally validated a nomogram for predicting the probability of biopsy Gleason sum upgrading in a cohort of 2,982 patients treated with radical prostatectomy *(91)*. Using pre-operative PSA, clinical stage, and primary and secondary biopsy Gleason grade, their model achieved a *c*-index of 0.80 and its predictions closely approximated the observed rate of Gleason sum upgrading between biopsy and final pathology.

## *Prediction of Biochemical Recurrence After Radical Prostatectomy*

Both before-treatment and after-treatment nomograms have been developed to predict the continuous probability of disease recurrence after radical prostatectomy *(13,14,119, 120)* (Table 6).

### BEFORE RADICAL PROSTATECTOMY

Clinical stage, biopsy Gleason sum, and pre-treatment PSA are strong predictors of pathologic stage. Although this endpoint is important for surgical planning, it often does not correlate with the risk of disease recurrence/progression *(121)*. Therefore, Kattan et al. developed a pre-treatment nomogram that predicts the 5-year biochemical recurrence for patients who chose radical prostatectomy based on clinical stage, biopsy-derived primary and secondary Gleason grades, and pre-treatment PSA levels (Fig. 1) *(14)*. Currently, it is the most widely used disease-specific prediction tool for the Palm™ handheld in oncology *(122)*. The model was based on 983 patients with clinically localized prostate cancer treated by one surgeon. Disease recurrence was defined as an initial PSA increase to $\geq 0.4$ ng/mL followed by any further rise above this level, evidence of clinical recurrence (local, regional, or distant), administration of adjuvant therapy, or death from prostate cancer. In addition, patients with lymph node metastasis in whom radical prostatectomy was aborted were classified as treatment failures at the time of surgery. The overall 5-year biochemical recurrence for this cohort was 73%. The nomogram was accurate and discriminating with a *c*-index of 0.75 when applied to an external validation cohort *(43,44)*. It was also validated in the African-American population, with a *c*-index of 0.74 *(123)*.

The 5-year endpoint is insufficient to predict the likelihood of cure after radical prostatectomy, as many patients are at risk of disease recurrence beyond 5 years *(121,124,125)*. However, after 10 years recurrence is rare *(120)*. Thus, the 10-year biochemical recurrence probability would appear to be a sufficient endpoint for estimating the likelihood that a man will be cured of his prostate cancer by radical prostatectomy alone. Therefore, Stephenson et al. recently updated the pre-operative nomogram by incorporating clinical stage, biopsy Gleason grade, pre-operative PSA, and number of positive and negative prostate biopsy cores to predict the 10-year probability of bio-chemical recurrence after radical prostatectomy (Fig. 5A) *(120)*. Inclusion of the number of positive and negative cores resulted in only a mild improvement in predictive accuracy over clinical stage, Gleason grade, and pre-operative PSA in an independent validation (*c*-index 0.79 vs 0.77). The model exhibited good calibration across the spectrum of predictions in internal validation but exhibited some optimism in external validation.

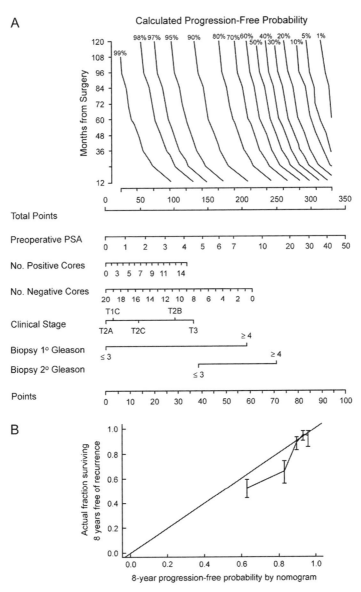

**Fig. 5.** (A) Pre-operative nomogram estimating the 1- to 10-year biochemical recurrence-free probability after radical prostatectomy alone. (B) Calibration plot of the nomogram in external validation. The 45° line represents an ideal model in which estimates of recurrence are perfectly calibrated with outcome. Vertical bars are 95% confidence intervals for quintiles in the validation set. Reprinted with permission from Stephenson et al. *(120)*.

An added feature of the nomogram is the ability to estimate the probability of recurrence at any point in time from 1 to 10 years after radical prostatectomy. Patients with an 8-year recurrence-free probability between 70% and 85% had an observed rate of freedom from biochemical recurrence of 57–72% (Fig. 5 B). The ability to predict the risk of early biochemical recurrence may be important for neo-adjuvant treatment strategies, because disease recurrence within 2–3 years of radical prostatectomy is associated with an increased risk of development of metastasis and cancer-specific death *(124,125)*.

## AFTER RADICAL PROSTATECTOMY

Kattan et al. also developed a nomogram to identify patients at high-risk for biochemical recurrence after radical prostatectomy using data from 996 men with clinically localized prostate cancer treated by a single surgeon *(13)*. This instrument uses preoperative PSA, prostatectomy Gleason sum, extracapsular extension, surgical margin status, seminal vesicle invasion, and lymph node involvement to predict the 7-year probability of biochemical recurrence. Treatment failure was defined as an initial PSA increase to $\geq 0.4$ ng/mL, followed by any further rise above this level, clinical evidence of disease recurrence (local or distant), initiation of adjuvant therapy, or death from prostate cancer. The 7-year biochemical recurrence-free probability for the cohort was 73%. The nomogram had a $c$-index of 0.80 when applied to an international validation cohort *(42)* and 0.83 when applied to a cohort of African-Americans *(123)*.

Despite the robust information contained within this nomogram, it has certain limitations. While the 7-year endpoint for disease recurrence is a reasonable estimate of the likelihood of cure, it is known that clinically significant prostate cancer recurrence can occur after 7 years *(121,124,125)*. In addition, in developing the nomogram, patients receiving adjuvant radiotherapy were considered as treatment failures. Thus, the predictions of the nomogram may be overly pessimistic, given that several of these patients would not have recurred without adjuvant therapy. Lastly, widespread PSA screening has resulted in a stage migration with a shift to more favorable pathologic features and prognosis *(126)*. The initial post-operative nomogram was developed on patients treated over a 14-year period beginning in 1984 (many of whom were treated before the introduction of the PSA assay), so the predictions may not be accurate for patients treated contemporaneously. Therefore, Stephenson et al. updated the post-operative nomogram by extending the predictions out to 10 years after radical prostatectomy (Fig. 6) *(119)*. They also enhanced the current version of the post-operative nomogram by adjusting the prediction for patients' treatment year and for the use of adjuvant radiotherapy (which was considered as a treatment failure in the original model). To account for the changing prognosis of patients who have maintained an undetectable PSA for specific time intervals after radical prostatectomy, they have enabled the 10-year biochemical recurrence prediction of the nomogram to be re-estimated based on the disease-free interval patients have achieved. The resulting new post-operative nomogram is a robust predictive model with a calculated $c$-index of 0.81 and 0.78 when applied to separate independent validation sets *(119)*.

## *Prediction of Biochemical Recurrence After External Beam Radiotherapy*

Kattan et al. developed a pre-treatment nomogram to predict the 5-year biochemical recurrence-free probability after treatment with three-dimensional conformal external

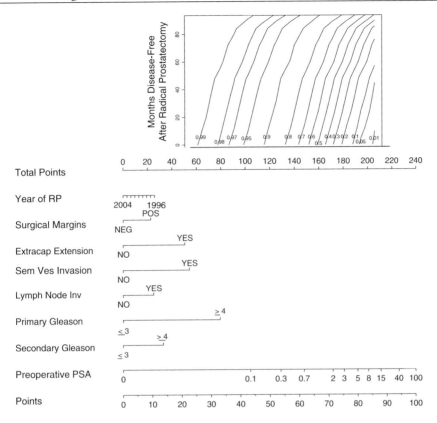

**Fig. 6.** Post-operative nomogram predicting 10-year biochemical recurrence-free probability after radical prostatectomy. RP, radical prostatectomy; extracap, extracapsular; sem ves, seminal vesicle; inv, involvement; PSA, prostate-specific antigen. Reprinted with permission from Stephenson et al. *(119).*

beam radiotherapy in a cohort of 1,042 men treated at the Memorial Sloan-Kettering Cancer Center between 1988 and 1998. This model is based on clinical stage, biopsy Gleason sum, pre-treatment PSA, use of neo-adjuvant androgen deprivation therapy, and radiation dose (Fig. 7) *(127).* The definition of the American Society for Therapeutic Radiology and Oncology (ASTRO) was applied for the determination of biochemical

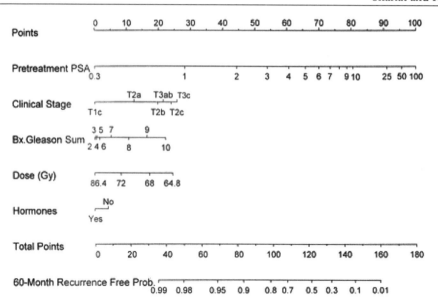

**Fig. 7.** Pre-treatment nomogram for predicting 5-year biochemical recurrence-free probability after three-dimensional conformal radiation therapy (3D-CRT). Reprinted with permission from Kattan et al. *(127)*.

failure (i.e., three cumulative increases in serum PSA level, with the failure date designated as the mid-point in time between the first rise and the PSA level immediately before this rise). Bootstrap analysis yielded a *c*-index of 0.73 and external validation with a cohort of 912 men treated at the Cleveland Clinic yielded a *c*-index of 0.76. The accuracy of this model is significantly better than the best risk-grouping model available *(72,73)* (Table 7).

### *Prediction of Biochemical Recurrence After Prostate Brachytherapy*

Kattan et al. developed a pre-treatment nomogram that predicts the 5-year biochemical recurrence-free probability after brachytherapy with [125]I-seeds in the absence of adjuvant hormonal therapy, based on pre-treatment PSA, clinical stage, biopsy Gleason sum, and the co-administration of external beam radiotherapy (Fig. 8) *(128)*. The model was based on 920 men treated for clinically T1-2 prostate cancer, with treatment failure defined by a modified version of the ASTRO criteria, the administration of adjuvant hormonal deprivation therapy, clinical evidence of disease progression (local, regional, or distant), or death from prostate cancer. External validation with 1,827 men treated at the Seattle Prostate Institute gave a *c*-index of 0.61, and further validation with 765 men treated at the Arizona Oncology Services yielded a *c*-index of 0.64 (Table 7).

### *Prediction of Metastasis*

Biochemical recurrence may result from local failure related to residual disease present after radical prostatectomy, occult nodal or distant metastatic disease present at the time of surgery, or a combination of these *(93,125,129–131)*. These forms of biochemical recurrence have variable progression rates with regard to metastases and

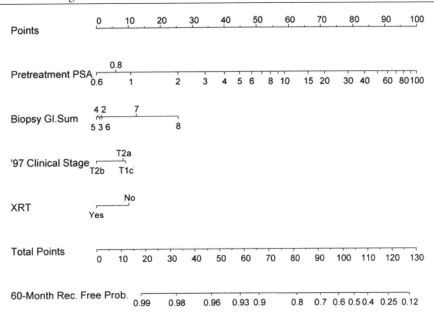

**Fig. 8.** Pre-treatment nomogram for predicting 5-year biochemical recurrence-free probability after permanent prostate brachytherapy without neo-adjuvant androgen ablative therapy. Reprinted with permission from Kattan et al. *(128)*.

eventual death. Therefore, prediction of metastasis is a more robust endpoint for management of prostate cancer patients than simple prediction of recurrence assessed by a rising PSA (Table 8).

Kattan et al. developed a nomogram for prediction of the probability of metastasis within 5 years following external beam radiotherapy, based on 1,677 patients treated at Memorial Sloan-Kettering Cancer Center *(79)*. The nomogram was externally validated in 1,626 men treated at the Cleveland Clinic Foundation and was found to have a *c*-index of 0.81.

Dotan et al. developed a nomogram for prediction of the probability of a positive bone scan using data from 239 men with a rising PSA after radical prostatectomy and no history of androgen deprivation therapy *(132)*. The nomogram relies upon pre-treatment and present PSA levels, surgical margin status, seminal vesicle invasion, pathologic Gleason sum, extraprostatic extension, and PSA velocity, and has a *c*-index of 0.93. This model allows the treating physician to predict the probability of a systemic progression according to the pre- and post-operative characteristics and pattern of PSA failure at any time during the patient's follow-up after the detection of an increasing PSA.

This nomogram will be useful in counseling patients with increasing PSA after radical prostatectomy before treatment with androgen deprivation therapy.

Similarly, Slovin et al. attempted to predict the time to radiographically detectable metastases in 148 patients who experienced biochemical recurrence after radical prostatectomy or radiation therapy and who had a PSA doubling time (PSADT) of less than 12 months *(133)*. This nomogram predicts the probability of metastases-free survival at 12 to 24 months after biochemical recurrence. However, validation was not performed to confirm its performance.

### Prediction of Survival in Patients with Prostate Cancer Metastasis

Smaletz et al. developed a nomogram to predict the median survival time and the probabilities of survival at 1- and 2-years after castration in 409 men with progressive metastatic prostate cancer *(134)*. The tool uses age, Karnofsky performance status, hemoglobin, PSA, lactate dehydrogenase, alkaline phosphatase, and albumin as predictors. External validation in a multicenter trial of suramin plus hydrocortisone versus hydrocortisone alone yielded a *c*-index of 0.67. Although the multicenter trial patients had worse median survival than the nomogram development population, the nomogram still predicted well by properly adjusting for the more severe case-mix of patients who enrolled in the trial (Table 8).

Halabi et al. developed a similar survival nomogram based on visceral disease, Gleason sum, performance status, PSA, lactate dehydrogenase, alkaline phosphatase, and hemoglobin in 1,101 patients *(135)*. The *c*-index of this model was 0.68.

Porter et al. developed a nomogram predicting prostate cancer-specific survival at 2-, 3-, 4-, and 5-years after start of hormone therapy for post-prostatectomy biochemical failure *(136)*. The *c*-index of this model was 0.66.

### Prediction of Life Expectancy

Patients diagnosed with a clinically localized prostate cancer may be offered an array of different treatment procedures. Life expectancy plays a crucial role in choosing the adequate treatment option. Cowen et al. developed a nomogram predicting the median life expectancy at 5, 10, and 15 years in men diagnosed with prostate cancer between the years of 1987 and 1989 *(137)*. Limitations of this model are the single institution nature of the patient cohort, the relevance of men treated between 1987 and –1989 to contemporary patients, and the interpretation of the treatment effect within the nomogram. Despite its limitations, this tool helps in patient counseling (Table 9).

### Nomograms of the Future-Inclusion of Novel Biomarkers and Imaging Tools

The accuracy of current predictive tools is not yet perfect. Better modeling of the data, assembling larger datasets, and collecting data more systematically and cleanly (e.g., by tightening the definition of symptom status) may yield some improvement. However, to date, the addition of other potentially informative clinical and pathologic features has not significantly improved the accuracy of these models *(138)*. This is largely due to the heterogeneous biologic behavior of tumors with the same clinical and/or pathologic features. Therefore, incorporation of novel biomarkers and/or imaging tools that are associated with the biologic behavior of prostate cancer may potentially improve nomogram predictions (Table 10).

Over the past two decades the molecular dissection of cancer has increased our understanding of the pathways that are altered in neoplastic cells. Protein expression profiling of prostate cancer offers an alternative means to distinguish aggressive tumor biology and may improve the accuracy of outcome prediction. In addition, the emergence of new therapeutic approaches for prostate cancer cannot flourish without a set of markers to serve as prognosticators and/or therapeutic targets. However, despite numerous reports of promising new biomarkers in the urological literature, only two studies have to date demonstrated a statistically significant improvement in predictive accuracy when biomarkers were added to established predictors in the nomogram setting *(47,139)*.

Kattan et al. developed and internally validated a prognostic model that incorporates pre-operative plasma levels of transforming growth factor-β1 and interleukin-6 soluble receptor in the standard pre-operative Kattan nomogram (based on pre-operative PSA, biopsy Gleason grade, and clinical stage) *(14)* to predict the probability of biochemical recurrence-free survival at 5 years after radical prostatectomy *(47)*. Addition of these biomarkers improved the predictive accuracy by a statistically and prognostically substantial margin relative to clinical variables alone (increase in $c$-index from 0.75 to 0.83). Before these promising findings can be used in routine clinical practice, they need to be validated in an independent external cohort.

Non-invasive diagnostic imaging, especially magnetic resonance imaging (MRI) and MR spectroscopic imaging (MRSI) has improved in recent years and is gaining widespread acceptance for aiding diagnosis, tumor localization, staging, assessment of tumor aggressiveness, treatment planning, and follow-up in patients with prostate cancer *(140–142)*. Wang et al. recently established the incremental value of MRI/MRSI to the staging nomograms for predicting organ-confined prostate cancer *(66)*. Pre-operative neural network software has also been developed using combined MRI variables, PSA level, and Gleason sum to predict biochemical recurrence after radical prostatectomy *(143)*. Another study demonstrated that MR findings are very accurate in predicting either definitely insignificant or definitely significant disease *(144)*. Although they could not determine the exact tumor volume, combined MRI and MRSI were capable of accurately separating tumors of $<0.5 \, cm^3$ from those of $>0.5 \, cm^3$, and improved the overall accuracy of a previously published nomogram *(87)* for predicting the probability of insignificant prostate cancer (from 0.73 to 0.85).

## CONCLUSIONS

At a minimum, prostate cancer patients need to be involved in the decision regarding management of their disease. They should know what their options are and what the consequences can be. Ideally, patients would make their own treatment decisions. At the core of any patient involvement is accurate prediction of consequences and, essentially, a spreadsheet of these predictions tailored to the individual. This spreadsheet represents informed consent for any medical decision. Providing this should reduce the likelihood of regret of treatment choice, particularly when complications arise.

Continuous, multivariable models such as nomograms are a highly appealing means of calculating accurate predictions with or without the use of a computer. Many nomograms have been constructed for patients with prostate cancer. Nomograms currently represent the most accurate and discriminating tools for predicting outcomes in patients with prostate cancer. When faced with the difficult decision of choosing among the treatment options for each clinical stage of prostate cancer, the nomograms provide patients with accurate estimates of outcomes. Equipped with this information, the patient is more likely to be confident in his treatment decision and less likely to experience regret in the future. However, it should be emphasized that nomogram predictions must be interpreted as such; they do not make treatment recommendations or act as a surrogate for physician–patient interactions, nor do they provide definitive information on symptomatic disease progression or complications associated with treatments.

Many more nomograms, as well as improvements to existing nomograms, are needed. For example, none of the nomograms predict with perfect accuracy. Novel biomarkers, larger datasets, better data collection methods, and more sophisticated modeling procedures are needed to improve predictive accuracy. In addition, better accuracy might be accomplished by modeling physician and/or hospital-specific data for patients being treated by that physician or at that hospital. Finally, nomograms that predict the likelihood of metastatic progression, cancer-specific mortality, and long-term urinary and sexual function are likely to have great utility for the patient and physician when exploring treatment alternatives. In summary, nomograms have empowered patients and physicians in their fight against prostate cancer by providing superior individualized disease-related risk estimations that facilitate management-related decisions.

## REFERENCES

1. Parkin DM, Bray F, Ferlay J, Pisani P. Global cancer statistics, 2002. CA: a cancer. J Clin 2005;55(2):74–108.
2. Jemal A, Siegel R, Ward E, Murray T, Xu J, Thun MJ. Cancer statistics, 2007. CA: a cancer. J Clin 2007;57(1):43–66.
3. Miles BJ, Giesler B, Kattan MW. Recall and attitudes in patients with prostate cancer. Urology 1999;53(1):169–74.
4. Clark JA, Wray NP, Ashton CM. Living with treatment decisions: regrets and quality of life among men treated for metastatic prostate cancer. J Clin Oncol 2001;19(1):72–80.
5. Elstein AS. Heuristics and biases: selected errors in clinical reasoning. Acad Med 1999;74(7):791–4.
6. Vlaev I, Chater N. Game relativity: how context influences strategic decision making. J Exp Psychol 2006;32(1):131–49.
7. Kattan M. Expert systems in medicine. In Smelser NJ, Baltes PB eds. International Encyclopedia of the Social and Behavioral Sciences Oxford: Pergamon 2001:5135–9.
8. Hogarth RM, Karelaia N. Heuristic and linear models of judgment: matching rules and environments. Psychol Rev 2007;114(3):733–58.
9. Kattan MW. Nomograms. Introduction. Semin Urol Oncol 2002;20(2):79–81.
10. Rabbani F, Stapleton AM, Kattan MW, Wheeler TM, Scardino PT. Factors predicting recovery of erections after radical prostatectomy. J Urol 2000;164(6):1929–34.
11. Ross PL, Gerigk C, Gonen M, et al. Comparisons of nomograms and urologists' predictions in prostate cancer. Semin Urol Oncol 2002;20(2):82–8.
12. Ross PL, Scardino PT, Kattan MW. A catalog of prostate cancer nomograms. J Urol 2001;165(5):1562–8.
13. Kattan MW, Wheeler TM, Scardino PT. Postoperative nomogram for disease recurrence after radical prostatectomy for prostate cancer. J Clin Oncol 1999;17(5):1499–507.
14. Kattan MW, Eastham JA, Stapleton AM, Wheeler TM, Scardino PT. A preoperative nomogram for disease recurrence following radical prostatectomy for prostate cancer. J Natl Cancer Inst 1998;90(10):766–71.
15. D'Amico AV, Whittington R, Malkowicz SB, et al. The combination of preoperative prostate specific antigen and postoperative pathological findings to predict prostate specific antigen outcome in clinically localized prostate cancer. J Urol 1998;160(6 Pt 1):2096–101.
16. D'Amico AV, Keshaviah A, Manola J, et al. Clinical utility of the percentage of positive prostate biopsies in predicting prostate cancer-specific and overall survival after radiotherapy for patients with localized prostate cancer. Int J Radiat Oncol Biol Phys 2002;53(3):581–7.
17. D'Amico AV, Whittington R, Malkowicz SB, et al. Pretreatment nomogram for prostate-specific antigen recurrence after radical prostatectomy or external-beam radiation therapy for clinically localized prostate cancer. J Clin Oncol 1999;17(1):168–72.
18. D'Amico AV, Whittington R, Malkowicz SB, et al. Combination of the preoperative PSA level, biopsy Gleason score, percentage of positive biopsies, and MRI T-stage to predict early PSA failure in men with clinically localized prostate cancer. Urology 2000;55(4):572–7.
19. Snow PB, Smith DS, Catalona WJ. Artificial neural networks in the diagnosis and prognosis of prostate cancer: a pilot study. J Urol 1994;152(5 Pt 2):1923–6.
20. Partin AW, Kattan MW, Subong EN, et al. Combination of prostate-specific antigen, clinical stage, and Gleason score to predict pathological stage of localized prostate cancer. A multi-institutional update

[see comments] [published erratum appears in JAMA 1997 Jul 9;278(2):118]. Jama 1997;277(18): 1445–51.

21. Makarov DV, Trock BJ, Humphreys EB, et al. Updated nomogram to predict pathologic stage of prostate cancer given prostate-specific antigen level, clinical stage, and biopsy Gleason score (Partin tables) based on cases from 2000 to 2005. Urology 2007;69(6):1095–101.

22. Conrad S, Graefen M, Pichlmeier U, et al. Prospective validation of an algorithm with systematic sextant biopsy to predict pelvic lymph node metastasis in patients with clinically localized prostatic carcinoma. J Urol 2002;167(2 Pt 1):521–5.

23. Graefen M, Haese A, Pichlmeier U, et al. A validated strategy for side specific prediction of organ confined prostate cancer: a tool to select for nerve sparing radical prostatectomy. J Urol 2001;165(3):857–63.

24. Bradley EaT, R.J. Monographs on statistics and applied probability: an introduction to the bootstrap: Champman and Hall/CRC; 1993.

25. Kattan MW. Comparison of Cox regression with other methods for determining prediction models and nomograms. J Urol 2003;170(6 Pt 2):S6–9; discussion S10.

26. Steyerberg EW, Bleeker SE, Moll HA, Grobbee DE, Moons KG. Internal and external validation of predictive models: a simulation study of bias and precision in small samples. J Clin Epidemiol 2003;56(5):441–7.

27. Steyerberg EW, Harrell FE, Jr., Borsboom GJ, Eijkemans MJ, Vergouwe Y, Habbema JD. Internal validation of predictive models: efficiency of some procedures for logistic regression analysis. J Clin Epidemiol 2001;54(8):774–81.

28. Steyerberg EW, Harrell FE, Jr., Goodman PH. Neural networks, logistic regression, and calibration. Med Decis Making 1998;18(3):349–50.

29. Steyerberg EW, Roobol MJ, Kattan MW, van der Kwast TH, de Koning HJ, Schroder FH. Prediction of indolent prostate cancer: validation and updating of a prognostic nomogram. J Urol 2007;177(1): 107–12; discussion 12.

30. Briganti A, Shariat SF, Chun FK, et al. Differences in the rate of lymph node invasion in men with clinically localized prostate cancer might be related to the continent of origin. BJU Int 2007;100(3):528–32.

31. Charlson ME, Ales KL, Simon R, MacKenzie CR. Why predictive indexes perform less well in validation studies. Is it magic or methods? Arch Intern Med 1987;147(12):2155–61.

32. Harrell FE, Jr., Lee KL, Mark DB. Multivariable prognostic models: issues in developing models, evaluating assumptions and adequacy, and measuring and reducing errors. Stat Med 1996;15(4): 361–87.

33. Justice AC, Covinsky KE, Berlin JA. Assessing the generalizability of prognostic information. Ann Intern Med 1999;130(6):515–24.

34. Yanke BV, Carver BS, Bianco FJ, Jr., et al. African-American race is a predictor of prostate cancer detection: incorporation into a pre-biopsy nomogram. BJU Int 2006;98(4):783–7.

35. Suzuki H, Komiya A, Kamiya N, et al. Development of a nomogram to predict probability of positive initial prostate biopsy among Japanese patients. Urology 2006;67(1):131–6.

36. Eastham JA, May R, Robertson JL, Sartor O, Kattan MW. Development of a nomogram that predicts the probability of a positive prostate biopsy in men with an abnormal digital rectal examination and a prostate-specific antigen between 0 and 4 ng/mL. Urology 1999;54(4):709–13.

37. Garzotto M, Hudson RG, Peters L, et al. Predictive modeling for the presence of prostate carcinoma using clinical, laboratory, and ultrasound parameters in patients with prostate specific antigen levels < or = 10 ng/mL. Cancer 2003;98(7):1417–22.

38. Porter CR, O'Donnell C, Crawford ED, et al. Predicting the outcome of prostate biopsy in a racially diverse population: a prospective study. Urology 2002;60(5):831–5.

39. Gamito EJ, Stone NN, Batuello JT, Crawford ED. Use of artificial neural networks in the clinical staging of prostate cancer: implications for prostate brachytherapy. Tech urol 2000;6(2):60–3.

40. Tewari A, Johnson CC, Divine G, et al. Long-term survival probability in men with clinically localized prostate cancer: a case-control, propensity modeling study stratified by race, age, treatment and comorbidities. J Urol 2004;171(4):1513–9.

41. Bauer JJ, Connelly RR, Sesterhenn IA, et al. Biostatistical modeling using traditional variables and genetic biomarkers for predicting the risk of prostate carcinoma recurrence after radical prostatectomy. Cancer 1997;79(5):952–62.

42. Graefen M, Karakiewicz PI, Cagiannos I, et al. Validation study of the accuracy of a postoperative nomogram for recurrence after radical prostatectomy for localized prostate cancer. J Clin Oncol 2002;20(4):951–6.

43. Graefen M, Karakiewicz PI, Cagiannos I, et al. International validation of a preoperative nomogram for prostate cancer recurrence after radical prostatectomy. J Clin Oncol 2002;20(15):3206–12.
44. Graefen M, Karakiewicz PI, Cagiannos I, et al. A validation of two preoperative nomograms predicting recurrence following radical prostatectomy in a cohort of European men. Urol Oncol 2002;7(4):141–6.
45. Shariat SF, Karakiewicz PI, Palapattu GS, et al. Nomograms provide improved accuracy for predicting survival after radical cystectomy. Clin Cancer Res 2006;12(22):6663–76.
46. Kattan MW. Nomograms are superior to staging and risk grouping systems for identifying high-risk patients: preoperative application in prostate cancer. Curr Opin Urol 2003;13(2):111–6.
47. Kattan MW, Shariat SF, Andrews B, et al. The addition of interleukin-6 soluble receptor and transforming growth factor beta1 improves a preoperative nomogram for predicting biochemical progression in patients with clinically localized prostate cancer. J Clin Oncol 2003;21(19):3573–9.
48. Chun FK, Graefen M, Briganti A, et al. Initial biopsy outcome prediction – head-to-head comparison of a logistic regression-based nomogram versus artificial neural network. Eur Urol 2007;51(5):1236–40; discussion 41–3.
49. Chun FK, Karakiewicz PI, Briganti A, et al. A critical appraisal of logistic regression-based nomograms, artificial neural networks, classification and regression-tree models, look-up tables and risk-group stratification models for prostate cancer. BJU Int 2007;99(4):794–800.
50. Begg CB, Riedel ER, Bach PB, et al. Variations in morbidity after radical prostatectomy. N Engl J Med 2002;346(15):1138–44.
51. Bianco FJ, Jr., Riedel ER, Begg CB, Kattan MW, Scardino PT. Variations among high volume surgeons in the rate of complications after radical prostatectomy: further evidence that technique matters. J Urol 2005;173(6):2099–103.
52. Eastham JA, Kattan MW, Riedel E, et al. Variations among individual surgeons in the rate of positive surgical margins in radical prostatectomy specimens. J Urol 2003;170(6 Pt 1):2292–5.
53. Hu JC, Gold KF, Pashos CL, Mehta SS, Litwin MS. Role of surgeon volume in radical prostatectomy outcomes. J Clin Oncol 2003;21(3):401–5.
54. Shariat SF, Canto EI, Kattan MW, Slawin KM. Beyond prostate-specific antigen: new serologic biomarkers for improved diagnosis and management of prostate cancer. Rev Urol 2004;6(2):58–72.
55. Stamey TA, Johnstone IM, McNeal JE, Lu AY, Yemoto CM. Preoperative serum prostate specific antigen levels between 2 and 22 ng./ml. correlate poorly with post-radical prostatectomy cancer morphology: prostate specific antigen cure rates appear constant between 2 and 9 ng./ml. J Urol 2002;167(1):103–11.
56. Noguchi M, Stamey TA, McNeal JE, Yemoto CM. Preoperative serum prostate specific antigen does not reflect biochemical failure rates after radical prostatectomy in men with large volume cancers. J Urol 2000;164(5):1596–600.
57. Shariat SF, Abdel-Aziz KF, Roehrborn CG, Lotan Y. Pre-operative percent free PSA predicts clinical outcomes in patients treated with radical prostatectomy with total PSA levels below 10 ng/ml. Eur Urol 2006;49(2):293–302.
58. Roehrborn CG, Boyle P, Gould AL, Waldstreicher J. Serum prostate-specific antigen as a predictor of prostate volume in men with benign prostatic hyperplasia. Urology 1999;53(3):581–9.
59. Roehrborn CG, McConnell J, Bonilla J, et al. Serum prostate specific antigen is a strong predictor of future prostate growth in men with benign prostatic hyperplasia. PROSCAR long-term efficacy and safety study. J Urol 2000;163(1):13–20.
60. Roehrborn CG, McConnell JD, Lieber M, et al. Serum prostate-specific antigen concentration is a powerful predictor of acute urinary retention and need for surgery in men with clinical benign prostatic hyperplasia. PLESS Study Group. Urology 1999;53(3):473–80.
61. Shariat SF, Karam JA, Roehrborn CG. Blood biomarkers for prostate cancer detection and prognosis. Future Oncol 2007;3(4):449–61.
62. Eichler K, Hempel S, Wilby J, Myers L, Bachmann LM, Kleijnen J. Diagnostic value of systematic biopsy methods in the investigation of prostate cancer: a systematic review. J Urol 2006;175(5):1605–12.
63. Albertsen PC, Hanley JA, Gleason DF, Barry MJ. Competing risk analysis of men aged 55 to 74 years at diagnosis managed conservatively for clinically localized prostate cancer. JAMA 1998;280(11):975–80.
64. Kattan MW, Giri D, Panageas KS, et al. A tool for predicting breast carcinoma mortality in women who do not receive adjuvant therapy. Cancer 2004;101(11):2509–15.
65. Kattan MW, Heller G, Brennan MF. A competing-risks nomogram for sarcoma-specific death following local recurrence. Stat Med 2003;22(22):3515–25.

66. Wang L, Hricak H, Kattan MW, et al. Prediction of seminal vesicle invasion in prostate cancer: incremental value of adding endorectal MR imaging to the Kattan nomogram. Radiology 2007;242(1): 182–8.

67. Wang L, Hricak H, Kattan MW, et al. Combined endorectal and phased-array MRI in the prediction of pelvic lymph node metastasis in prostate cancer. Ajr 2006;186(3):743–8.

68. Khoddami SM, Shariat SF, Lotan Y, et al. Predictive value of primary Gleason pattern 4 in patients with Gleason score 7 tumours treated with radical prostatectomy. BJU Int 2004;94(1):42–6.

69. Begg CB, Cramer LD, Venkatraman ES, Rosai J. Comparing tumour staging and grading systems: a case study and a review of the issues, using thymoma as a model. Stat Med 2000;19(15): 1997–2014.

70. D'Amico AV, Cote K, Loffredo M, Renshaw AA, Schultz D. Determinants of prostate cancer-specific survival after radiation therapy for patients with clinically localized prostate cancer. J Clin Oncol 2002;20(23):4567–73.

71. D'Amico AV, Cote K, Loffredo M, Renshaw AA, Schultz D. Determinants of prostate cancer specific survival following radiation therapy during the prostate specific antigen era. J Urol 2003;170(6 Pt 2):S42–6; discussion S6–7.

72. D'Amico AV, Whittington R, Malkowicz SB, et al. Biochemical outcome after radical prostatectomy or external beam radiation therapy for patients with clinically localized prostate carcinoma in the prostate specific antigen era. Cancer 2002;95(2):281–6.

73. D'Amico AV, Whittington R, Malkowicz SB, et al. Biochemical outcome after radical prostatectomy, external beam radiation therapy, or interstitial radiation therapy for clinically localized prostate cancer. JAMA 1998;280(11):969–74.

74. D'Amico AV, Moul J, Carroll PR, Sun L, Lubeck D, Chen MH. Cancer-specific mortality after surgery or radiation for patients with clinically localized prostate cancer managed during the prostate-specific antigen era. J Clin Oncol 2003;21(11):2163–72.

75. Karakiewicz PI, Shariat SF, Palapattu GS, et al. Nomogram for predicting disease recurrence after radical cystectomy for transitional cell carcinoma of the bladder. J Urol 2006;176(4 Pt 1):1354–61; discussion 61–2.

76. Kattan MW, Karpeh MS, Mazumdar M, Brennan MF. Postoperative nomogram for disease-specific survival after an R0 resection for gastric carcinoma. J Clin Oncol 2003;21(19):3647–50.

77. Kattan MW, Leung DH, Brennan MF. Postoperative nomogram for 12-year sarcoma-specific death. J Clin Oncol 2002;20(3):791–6.

78. Kattan MW, Reuter V, Motzer RJ, Katz J, Russo P. A postoperative prognostic nomogram for renal cell carcinoma. J Urol 2001;166(1):63–7.

79. Kattan MW, Zelefsky MJ, Kupelian PA, et al. Pretreatment nomogram that predicts 5-year probability of metastasis following three-dimensional conformal radiation therapy for localized prostate cancer. J Clin Oncol 2003;21(24):4568–71.

80. Mitchell JA, Cooperberg MR, Elkin EP, et al. Ability of 2 pretreatment risk assessment methods to predict prostate cancer recurrence after radical prostatectomy: data from CaPSURE. J Urol 2005;173(4):1126–31.

81. Meehl PE. Causes and effects of my disturbing little book. J Pers Assess 1986;50(3):370–5.

82. Antman EM, Cohen M, Bernink PJ, et al. The TIMI risk score for unstable angina/non-ST elevation MI: A method for prognostication and therapeutic decision making. JAMA 2000;284(7):835–42.

83. Cooperberg MR, Freedland SJ, Pasta DJ, et al. Multiinstitutional validation of the UCSF cancer of the prostate risk assessment for prediction of recurrence after radical prostatectomy. Cancer 2006;107(10):2384–91.

84. Cooperberg MR, Pasta DJ, Elkin EP, et al. The University of California, San Francisco Cancer of the Prostate Risk Assessment score: a straightforward and reliable preoperative predictor of disease recurrence after radical prostatectomy. J Urol 2005;173(6):1938–42.

85. Partin AW, Yoo J, Carter HB, et al. The use of prostate specific antigen, clinical stage and Gleason score to predict pathological stage in men with localized prostate cancer [see comments]. J Urol 1993;150(1):110–4.

86. Cagiannos I, Karakiewicz P, Eastham JA, et al. A preoperative nomogram identifying decreased risk of positive pelvic lymph nodes in patients with prostate cancer. J Urol 2003;170(5):1798–803.

87. Kattan MW, Eastham JA, Wheeler TM, et al. Counseling men with prostate cancer: a nomogram for predicting the presence of small, moderately differentiated, confined tumors. J Urol 2003;170(5):1792–7.

88. Koh H, Kattan MW, Scardino PT, et al. A nomogram to predict seminal vesicle invasion by the extent and location of cancer in systematic biopsy results. J Urol 2003;170(4 Pt 1):1203–8.

89. Briganti A, Chun FK, Salonia A, et al. Validation of a nomogram predicting the probability of lymph node invasion based on the extent of pelvic lymphadenectomy in patients with clinically localized prostate cancer. BJU Int 2006;98(4):788–93.

90. Gallina A, Chun FK, Briganti A, et al. Development and split-sample validation of a nomogram predicting the probability of seminal vesicle invasion at radical prostatectomy. Eur Urol 2007;52(1):98–105.

91. Chun FK, Steuber T, Erbersdobler A, et al. Development and internal validation of a nomogram predicting the probability of prostate cancer Gleason sum upgrading between biopsy and radical prostatectomy pathology. Eur Urol 2006;49(5):820–6.

92. D'Amico AV, Renshaw AA, Arsenault L, Schultz D, Richie JP. Clinical predictors of upgrading to Gleason grade 4 or 5 disease at radical prostatectomy: potential implications for patient selection for radiation and androgen suppression therapy. Int J Radiat Oncol Biol Phys 1999;45(4):841–6.

93. Stephenson AJ, Shariat SF, Zelefsky MJ, et al. Salvage radiotherapy for recurrent prostate cancer after radical prostatectomy. JAMA 2004;291(11):1325–32.

94. Kattan MW, Cooper RB. A simulation of factors affecting machine learning techniques: an examination of partitioning and class proportions. Onmega Int J Mgmt Sci 2000;28:501.

95. Marshall RJ. The use of classification and regression trees in clinical epidemiology. J Clin Epidemiol 2001;54(6):603–9.

96. Ohori M, Kattan MW, Koh H, et al. Predicting the presence and side of extracapsular extension: a nomogram for staging prostate cancer. J Urol 2004;171(5):1844–9; discussion 9.

97. Steuber T, Graefen M, Haese A, et al. Validation of a nomogram for prediction of side specific extracapsular extension at radical prostatectomy. J Urol 2006;175(3 Pt 1):939–44; discussion 44.

98. Dayhoff JE, DeLeo JM. Artificial neural networks: opening the black box. Cancer 2001;91(8 Suppl):1615–35.

99. Sargent DJ. Comparison of artificial neural networks with other statistical approaches: results from medical data sets. Cancer 2001;91(8 Suppl):1636–42.

100. Schwarzer G, Schumacher M. Artificial neural networks for diagnosis and prognosis in prostate cancer. Semin Urol Oncol 2002;20(2):89–95.

101. Terrin N, Schmid CH, Griffith JL, D'Agostino RB, Selker HP. External validity of predictive models: a comparison of logistic regression, classification trees, and neural networks. J Clin Epidemiol 2003;56(8):721–9.

102. Stephan C, Cammann H, Semjonow A, et al. Multicenter evaluation of an artificial neural network to increase the prostate cancer detection rate and reduce unnecessary biopsies. Clin Chem 2002;48(8):1279–87.

103. Karakiewicz PI, Benayoun S, Kattan MW, et al. Development and validation of a nomogram predicting the outcome of prostate biopsy based on patient age, digital rectal examination and serum prostate specific antigen. J Urol 2005;173(6):1930–4.

104. Chun FK, Briganti A, Graefen M, et al. Development and external validation of an extended 10-core biopsy nomogram. Eur Urol 2007;52(2):436–45.

105. Chun FK, Briganti A, Graefen M, et al. Development and external validation of an extended repeat biopsy nomogram. J Urol 2007;177(2):510–5.

106. O'Dowd G J, Miller MC, Orozco R, Veltri RW. Analysis of repeated biopsy results within 1 year after a noncancer diagnosis. Urology 2000;55(4):553–9.

107. Lopez-Corona E, Ohori M, Scardino PT, Reuter VE, Gonen M, Kattan MW. A nomogram for predicting a positive repeat prostate biopsy in patients with a previous negative biopsy session. J Urol 2003;170(4 Pt 1):1184–8; discussion 8.

108. Yanke BV, Gonen M, Scardino PT, Kattan MW. Validation of a nomogram for predicting positive repeat biopsy for prostate cancer. J Urol 2005;173(2):421–4.

109. Penson DF, Grossfeld GD, Li YP, Henning JM, Lubeck DP, Carroll PR. How well does the Partin nomogram predict pathological stage after radical prostatectomy in a community based population? Results of the cancer of the prostate strategic urological research endeavor. J Urol 2002;167(4):1653–7; discussion 7–8.

110. Augustin H, Eggert T, Wenske S, et al. Comparison of accuracy between the Partin tables of 1997 and 2001 to predict final pathological stage in clinically localized prostate cancer. J Urol 2004;171(1):177–81.

111. Partin AW, Mangold LA, Lamm DM, Walsh PC, Epstein JI, Pearson JD. Contemporary update of prostate cancer staging nomograms (Partin Tables) for the new millennium. Urology 2001;58(6):843–8.

112. Heidenreich A, Varga Z, Von Knobloch R. Extended pelvic lymphadenectomy in patients undergoing radical prostatectomy: high incidence of lymph node metastasis. J Urol 2002;167(4):1681–6.

113. Bader P, Burkhard FC, Markwalder R, Studer UE. Is a limited lymph node dissection an adequate staging procedure for prostate cancer? J Urol 2002;168(2):514–8; discussion 8.

114. Briganti A, Chun FK, Salonia A, et al. Validation of a nomogram predicting the probability of lymph node invasion among patients undergoing radical prostatectomy and an extended pelvic lymphadenectomy. Eur Urol 2006;49(6):1019–26; discussion 26–7.

115. Briganti A, Chun FK, Salonia A, et al. A nomogram for staging of exclusive nonobturator lymph node metastases in men with localized prostate cancer. Eur Urol 2007;51(1):112–9; discussion 9–20.

116. Johansson JE, Andren O, Andersson SO, et al. Natural history of early, localized prostate cancer. JAMA 2004;291(22):2713–9.

117. Schroder FH. Prostate cancer: to screen or not to screen? BMJ (Clinical research ed) 1993;306(6875):407–8.

118. Steuber T, Chun FK, Erbersdobler A, et al. Development and internal validation of preoperative transition zone prostate cancer nomogram. Urology 2006;68(6):1295–300.

119. Stephenson AJ, Scardino PT, Eastham JA, et al. Postoperative nomogram predicting the 10-year probability of prostate cancer recurrence after radical prostatectomy. J Clin Oncol 2005;23(28):7005–12.

120. Stephenson AJ, Scardino PT, Eastham JA, et al. Preoperative nomogram predicting the 10-year probability of prostate cancer recurrence after radical prostatectomy. J Natl Cancer Inst 2006;98(10):715–7.

121. Hull GW, Rabbani F, Abbas F, Wheeler TM, Kattan MW, Scardino PT. Cancer control with radical prostatectomy alone in 1,000 consecutive patients. J Urol 2002;167(2 Pt 1):528–34.

122. Blumberg J. PDA applications for physicians. ASCO News 2004 2004;16:S4–6.

123. Bianco FJ, Jr., Kattan MW, Scardino PT, Powell IJ, Pontes JE, Wood DP, Jr. Radical prostatectomy nomograms in black American men: accuracy and applicability. J Urol 2003;170(1):73–6; discussion 6–7.

124. Pound CR, Partin AW, Eisenberger MA, Chan DW, Pearson JD, Walsh PC. Natural history of progression after PSA elevation following radical prostatectomy [see comments]. JAMA 1999;281(17):1591–7.

125. Freedland SJ, Humphreys EB, Mangold LA, et al. Risk of prostate cancer-specific mortality following biochemical recurrence after radical prostatectomy. JAMA 2005;294(4):433–9.

126. Cagiannos I, Karakiewicz P, Graefen M, et al. Is year of radical prostatectomy a predictor of outcome in prostate cancer? J Urol 2004;171(2 Pt 1):692–6.

127. Kattan MW, Zelefsky MJ, Kupelian PA, Scardino PT, Fuks Z, Leibel SA. Pretreatment nomogram for predicting the outcome of three-dimensional conformal radiotherapy in prostate cancer. J Clin Oncol 2000;18(19):3352–9.

128. Kattan MW, Potters L, Blasko JC, et al. Pretreatment nomogram for predicting freedom from recurrence after permanent prostate brachytherapy in prostate cancer. Urology 2001;58(3):393–9.

129. Pound CR, Partin AW, Eisenberger MA, Chan DW, Pearson JD, Walsh PC. Natural history of progression after PSA elevation following radical prostatectomy. JAMA 1999;281(17):1591–7.

130. Leventis AK, Shariat SF, Kattan MW, Butler EB, Wheeler TM, Slawin KM. Prediction of response to salvage radiation therapy in patients with prostate cancer recurrence after radical prostatectomy. J Clin Oncol 2001;19(4):1030–9.

131. Lee AK, D'Amico AV. Utility of prostate-specific antigen kinetics in addition to clinical factors in the selection of patients for salvage local therapy. J Clin Oncol 2005;23(32):8192–7.

132. Dotan ZA, Bianco FJ, Jr., Rabbani F, et al. Pattern of prostate-specific antigen (PSA) failure dictates the probability of a positive bone scan in patients with an increasing PSA after radical prostatectomy. J Clin Oncol 2005;23(9):1962–8.

133. Slovin SF, Wilton AS, Heller G, Scher HI. Time to detectable metastatic disease in patients with rising prostate-specific antigen values following surgery or radiation therapy. Clin Cancer Res 2005;11(24 Pt 1):8669–73.

134. Smaletz O, Scher HI, Small EJ, et al. Nomogram for overall survival of patients with progressive metastatic prostate cancer after castration. J Clin Oncol 2002;20(19):3972–82.

135. Halabi S, Small EJ, Kantoff PW, et al. Prognostic model for predicting survival in men with hormone-refractory metastatic prostate cancer. J Clin Oncol 2003;21(7):1232–7.

136. Porter CR, Gallina A, Kodama K, et al. Prostate cancer-specific survival in men treated with hormonal therapy after failure of radical prostatectomy. Eur Urol 2007;52(2):446–54.

137. Cowen ME, Halasyamani LK, Kattan MW. Predicting life expectancy in men with clinically localized prostate cancer. J Urol 2006;175(1):99–103.

138. Chun FK, Briganti A, Jeldres C, et al. Tumour volume and high grade tumour volume are the best predictors of pathologic stage and biochemical recurrence after radical prostatectomy. Eur J Cancer 2007;43(3):536–43.

139. Stephenson AJ, Smith A, Kattan MW, et al. Integration of gene expression profiling and clinical variables to predict prostate carcinoma recurrence after radical prostatectomy. Cancer 2005;104(2):290–8.

140. Hricak H, Choyke PL, Eberhardt SC, Leibel SA, Scardino PT. Imaging prostate cancer: a multidisciplinary perspective. Radiology 2007;243(1):28–53.

141. Hricak H, Wang L, Wei DC, et al. The role of preoperative endorectal magnetic resonance imaging in the decision regarding whether to preserve or resect neurovascular bundles during radical retropubic prostatectomy. Cancer 2004;100(12):2655–63.

142. Zakian KL, Sircar K, Hricak H, et al. Correlation of proton MR spectroscopic imaging with Gleason score based on step-section pathologic analysis after radical prostatectomy. Radiology 2005;234(3):804–14.

143. Poulakis V, Witzsch U, de Vries R, et al. Preoperative neural network using combined magnetic resonance imaging variables, prostate-specific antigen, and Gleason score for predicting prostate cancer biochemical recurrence after radical prostatectomy. Urology 2004;64(6):1165–70.

144. Shukla-Dave A, Hricak H, Kattan MW, et al. The utility of magnetic resonance imaging and spectroscopy for predicting insignificant prostate cancer: an initial analysis. BJU Int 2007;99(4):786–93.

145. Babaian RJ, Fritsche HA, Zhang Z, Zhang KH, Madyastha KR, Barnhill SD. Evaluation of prostasure index in the detection of prostate cancer: a preliminary report. Urology 1998;51(1):132–6.

146. Virtanen A, Gomari M, Kranse R, Stenman UH. Estimation of prostate cancer probability by logistic regression: free and total prostate-specific antigen, digital rectal examination, and heredity are significant variables. Clin Chem 1999;45(7):987–94.

147. Finne P, Finne R, Auvinen A, et al. Predicting the outcome of prostate biopsy in screen-positive men by a multilayer perceptron network. Urology 2000;56(3):418–22.

148. Horninger W, Bartsch G, Snow PB, Brandt JM, Partin AW. The problem of cutoff levels in a screened population: appropriateness of informing screenees about their risk of having prostate carcinoma. Cancer 2001;91(8 Suppl):1667–72.

149. Kalra P, Togami J, Bansal BSG, et al. A neurocomputational model for prostate carcinoma detection. Cancer 2003;98(9):1849–54.

150. Finne P, Finne R, Bangma C, et al. Algorithms based on prostate-specific antigen (PSA), free PSA, digital rectal examination and prostate volume reduce false-positive PSA results in prostate cancer screening. Int J Cancer 2004;111(2):310–5.

151. Porter CR, Gamito EJ, Crawford ED, et al. Model to predict prostate biopsy outcome in large screening population with independent validation in referral setting. Urology 2005;65(5):937–41.

152. Remzi M, Anagnostou T, Ravery V, et al. An artificial neural network to predict the outcome of repeat prostate biopsies. Urology 2003;62(3):456–60.

153. Walz J, Graefen M, Chun FK, et al. High incidence of prostate cancer detected by saturation biopsy after previous negative biopsy series. Eur Urol 2006;50(3):498–505.

154. Carlson GD, Calvanese CB, Partin AW. An algorithm combining age, total prostate-specific antigen (PSA), and percent free PSA to predict prostate cancer: results on 4298 cases. Urology 1998;52(3):455–61.

155. Djavan B, Remzi M, Zlotta A, Seitz C, Snow P, Marberger M. Novel artificial neural network for early detection of prostate cancer. J Clin Oncol 2002;20(4):921–9.

156. Matsui Y, Utsunomiya N, Ichioka K, et al. The use of artificial neural network analysis to improve the predictive accuracy of prostate biopsy in the Japanese population. Jpn J Clin Oncol 2004;34(10):602–7.

157. Benecchi L. Neuro-fuzzy system for prostate cancer diagnosis. Urology 2006;68(2):357–61.

158. Kattan MW, Stapleton AM, Wheeler TM, Scardino PT. Evaluation of a nomogram used to predict the pathologic stage of clinically localized prostate carcinoma. Cancer 1997;79(3):528–37.

159. Narayan P, Gajendran V, Taylor SP, et al. The role of transrectal ultrasound-guided biopsy-based staging, preoperative serum prostate-specific antigen, and biopsy Gleason score in prediction of final pathologic diagnosis in prostate cancer. Urology 1995;46(2):205–12.

160. Blute ML, Bergstralh EJ, Partin AW, et al. Validation of Partin tables for predicting pathological stage of clinically localized prostate cancer. J Urol 2000;164(5):1591–5.

161. Epstein JI, Walsh PC, Carmichael M, Brendler CB. Pathologic and clinical findings to predict tumor extent of nonpalpable (stage T1c) prostate cancer. JAMA 1994;271(5):368–74.

162. Carter HB, Epstein JI. Prediction of significant cancer in men with stage T1c adenocarcinoma of the prostate. World J Urol 1997;15(6):359–63.

163. Goto Y, Ohori M, Arakawa A, Kattan MW, Wheeler TM, Scardino PT. Distinguishing clinically important from unimportant prostate cancers before treatment: value of systematic biopsies. J Urol 1996;156(3):1059–63.

164. Chun FK, Briganti A, Shariat SF, et al. Significant upgrading affects a third of men diagnosed with prostate cancer: predictive nomogram and internal validation. BJU Int 2006;98(2):329–34.

165. Peller PA, Young DC, Marmaduke DP, Marsh WL, Badalament RA. Sextant prostate biopsies. A histopathologic correlation with radical prostatectomy specimens. Cancer 1995;75(2):530–8.

166. Ackerman DA, Barry JM, Wicklund RA, Olson N, Lowe BA. Analysis of risk factors associated with prostate cancer extension to the surgical margin and pelvic node metastasis at radical prostatectomy. J Urol 1993;150(6):1845–50.

167. Rabbani F, Bastar A, Fair WR. Site specific predictors of positive margins at radical prostatectomy: an argument for risk based modification of technique. J Urol 1998;160(5):1727–33.

168. Bostwick DG, Qian J, Bergstralh E, et al. Prediction of capsular perforation and seminal vesicle invasion in prostate cancer. J Urol 1996;155(4):1361–7.

169. Gilliland FD, Hoffman RM, Hamilton A, et al. Predicting extracapsular extension of prostate cancer in men treated with radical prostatectomy: results from the population based prostate cancer outcomes study. J Urol 1999;162(4):1341–5.

170. Badalament RA, Miller MC, Peller PA, et al. An algorithm for predicting nonorgan confined prostate cancer using the results obtained from sextant core biopsies with prostate specific antigen level. J Urol 1996;156(4):1375–80.

171. Pisansky TM, Blute ML, Suman VJ, Bostwick DG, Earle JD, Zincke H. Correlation of pretherapy prostate cancer characteristics with seminal vesicle invasion in radical prostatectomy specimens. Int J Radiat Oncol Biol Phys 1996;36(3):585–91.

172. Baccala A, Jr., Reuther AM, Bianco FJ, Jr., Scardino PT, Kattan MW, Klein EA. Complete resection of seminal vesicles at radical prostatectomy results in substantial long-term disease-free survival: multi-institutional study of 6740 patients. Urology 2007;69(3):536–40.

173. Bluestein DL, Bostwick DG, Bergstralh EJ, Oesterling JE. Eliminating the need for bilateral pelvic lymphadenectomy in select patients with prostate cancer. J Urol 1994;151(5):1315–20.

174. Roach M, 3rd, Marquez C, Yuo HS, et al. Predicting the risk of lymph node involvement using the pre-treatment prostate specific antigen and Gleason score in men with clinically localized prostate cancer. Int J Radiat Oncol Biol Phys 1994;28(1):33–7.

175. Batuello JT, Gamito EJ, Crawford ED, et al. Artificial neural network model for the assessment of lymph node spread in patients with clinically localized prostate cancer. Urology 2001;57(3):481–5.

176. Briganti A, Karakiewicz PI, Chun FK, et al. Percentage of positive biopsy cores can improve the ability to predict lymph node invasion in patients undergoing radical prostatectomy and extended pelvic lymph node dissection. Eur Urol 2007;51(6):1573–81.

177. Greene KL, Meng MV, Elkin EP, et al. Validation of the Kattan preoperative nomogram for prostate cancer recurrence using a community based cohort: results from cancer of the prostate strategic urological research endeavor (capsure). J Urol 2004;171(6 Pt 1):2255–9.

178. Graefen M, Augustin H, Karakiewicz PI, et al. [Can nomograms derived in the U.S. applied to German patients? A study about the validation of preoperative nomograms predicting the risk of recurrence after radical prostatectomy]. Urologe A 2003;42(5):685–92.

179. Graefen M, Noldus J, Pichlmeier U, et al. Early prostate-specific antigen relapse after radical retropubic prostatectomy: prediction on the basis of preoperative and postoperative tumor characteristics. Eur Urol 1999;36(1):21–30.

180. Tewari A, Issa M, El-Galley R, et al. Genetic adaptive neural network to predict biochemical failure after radical prostatectomy: a multi-institutional study. Mol urol 2001;5(4):163–9.

181. Bauer JJ, Connelly RR, Seterhenn IA, et al. Biostatistical modeling using traditional preoperative and pathological prognostic variables in the selection of men at high risk for disease recurrence after radical prostatectomy for prostate cancer. J Urol 1998;159(3):929–33.

182. Moul JW, Connelly RR, Lubeck DP, et al. Predicting risk of prostate specific antigen recurrence after radical prostatectomy with the Center for Prostate Disease Research and Cancer of the Prostate Strategic Urologic Research Endeavor databases. J Urol 2001;166(4):1322–7.

183. Potter SR, Miller MC, Mangold LA, et al. Genetically engineered neural networks for predicting prostate cancer progression after radical prostatectomy. Urology 1999;54(5):791–5.

184. Ramsden AR, Chodak G. An analysis of risk factors for biochemical progression in patients with seminal vesicle invasion: validation of Kattan's nomogram in a pathological subgroup. BJU Int 2004;93(7):961–4.

185. Stamey TA, Yemoto CM, McNeal JE, Sigal BM, Johnstone IM. Prostate cancer is highly predictable: a prognostic equation based on all morphological variables in radical prostatectomy specimens. J Urol 2000;163(4):1155–60.

186. McAleer SJ, Schultz D, Whittington R, et al. PSA outcome following radical prostatectomy for patients with localized prostate cancer stratified by prostatectomy findings and the preoperative PSA level. Urol Oncol 2005;23(5):311–7.

187. Duchesne GM, Bloomfield D, Wall P. Identification of intermediate-risk prostate cancer patients treated with radiotherapy suitable for neoadjuvant hormone studies. Radiother Oncol 1996;38(1):7–12.

188. Pisansky TM, Kahn MJ, Bostwick DG. An enhanced prognostic system for clinically localized carcinoma of the prostate. Cancer 1997;79(11):2154–61.

189. Zagars GK, Pollack A, von Eschenbach AC. Prognostic factors for clinically localized prostate carcinoma: analysis of 938 patients irradiated in the prostate specific antigen era. Cancer 1997;79(7):1370–80.

190. Shipley WU, Thames HD, Sandler HM, et al. Radiation therapy for clinically localized prostate cancer: a multi-institutional pooled analysis. JAMA 1999;281(17):1598–604.

191. Potters L, Morgenstern C, Calugaru E, et al. 12-year outcomes following permanent prostate brachytherapy in patients with clinically localized prostate cancer. J Urol 2005;173(5):1562–6.

192. Ragde H, Elgamal AA, Snow PB, et al. Ten-year disease free survival after transperineal sonography-guided iodine-125 brachytherapy with or without 45-gray external beam irradiation in the treatment of patients with clinically localized, low to high Gleason grade prostate carcinoma. Cancer 1998;83(5):989–1001.

193. Stephenson AJ, Scardino PT, Kattan MW, et al. Predicting the outcome of salvage radiation therapy for recurrent prostate cancer after radical prostatectomy. J Clin Oncol 2007;25(15):2035–41.

194. Partin AW, Pearson JD, Landis PK, et al. Evaluation of serum prostate-specific antigen velocity after radical prostatectomy to distinguish local recurrence from distant metastases. Urology 1994;43(5):649–59.

195. Zhou P, Chen MH, McLeod D, Carroll PR, Moul JW, D'Amico AV. Predictors of prostate cancer-specific mortality after radical prostatectomy or radiation therapy. J Clin Oncol 2005;23(28):6992–8.

196. Svatek R, Karakiewicz PI, Shulman M, Karam J, Perrotte P, Benaim E. Pre-treatment nomogram for disease-specific survival of patients with chemotherapy-naive androgen independent prostate cancer. Eur Urol 2006;49(4):666–74.

197. Albertsen PC, Fryback DG, Storer BE, Kolon TF, Fine J. The impact of co-morbidity on life expectancy among men with localized prostate cancer. J Urol 1996;156(1):127–32.

198. Walz J, Gallina A, Saad F, et al. A nomogram predicting 10-year life expectancy in candidates for radical prostatectomy or radiotherapy for prostate cancer. J Clin Oncol 2007;25(24):3576–81.

199. Shariat SF, Walz J, Roehrborn CG, et al. External validation of a biomarker-based preoperative nomogram predicts biochemical recurrence after radical prostatectomy. J Clin Oncol 2008;26(9):1526–31.

200. Shariat SF, Park S, Trinh QD, Roehrborn CG, Slawin KM, Karakiewicz PI. Plasminogen activation inhibitor-1 improves the predictive accuracy of prostate cancer nomograms. J Urol 2007;178(4 Pt 1):1229–36; discussion 36–7.

# 11 Decision Aid Criteria and Artificial Neural Networks for Optimizing Prostate Cancer Risk Prediction

*Felix K.-H. Chun and Pierre I. Karakiewicz*

## CONTENTS

## SUMMARY

Artificial neural networks (ANN) represent an interesting alternative methodological approach to predict prostate cancer related outcomes on an individual basis. Constructed by flexible, nonlinear regression models, they have the potential to offer enhanced goodness-of-fit and predictive ability over traditional linear models. However, this potential comes at the price of increased complexity in modeling building and validation. Therefore, despite their promotion in the field of prostate cancer since the early 1990s, due to less transparency and the need for computational infrastructure, ANNs have become less popular. Their utility hinges on appropriate implementation and validation, which unfortunately is only recently being recognized and addressed. In this chapter, the reader is provided with a descriptive and an analytic tabulation of decision aid criteria for ANNs for prostate cancer detection.

**Key Words:** Artificial neural network, Prostate cancer, Prediction models, Decision aid, Nomogram.

From: *Current Clinical Urology: Prostate Cancer Screening*, Edited by: D. P. Ankerst et al.
DOI 10.1007/978-1-60327-281-0_11 © Humana Press, a part of Springer Science+Business Media, LLC 2009

Artificial neural network (ANN) models represent an interesting alternative to traditional regression modeling approaches. They may assist the clinician on an individual level as a predictive or prognostic tool for medical decision-making in the most evidence-based and bias-free fashion *(1–3)*. In fact, they address numerous outcomes, ranging from prediction of biopsy outcome *(4)* in men considered at risk of prostate cancer (PCa) to the probability of mortality from hormone-refractory PCa *(5)*. Despite apparent differences in the methodological approaches underlying decision aids, standard assessment criteria may be applied to assess the qualities and/or weaknesses of decision aids. In the current chapter we outline criteria for decision aids and how these affect the application of ANNs.

# CRITERIA FOR DECISION AIDS
## *Discrimination*

Discrimination, or the ability to correctly identify the individuals with the endpoint of interest, represents the most important characteristic of all predictive and prognostic models. Discrimination is synonymous with model accuracy or predictive accuracy and plays a primary role in model validation.

Current statistical methods offer the possibility of quantifying a model's predictive accuracy. This is usually performed within an external cohort, which represents the gold-standard method for quantifying models' accuracy. Alternatively, statistical methods such as bootstrapping, split sample, or leave-one-out methods may be used. These methods rely on the same sample that was used for the model development and are termed internal validation. The use of the same sample to develop and validate a model may be associated with an inflated accuracy. Therefore external validation is preferred, except for excessively rare pathologies where sample sizes are critically small *(1,6–14)*.

In analyses where time to event is not considered, the discriminatory ability of predictive accuracy is summarized by the area underneath the receiver operating characteristic (ROC) curve (AUC), expressed as a percentage. In models that rely on time to event analyses and are subject to data censoring, the AUC method is replaced with Harrell's concordance index *(15)*. For both methods, predictive accuracy ranges from 50 to 100%, where 50% is equivalent to a flip of a coin and 100% represents perfect prediction. No model is perfect; most commonly reported predictive accuracy values range from 70 to 85%.

## *Model Calibration*

Discrimination or accuracy indicates the overall ability of the model to predict the outcome of interest. However, neither the AUC nor Harrell's index provide information about the ability to correctly predict the probability of a given outcome of interest in specific patient subgroups. For example, some models may be ideally suited to predict in high-risk patients, but may predict poorly in low-risk patients. Other models may predict well throughout the entire range of predictions. Calibration plots graphically display the relationship between the model's predicted rate and the observed rate of the outcome of interest. A 1:1 ratio between predicted and observed, which corresponds to a 45 degree line, would be expected from an ideal model *(6,13,16–18)*.

## Generalizability

Decision aids depend heavily on their development cohort and reflect the characteristics of these cohorts. Thus prior to implementing a new or established tool, the clinician should ensure that it was validated in patients with similar disease characteristics as those in the target population *(6,13,16,17)*. For example, since ethnicity is a known confounder of PCa rate at needle biopsy, Suzuki et al. *(18)* pioneered the first race-specific initial prostate biopsy nomogram. Yanke et al. *(19)* developed a PCa risk-prediction tool for African-Americans.

## Level of Complexity

Excessively complex models that rely on a variety of predictors that are difficult to access are clearly impractical in busy clinical practice. Similarly, models that depend on complex computational infrastructure might pose applicability problems. For example, ANNs may accurately predict several outcomes of interest but their use might be restricted due to lack of access to their code or lack of computer infrastructure, which provides their formulae. Probability tables, decision-trees, and nomograms are user-friendly, paper-based alternatives, which circumvent these problems *(12,20–28)*.

## Head-to-Head Comparisons

For comparing decision aids' characteristics one should ensure that accuracy, calibration, and generalizability are adequate, and that the level of adequacy or inadequacy be judged according to established models, with the intent of determining whether the new model offers advantages relative to available alternatives *(1,6,10,12–14)*. The most valid comparisons are obtained when two or more models of interest are tested in parallel applied to the same target population, which is termed a head-to-head comparison. Head-to-head comparisons of clinicians' and nomogram predictions have been completed and showed that decision aids (specifically nomograms) predict more accurately than clinicians *(29,30)*. In PCa, Ross et al. *(29)* showed that urologists' predictions of biochemical recurrence (BCR) after radical prostatectomy (RP) were inferior to those of a nomogram (concordance-index decreased from 67 to 55%, $-12\%$, $p<0.05$).

## LIMITATIONS OF DECISION AIDS

Despite their advantages, decision aids also have limitations. Most PCa decision aids are based on either single center series and/or represent data of high-volume surgeons/pathologists from highly specialized tertiary care centers. These characteristics may bias the data toward better results. Therefore, population-specific external validations are very important, before model implementation. Other limitations of existing models consist of the following *(7,28,31–34)*:

- Despite prospective data collection, decision-aid modeling itself represents a retrospective statistical methodological approach.
- Patient selection criteria need to be considered. For example, patients who received neoadjuvant hormonal therapy are excluded in many prognostic models for outcomes following therapy. Consequently, such models cannot be applied for predictions for patients receiving hormonal therapy.

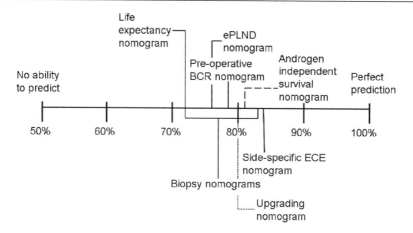

**Fig. 1.** Predictive accuracy levels of prostate cancer nomograms.
ePLND: extended pelvic lymph node dissection BCR; biochemical recurrence ECE; extracapsular extension

- Variable inclusion criteria are equally important. For example, most decision aids use total PSA. Other PSA isoforms may be more informative. Different PSA assays may affect the discriminant properties of various nomograms, for example, type of PSA assay affected performance of nomograms predicting the outcome of prostate biopsy *(35)*.
- Contemporaneity. Stage and grade migration may affect the accuracy and calibration of older tools. Constant updating is therefore necessary to ensure validity *(36)*.
- Surrogate versus clinically proven endpoints. Prognostic models predict a range of outcomes, from PSA recurrence to PCa mortality. Models predicting surrogate endpoints, such as PSA recurrence, are usually considered less valuable than models predicting clinically proven endpoints, such as mortality. Nonetheless, both are important. PSA recurrence predictions may help with early identification of individuals at risk of rapid disease progression in whom early hormonal therapy might be particularly indicated *(5,37–39)*.
- Suboptimal predictive accuracy. To date there are no perfect predictive or prognostic models (100% accuracy). Due to several sources of variability in both predictor variables and in the outcomes, models are usually between 70 and 85% accurate as demonstrated in Fig. 1 *(10)*. Biomarkers may improve the accuracy of standard predictor variables *(40)*.

## CLINICAL VALUE OF DECISION AIDS

Controversy surrounds the question of the clinical value of decision aids. Increases in predictive accuracy related to decision aids may not only be of statistical significance but more importantly, clinically meaningful. For example, in a cohort of 1,000 patients, an increase in predictive accuracy of 3% is synonymous with 30 additional correctly classified patients. These patients may then be provided with the most appropriate follow-up or treatment. The use of decision aids may better classify patients between those with or without disease, for example. To date it is not known whether the use of statistical models contributes to better population health, but despite this lack of proven effect on population health, the use of predictive and/or prognostic models results in most accurate risk prediction. Patients and physicians deserve to be provided with the most accurate risk estimates at all times *(1,30)*. Specific triggers for more frequent use of predictive and prognostic tools include the following:

1. Advances in therapeutics have opened numerous treatment options and men no longer accept paternalistic physician-centered treatment decision-making. Instead, they demand to know the efficacy and detailed side effect profiles of treatment alternatives.
2. The patient, and not the physician, is increasingly recognized as a pivotal player in medical decision-making. For example, the American Urological Association recommends detailed informed consent prior to PSA testing.
3. Health care "consumerism" is a growing phenomenon in North America and Europe. Patients select what option of health care to purchase, rather than passively receiving a given treatment modality.
4. Attention to bioethical considerations has greatly increased over the past decade and has promoted autonomous decision-making.

These considerations may further motivate clinicians to use decision tools. Their motivation may also stem from the wealth of clinical data that are used for the development and validation of each model. Most decision tools are based on thousands of observations, and it is virtually impossible to achieve that level of clinical exposure and expertise on an individual level. Moreover, most clinicians do not have the capacity to systematically record or remember the risk characteristics of several thousands of patients. Additionally, unlike computers, clinicians are incapable of systematically and cumulatively processing the recorded risk characteristics and outcomes of historic cases and to derive an estimated probability of outcome for a new case at hand. Thus, it may be expected that the majority of physician-derived estimates are not as accurate as computer-derived decision models. Despite this advantage, decision tools are not meant to replace clinical judgment. Their input needs to be weighed against the pros and cons of several other considerations, such as comorbidity, cost, social, religious, or emotional considerations *(7,10,17,29,41)*.

Within this context, promising methodologies in urologic oncology such as ANNs need to be critically assessed. Herein based on a literature review and on own data, we critically assess the ability of ANNs for risk stratification of prostate cancer patients.

## ARTIFICIAL NEURAL NETWORKS

ANNs have been an area of research for the past 50 years. Rosenblatt, McCulloch and Rumelhart pioneered this approach *(20,41)*. In 1994 Snow and co-workers pioneered the first ANNs to predict prostate biopsy outcome with data from 1,787 men with a PSA in excess of 4 ng/ml *(21)*.

## DEFINITION OF ARTIFICIAL NEURAL NETWORKS

Artificial (feed forward) neural networks (ANN), synonymously called multilayer perceptrons, are named according to the physiologic neuronal arrangement, where neurons, as specialized entities, are interconnected, receiving signals propagated throughout the system. The nervous system has the capacity to learn by receiving weighted signals from specialized systems. A typical ANN consists of an input layer, at least one hidden layer and an output layer (Fig. 2). Each layer is represented by a various number

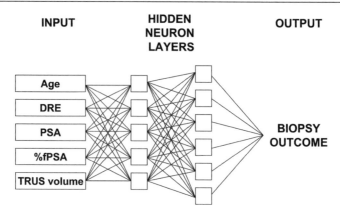

**Fig. 2.** Schematic display of an ANN.

DRE; digital rectal examination PSA; prostate-specific antigen %fPSA; percent-free prostate-specific antigen TRUS; transrectal ultrasound derived total prostate volume

of units, which are called neurons or intelligent nodes. These units form a layer and are, like human neurons, interconnected. The units in the input layer relate to the available information (i.e., risk factors) to predict a certain outcome of interest. Increasing the number of hidden neuron layers and units increases complexity and determines the ANNs ability to learn. Output layers in the field of prostate cancer predictions are mainly binary, e.g., positive versus negative biopsy outcome *(8,14,20,21,41–48)*.

For example as displayed in Fig. 2, input or risk factors such as age, digital rectal examination, prostate-specific antigen (PSA), percent-free PSA (%fPSA), and transrectal ultrasound derived prostate volume (TRUS volume) represent the input layer variables. These are combined to form hidden neuron layers or intermediate predictions, which are again combined to derive a probability for whether or not an individual patient needs to undergo a prostate biopsy.

## ADVANTAGES OF ARTIFICIAL NEURAL NETWORKS

Compared to other modeling techniques the advantage of ANNs is their ability to allow nonlinear relations between the dependent and independent risk factors. This flexibility promotes their theoretical superiority compared to standard risk-stratification models based on logistic or Cox regression analyses. Ultimately, this advantage should translate into superior predictive accuracy, such as increased AUC, sensitivity, specificity, and other measures of model generalizability or performance *(41)*.

## MODELING OF ARTIFICIAL NEURAL NETWORKS

Typically, modeling of an ANN consists of three distinct steps: training, testing, and validation, each relying on its own distinct independent sample of patients. Within the training process number of hidden layers (i.e., model complexity, correlated with overfitting) as well as estimation of weights summarizing individual predictors' contributions are determined. The ANN "learns" within this testing process by optimizing predictions to outcomes in the test set. Thus, this step ideally minimizes error and tells the model when to stop training. The last step consists of model generalization, also called validation, which displays its performance. This step uses an independent patient sample which is fed-forward within the new model to derive its predictive accuracy, AUC, sensitivity, or specificity. As suggested by Schwarzer et al. *(41)* cross-validation optimizes the efficiency of the analysis over single validation. Although, the structure of neural networks can be presented in schematic form (Fig. 2), the actual effect of the input variables on the output cannot. This is due to the numerous interactions that are allowed when data are processed from the input units toward hidden neuron layers and then eventually to one or several output units. For example, ANNs predicting the outcome of needle biopsy have been generally limited to one layer of hidden neurons. The use of several layers of hidden neurons renders the computational data manipulations highly complex and lacks transparency, which results in the black box connotation that is associated with ANNs *(19,20)*.

Multiple interactions are allowed between input variables at each level, which are weighted to promote the most accurate prediction of the outcome of interest. At each hidden neuron, binary outputs are transmitted to the next level of hidden neurons. These resemble multiple outputs within a logistic regression model. Interactions between these outputs, which can again be weighted to further promote accuracy, increase the complexity of the model. The process contributes to highly accurate prediction of the outcome of interest, which in several reported prostate biopsy ANNs, closely approximates the 74–91% range. Although accuracy is of key importance, models that underlie predictions need to be tested before their discriminant ability can be taken at face value. Unfortunately, lack of familiarity with biostatistical considerations frequently severely undermines the validity of reported predicted accuracy estimates, which are exaggerated and reported in a biased and methodologically incorrect way. Thus, despite good intentions, many investigators report spuriously high ability to predict the outcome of interest, for example, due to unintentional omission of the training set *(40–47)*.

## CONCERNS WITH CURRENT NEURAL NETWORK APPLICATIONS

Several important problems have been identified with the methodology of ANNs. The potential for the emergence of these problems was signaled as early as 1977, when statistical packages, such as SPSS, SAS, and others became widely available for nonspecialists. Despite these early and continuing warnings, a recent review of existing ANNs for prediction and diagnostic classification in oncology found numerous crucial methodological mistakes in 43 identified articles *(20)*. These were summarized as follows:

1. biased and/or inefficient estimation,
2. overfitting and fitting of implausible functions,
3. incorrect or missing description of the complexity of the network,
4. use of inadequate statistical competitors or insufficient statistical comparisons, and
5. naive and inappropriate application to survival data.

(1) Mistakes in the estimation of predictive accuracy represent without doubt the most dangerous flaw of many ANNs in oncology. Most relate to inappropriate use of data sets to estimate the predictive ability of these models. For example, many reports on ANNs divided the data sets only into learning and validation sets, omitting the test set. While such methodology may be appropriate for reporting the accuracy of regression

models, ANNs behave differently—they require a distinct test set from the validation set. Therefore, due to a missing test set, validations demonstrate excessively optimistic predicted accuracy, relative to regression models. The degree of overoptimism of ANNs fit in this manner has been estimated at between 9 and 13% *(20)*. Thus, an ANN model may be reported to predict accurately 90% of the time, while in reality only 80% of predictions are correct.

Appropriate assessment of predictive accuracy requires the use of training, test, and validation sets. While these can be derived from the original cohort, such approach results in fewer observations that can be used for learning and validation. Alternatively, cross-validation techniques can be used, whereby the test set is generated from a randomly drawn proportion of the population (e.g., K-fold or leave-one-out cross-validation). Another test set can then be randomly identified and the process may be repeated several times. Each time the predictive accuracy of the neural network is determined. Once all repetitions have been completed, an average predictive accuracy is determined. This method is more sophisticated than simple splitting of the data set between learning, test, and validation sets. It allows testing of the unbiasedness of the ANN on substantially larger test sets, relative to when the cohort is split into three subsets. The most efficient validation may be provided by a computer-intensive resampling technique called bootstrapping *(6,13)*. This methodology replicates the process of test set generation from an underlying validation set by drawing sample sizes with replacement from the original validation data set. Each resample is of the same size as the original validation set. Use of resampling maximizes the efficiency of predictive accuracy testing. Thus, instead of dividing the population between three subsets, only the learning and validation sets are required. Use of cross-validation or bootstrapping techniques may allow fewer instances of overfitting, where ANN learning sets rely on a few dozen observations and numerous input nodes. It is of note that regression models do not require a test set. Instead, their validation may be achieved by using either split sample, cross-validation, or bootstrapping methodologies. For all tools, external validation samples still represent the gold standard.

(2) Overfitting may undermine the validity of neural networks because of their potential to overly mirror the underlying data. For example, ANNs based on few observations but numerous hidden units have a tendency to result in implausible functions describing the relation between the input nodes and the output nodes. Such models may be associated with spuriously high accuracy, which may be difficult to confirm in a validation set. Despite great ability to replicate relationships between input and output nodes, ANNs do require between 5 and 10 observations for each parameter to be estimated. Thus, readers are cautioned about taking at face value the predictive ability of ANNs that bypass that key consideration.

(3) Incorrect or incomplete description of reported ANNs represents a common limitation in the ability of the reader to independently assess the properties of the network at hand as well as the learning, testing, and validation steps. For example, it is not uncommon that multiple hidden layers are mentioned, without specifying how many.

(4) Excessively optimistic performance of ANNs may be due to comparisons with inappropriate, insufficient, or inadequate statistical competitors. For example, ANNs are frequently compared to logistic regression models. Although we have demonstrated that in specific circumstances logistic regression-based models can favorably out-compete neural networks, this is not invariably the case. The advantage of ANNs resides in their complexity relative to straightforward regression models, which rely on linear relations

between predictors and the outcome of interest. In order to provide comparable conditions, regression models should be fitted with multiple interaction terms and with cubic as well as quadratic predictor terms. Such methodology would result in comparable ability of the predictors to interact with one another in a nonlinear fashion, as in ANNs.

(5) The above methodological problems are compounded by inappropriate applications of ANNs. For example, the statistical assumptions governing ANNs do not allow the use of censored data. Thus, ANNs are not amenable to modeling of survival data. Many investigators have attempted to circumvent this methodological limitation by either ignoring, omitting, or imputing censored cases, or finally by using time to event data as an additional input. All these approaches are methodologically flawed and are known to results in biased estimates of the outcome of interest (20,41).

Finally, ANNs have been popularized in the medical literature by overinflated praises, such as "ability to learn...makes them formidable tools in the fight against cancer" and "neural computation may be as beneficial to medicine and urology in the twenty-first century as molecular biology has been in the twentieth." Despite these praises, ANNs have made little difference in the diagnosis or management of localized PCa since their introduction in the early 1990s (21). Besides severely limited availability, practical considerations related to the misuses of ANN methodology have without doubt contributed to the observed marginal use of these tools in clinical practice.

## HEAD-TO-HEAD COMPARISON OF AN ARTIFICIAL NEURAL NETWORK AND A NOMOGRAM

To substantiate the claim that ANN predictions are less accurate when they are subjected to strict external validity tests, we compared the ability to predict presence of cancer on biopsy between our nomogram and an ANN model that was made available by investigators at the Charité Hospital in Berlin, Germany. The nomogram was based on four input variables, namely, age, DRE findings, serum PSA, and %fPSA and its maximum predictive accuracy was estimated at 78% (49). The ANN additionally included prostate volume as a risk variable and its predictive accuracy was estimated at 84%. Prostate volume has been proven to be an important predictor of PCa risk on needle biopsy in several contemporary analyses (4,50–54). Thus, its inclusion should bias the ability of the network to predict more accurately than the nomogram, where this variable is not considered. Moreover, unlike the neural network, the nomogram variables were not allowed to interact with one another, which further undermined their predictive ability.

Both models were tested on an external cohort of 3,980 patients subjected to at least an 8-core initial biopsy. Despite the a priori disadvantages of the nomogram the results indicated that the nomogram (AUC = 70.6%) had an increase in the AUC of 3.6% compared to the neural network (AUC = 67.0%). Both models predicted less accurately than in the original studies where they were described (49,55). The decrease in discrimination relative to original data could be related to development of both tools on populations subjected to virtually exclusive sextant biopsies, while their head-to-head comparison was performed on a cohort exposed to extended biopsy schemes. In addition to the AUC we compared the nomogram and ANN in terms of agreement of predicted versus observed rates of PCa. As shown in Fig. 3A, the calibration curve of the nomogram virtually paralleled the ideal 45° prediction line implying high agreement. Conversely, the ANN demonstrated important departures from ideal predictions (Fig. 3B), which were

**A**

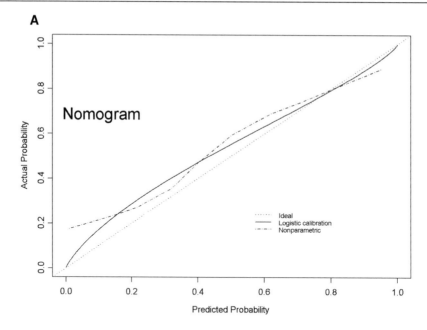

**B**

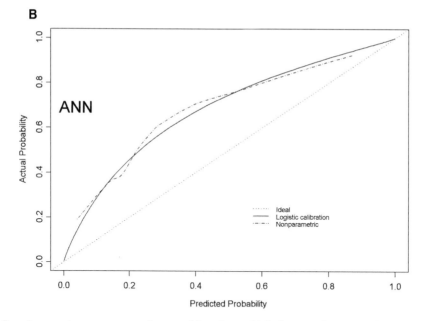

**Fig. 3.** Local regression nonparametric smoothing plots which show performance characteristics of a sextant biopsy nomogram *(55)* and an artificial neural network *(49)* in a cohort of 4,093 men at initial biopsy. **A.** External calibration plot of a logistic regression-based nomogram based on age, DRE, PSA, and %fPSA in a cohort of 3,980 men at initial biopsy *(55)*. **B.** External calibration plot of an artificial neural network based on age, DRE, PSA, %fPSA, and prostate volume in a cohort of 3,980 men at initial biopsy *(49)*.

manifested by severe underestimation throughout the range of predicted probabilities. The most important departures were recorded for predicted probabilities between 20 and 80%. This example of a head-to-head comparison showed that nomograms can be more accurate and achieve better performance characteristics than ANNs, directly contradicting several urological publications where the accuracy of ANNs was reported as substantially higher than that of nomograms. Moreover, this example illustrates some of the concerns that experts in prognostics have voiced about the true predictive ability of ANNs.

Nonetheless, our findings and their interpretation are not meant to suggest that the ANN methodology should be abandoned. Instead, they indicate the need for methodologically sound application and critical appraisal of the approach.

## CONCLUSIONS

Prediction of several PCa related outcomes can be optimized with different methodological approaches such as nomograms, look-up tables or ANNs. While look-up tables represent a simplification of logistic regression, nomograms and ANNs represent two distinct methodological approaches toward individualized prediction of clinical outcomes. Accuracy and performance characteristics of nomograms can be as good as those of ANNs. Due to these properties and a paper-based format, nomograms have been adopted in clinical practice across several continents. Conversely, despite promotion in the field of prostate cancer since the early 1990s, due to less transparency and the need for computational infrastructure ANNs are less popular. However, ANNs represent a valid alternative as long as their methodology is used with scrutiny to optimize prostate cancer risk prediction.

## REFERENCES

 1. Chun FK, Karakiewicz PI, Briganti A, et al. Prostate cancer nomograms: an update. Eur Urol 2006;50(5):914–26; discussion 26.
 2. Karakiewicz PI, Briganti A, Chun FK, Valiquette L. Outcomes Research: A Methodologic Review. Eur Urol 2006.
 3. Ross PL, Scardino PT, Kattan MW. A catalog of prostate cancer nomograms. J Urol 2001;165(5):1562–8.
 4. Chun FK, Briganti A, Graefen M, et al. Development and external validation of an extended 10-core biopsy nomogram. Eur Urol 2007;52(2):436–45.
 5. Svatek R, Karakiewicz PI, Shulman M, Karam J, Perrotte P, Benaim E. Pre-treatment nomogram for disease-specific survival of patients with chemotherapy-naive androgen independent prostate cancer. Eur Urol 2006;49(4):666–74.
 6. Bradley E, Tibshirani RJ. Monographs on statistics and applied probability: An introduction to the bootstrap. Champman and Hall/CRC 1993:275.
 7. Eastham JA, Kattan MW, Scardino PT. Nomograms as predictive models. Semin Urol Oncol 2002;20(2):108–15.
 8. Karakiewicz PI, Chun FK, Briganti A, et al. Prostate cancer nomograms are superior to neural networks. Can J Urol 2006;13 Suppl 2:18–25.
 9. Kattan M. Statistical prediction models, artificial neural networks, and the sophism "I am a patient, not a statistic".J Clin Oncol 2002;20(4):885–7.
10. Kattan MW. Nomograms. Introduction. Semin Urol Oncol 2002;20(2):79–81.
11. Kattan MW. Judging new markers by their ability to improve predictive accuracy. J Natl Cancer Inst 2003;95(9):634–5.
12. Kattan MW. Comparison of Cox regression with other methods for determining prediction models and nomograms. J Urol 2003;170(6 Pt 2):S6–9; discussion S10.

13. Steyerberg EW, Harrell FE, Jr., Borsboom GJ, Eijkemans MJ, Vergouwe Y, Habbema JD. Internal validation of predictive models: efficiency of some procedures for logistic regression analysis. J Clin Epidemiol 2001;54(8):774–81.

14. Steyerberg EW, Harrell FE, Jr., Goodman PH. Neural networks, logistic regression, and calibration. Med Decis Making 1998;18(3):349–50.

15. Harrell FEJ. Regression Modelling Strategies with Applications to Linear Models, Logistic Regression, and Survival Analysis. In. New York: Springer; 2001.

16. Kattan MW. Validating a prognostic model. Cancer 2006;107(11):2523–4.

17. Vergouwe Y, Steyerberg EW, Eijkemans MJ, Habbema JD. Validity of prognostic models: when is a model clinically useful? Semin Urol Oncol 2002;20(2):96–107.

18. Suzuki H, Komiya A, Kamiya N, et al. Development of a nomogram to predict probability of positive initial prostate biopsy among Japanese patients. Urology 2006;67(1):131–6.

19. Yanke BV, Carver BS, Bianco FJ, Jr., et al. African-American race is a predictor of prostate cancer detection: incorporation into a pre-biopsy nomogram. fg 2006;98(4):783–7.

20. Schwarzer G, Vach W, Schumacher M. On the misuses of artificial neural networks for prognostic and diagnostic classification in oncology. Stat Med 2000;19(4):541–61.

21. Snow PB, Smith DS, Catalona WJ. Artificial neural networks in the diagnosis and prognosis of prostate cancer: a pilot study. J Urol 1994;152(5 Pt 2):1923–6.

22. Partin AW, Kattan MW, Subong EN, et al. Combination of prostate-specific antigen, clinical stage, and Gleason score to predict pathological stage of localized prostate cancer. A multi-institutional update. Jama 1997;277(18):1445–51.

23. Partin AW, Mangold LA, Lamm DM, Walsh PC, Epstein JI, Pearson JD. Contemporary update of prostate cancer staging nomograms (Partin Tables) for the new millennium. Urology 2001;58(6):843–8.

24. Conrad S, Graefen M, Pichlmeier U, et al. Prospective validation of an algorithm with systematic sextant biopsy to predict pelvic lymph node metastasis in patients with clinically localized prostatic carcinoma. J Urol 2002;167(2 Pt 1):521–5.

25. Graefen M, Haese A, Pichlmeier U, et al. A validated strategy for side specific prediction of organ confined prostate cancer: a tool to select for nerve sparing radical prostatectomy. J Urol 2001;165(3):857–63.

26. Chun FK, Briganti A, Graefen M, Porter C, Montorsi F, Haese A, Scattoni V, Borden L, Steuber T, Salonia A, Schlomm T, Latchemsetty K, Walz J, Kim J, Eichelberg C, Currlin E, Ahyai SA, Erbersdobler A, Valiquette L, Heinzer H, Rigatti P, Huland H, Karakiewicz PI. Development and External Validation of an Extended Repeat Biopsy Nomogram. J Urol. 2007 Feb;177(2):510–515.

27. Chun FK, Briganti A, Graefen M, Montorsi F, Porter C, Scattoni V, Gallina A, Walz J, Haese A, Steuber T, Erbersdobler A, Schlomm T, Ahyai SA, Currlin E, Valiquette L, Heinzer H, Rigatti P, Huland H, Karakiewicz PI. Development and external validation of an extended 10-core biopsy nomogram. Eur Urol. 2007 Aug;52(2):436–44.

28. Chun FK, Steuber T, Erbersdobler A, et al. Development and internal validation of a nomogram predicting the probability of prostate cancer Gleason sum upgrading between biopsy and radical prostatectomy pathology. Eur Urol 2006;49(5):820–6.

29. Ross PL, Gerigk C, Gonen M, et al. Comparisons of nomograms and urologists' predictions in prostate cancer. Semin Urol Oncol 2002;20(2):82–8.

30. Specht MC, Kattan MW, Gonen M, Fey J, Van Zee KJ. Predicting nonsentinel node status after positive sentinel lymph biopsy for breast cancer: clinicians versus nomogram. Ann Surg Oncol 2005;12(8):654–9.

31. Chun FK, Briganti A, Antebi E, Graefen M, Currlin E, Steuber T, Schlomm T, Walz J, Haese A, Friedrich MG, Ahyai SA, Eichelberg C, Salomon G, Gallina A, Erbersdobler A, Perrotte P, Heinzer H, Huland H, Karakiewicz PI. Surgical volume is related to the rate of positive surgical margins at radical prostatectomy in European patients. BJU Int. 2006 Dec;98(6):1204–9.

32. Eastham JA, Kattan MW, Riedel E, et al. Variations among individual surgeons in the rate of positive surgical margins in radical prostatectomy specimens. J Urol 2003;170(6 Pt 1):2292–5.

33. Kattan MW, Eastham JA, Stapleton AM, Wheeler TM, Scardino PT. A preoperative nomogram for disease recurrence following radical prostatectomy for prostate cancer. J Natl Cancer Inst 1998;90(10):766–71.

34. Kattan MW, Wheeler TM, Scardino PT. Postoperative nomogram for disease recurrence after radical prostatectomy for prostate cancer. J Clin Oncol 1999;17(5):1499–507.

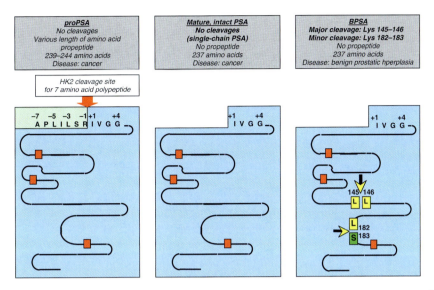

**Color Plate 1** Depiction of isoforms of free PSA (Chapter 8, Fig. 1; *see* discussion on p. 87).

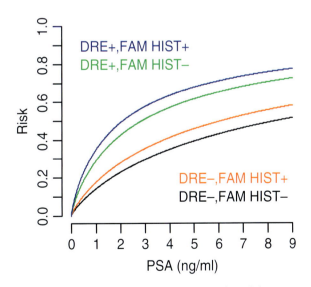

**Color Plate 2** Risk of prostate cancer by PSA for four groups of participants according to their DRE and family history status; + denotes abnormal for DRE and positive for family history, – denotes normal for DRE and negative for family history. Assumes no prior negative biopsy (Chapter 12, Fig. 1; *see* discussion on p. 198).

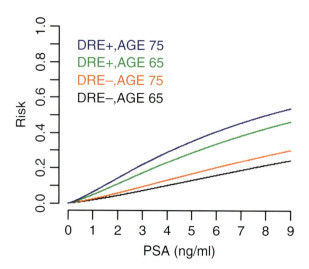

**Color Plate 3** Risk of high-grade prostate cancer by PSA for four groups of caucasian participants according to DRE age and; + abnormal DRE, − normal DRE. Assumes no prior negative biopsy (Chapter 12, Fig. 2; *see* discussion on p. 199).

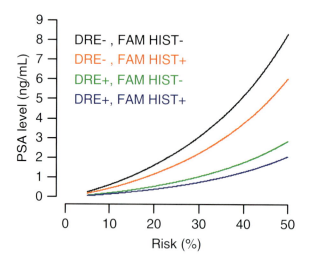

**Color Plate 4** Prostate-specific antigen levels achieving specified risks of prostate cancer adjusted for risk factors DRE and family history of prostate cancer (Chapter 12, Fig. 5; *see* discussion on p. 201).

(a)

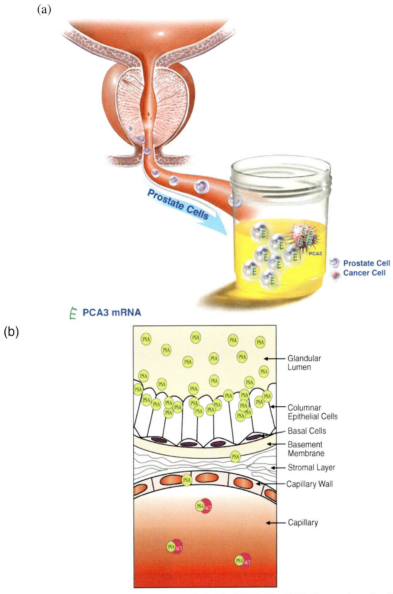

Ɛ **PCA3 mRNA**

(b)

Prostate Cell
Cancer Cell

Glandular
Lumen

Columnar
Epithelial Cells

Basal Cells

Basement
Membrane

Stromal Layer

Capillary Wall

Capillary

*Rittenhouse et al., Crit.Rev.Clin.Lab Sci, 35, 275-368, 1998. Reproduced with permission of the publisher (Taylor and Francis, Ltd, http://www.tandf.co.uk/journals)*

**Color Plate 5** Release of prostate cells into the urethra following DRE (**a**) vs. release of PSA protein into the bloodstream (**b**) (Chapter 16, Fig. 1; *see* discussion on p. 235).

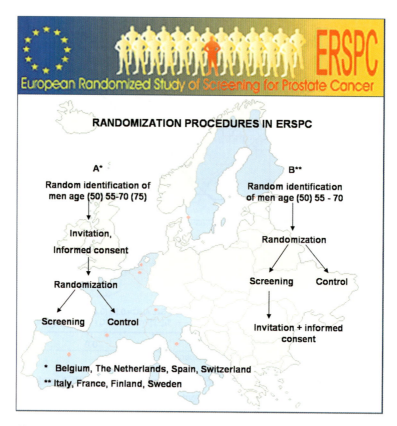

**Color Plate 14** Randomization procedures in ERSPC (Chapter 27, Fig. 1; *see* discussion on p. 376).

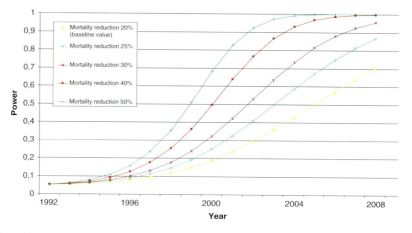

**Color Plate 15** Effect of different assumptions on the power of the ERSPC trial by follow-up year (Chapter 27, Fig. 2; *see* discussion on p. 383).

(Source: H. de Koning (2002). International Journal of Cancer 98: 268–73.)

35. Sotelo RJ, Mora KE, Perez LH, et al. Assay standardization bias: different prostate cancer detection rates and clinical outcomes resulting from different assays for free and total prostate-specific antigen. Urology 2007;69(6):1143–6.

36. Chun FK, Karakiewicz PI, Huland H, Graefen M. Role of nomograms for prostate cancer in 2007. World J Urol 2007;25(2):131–42.

37. Dotan ZA, Bianco FJ, Jr., Rabbani F, et al. Pattern of prostate-specific antigen (PSA) failure dictates the probability of a positive bone scan in patients with an increasing PSA after radical prostatectomy. J Clin Oncol 2005;23(9):1962–8.

38. Slovin SF, Wilton AS, Heller G, Scher HI. Time to detectable metastatic disease in patients with rising prostate-specific antigen values following surgery or radiation therapy. Clin Cancer Res 2005;11(24 Pt 1):8669–73.

39. Smaletz O, Scher HI, Small EJ, et al. Nomogram for overall survival of patients with progressive metastatic prostate cancer after castration. J Clin Oncol 2002;20(19):3972–82.

40. Shariat SF, Karakiewicz PI, Margulis V, Kattan MW. Inventory of prostate cancer predictive tools. Curr Opin Urol 2008;18(3):279–96.

41. Schwarzer G, Schumacher M. Artificial neural networks for diagnosis and prognosis in prostate cancer. Semin Urol Oncol 2002;20(2):89–95.

42. Chun FK, Karakiewicz PI, Briganti A, et al. A critical appraisal of logistic regression-based nomograms, artificial neural networks, classification and regression-tree models, look-up tables and risk-group stratification models for prostate cancer. fg 2007;99(4):794–800.

43. Schwartz E, Albertsen P. Nomograms for clinically localized disease. Part III: watchful waiting. Semin Urol Oncol 2002;20(2):140–5.

44. Ohori M, Swindle P. Nomograms and instruments for the initial prostate evaluation: the ability to estimate the likelihood of identifying prostate cancer. Semin Urol Oncol 2002;20(2):116–22.

45. Revold DM, McLeod, D.G., Brandt, J.M., Snow, P.B., Murphy, G.P. Introduction to artificial neural networks for physicians: taking the lid off the black box. Prostate 46(1), p 39–44 2001.

46. Wei JT, Zhang Z, Barnhill SD, Madyastha KR, Zhang H, Oesterling JE. Understanding artificial neural networks and exploring their potential applications for the practicing urologist. Urology 1998;52(2):161–72.

47. Kattan MW, Cowen ME, Miles BJ. Computer modeling in urology. Urology 1996;47(1):14–21.

48. Kattan MW, Beck JR. Artificial neural networks for medical classification decisions. Arch Pathol Lab Med 1995;119(8):672–7.

49. Stephan C, Cammann H, Semjonow A, et al. Multicenter evaluation of an artificial neural network to increase the prostate cancer detection rate and reduce unnecessary biopsies. Clin Chem 2002;48(8):1279–87.

50. Briganti A, Chun FK, Suardi N, et al. Prostate volume and adverse prostate cancer features: fact not artifact. Eur J Cancer 2007;43(18):2669–77.

51. Bianco FJ, Jr., Mallah KN, Korets R, Hricak H, Scardino PT, Kattan MW. Prostate volume measured preoperatively predicts for organ-confined disease in men with clinically localized prostate cancer. Urology 2007;69(2):343–6.

52. Freedland SJ, Isaacs WB, Platz EA, et al. Prostate size and risk of high-grade, advanced prostate cancer and biochemical progression after radical prostatectomy: a search database study. J Clin Oncol 2005;23(30):7546–54.

53. Karakiewicz PI, Bazinet M, Aprikian AG, et al. Outcome of sextant biopsy according to gland volume. Urology 1997;49(1):55–9.

54. Chun FK, Briganti A, Graefen M, et al. Development and external validation of an extended repeat biopsy nomogram. J Urol 2007;177(2):510–5.

55. Karakiewicz PI, Benayoun S, Kattan MW, et al. Development and validation of a nomogram predicting the outcome of prostate biopsy based on patient age, digital rectal examination and serum prostate specific antigen. J Urol 2005;173(6):1930–4.

# 12 Development of the Prostate Cancer Prevention Trial Prostate Cancer Risk Calculator

*Donna P. Ankerst and Ian M. Thompson*

## CONTENTS

## SUMMARY

The Prostate Cancer Prevention Trial (PCPT) Prostate Cancer Risk Calculator provides a single probability of prostate cancer and of high-grade disease (Gleason grade $\geq 7$) based on a man's serum prostate-specific antigen (PSA) level, digital rectal examination (DRE) result, family history, age, race, and history of a prior prostate biopsy. Incorporating the panel of risk factors in addition to PSA, it is recommended for individually tailored biopsy discussions between doctors and patients. This chapter reviews the development of the PCPT Risk Calculator, the algorithm behind the calculator, ongoing validation studies, and proposed modifications.

**Key Words:** Prostate cancer risk, Calculator, Prostate-specific antigen, External validation.

From: *Current Clinical Urology: Prostate Cancer Screening*, Edited by: D. P. Ankerst et al.
DOI 10.1007/978-1-60327-281-0_12 © Humana Press, a part of Springer Science+Business Media, LLC 2009

# INTRODUCTION

In 2006 the Prostate Cancer Prevention Trial (PCPT) Prostate Cancer Risk Calculator was posted on the Internet and its algorithm simultaneously published in the *Journal of the National Cancer Institute (1)*. Based on 5,519 healthy men over the age of 55 years prospectively enrolled in the 7-year PCPT who had definitive prostate cancer ascertainment by prostate biopsy, the PCPT Risk Calculator provides the most accurate assessment tool for prostate cancer and high-grade disease (Gleason grade $\geq 7$) risk estimation. The algorithm amalgamates the currently established risk factors for prostate cancer: serum prostate-specific antigen (PSA) level, digital rectal examination (DRE) result, family history, age, race, and history of a prior prostate biopsy into a single composite risk score. The PCPT Risk Calculator is recommended for use for biopsy diagnostic discussions between doctors and patients and for risk stratification in prevention trials.

Since its institution on the Internet, the PCPT Risk Calculator has been validated in several external populations and refinements are currently underway on the website to enhance further validation. Recognizing the shortcomings of prostate-specific-antigen (PSA) and the combined portfolio of PCPT risk factors for prostate cancer screening (an out-of-sample estimate of the area underneath the receiver-operating characteristic curve (AUC) is 70%), methods are being developed to integrate new biomarkers and further established risk factors, including detailed family history of prostate cancer and body mass index, into the calculator. This chapter reviews the development of the PCPT Risk Calculator, provides an update on validations of the calculator performed since its inception, and methodologies in progress for incorporating new markers into the calculator.

# THE PCPT PROSTATE CANCER AND HIGH-GRADE DISEASE RISK MODEL

To develop the PCPT Risk Calculator, a subset of 5,519 PCPT placebo arm participants were included in the analysis who had at least one prostate biopsy performed during the course of the trial and complete measurements for all risk factors *(1)*. The risk factors considered for analysis were family history (1 if father, brother, or son ever had prostate cancer; 0 otherwise), DRE result (1 abnormal; 0 normal), PSA transformed to the natural logarithmic scale, log ng/mL), age at biopsy, history of prior biopsy (1 if one or more prior biopsies were performed, all negative for prostate cancer; 0 otherwise), and PSA velocity (log ng/mL/year). PSA velocity was calculated based on all PSA values measured within 3 years prior to biopsy as the slope of log PSA per year using linear regression; this definition of velocity was chosen for optimal performance after examining a multitude of commonly used definitions *(1)*. If a participant only had two PSA measures prior to biopsy, PSA velocity was defined as the ratio of the difference in log PSA values to the difference in time of measurement of the two PSA values. Logistic regression was used to model the risk of prostate cancer given the predictors and a model search was performed to identify the optimal model considering every possible combination of main effects and two-way interactions of the risk factors which maximized cross-validated prediction. The risk modeling procedure was repeated for high-grade disease, defined as prostate cancer with Gleason grade $\geq 7$.

Table 1
Characteristics of the 5,519 PCPT Placebo Arm Participants
Used to Create the PCPT Risk Model

| Age at biopsy | Number (percent) |
|---|---|
| 55–60 | 38 (0.7%) |
| 60–64 | 1,143 (20.7%) |
| 65–69 | 1,741 (31.5%) |
| ≥ 70 | 2,597 (47.1%) |
| Family history | |
| No | 4,599 (83.3%) |
| Yes | 920 (16.7%) |
| Race | |
| White | 5,276 (95.6%) |
| African American | 175 (3.2%) |
| Other | 68 (1.2%) |
| Number of previous biopsies at time of biopsy used for the analysis | |
| ≥ 1 | 646 (11.7%) |
| ≥ 2 | 107 (1.9%) |

Characteristics of the 5,519 participants used in the analysis are given in Table 1. Nearly half of the participants were over 70 years old at the time of biopsy. The population was primarily Caucasian with only 3% African Americans. Approximately 17% had a family history of prostate cancer and 10% had at least one prior biopsy to that used for analysis. The median PSA value (last PSA prior to biopsy) was 1.5 ng/mL and 88% of the men had PSA < 4 ng/mL, which is a lower distribution of PSA than in general because the PCPT was a screened cohort with a requirement of PSA less than 3 ng/mL at study entry. There was an increase in risk of prostate cancer and high-grade disease for increasing PSA.

Table 2 shows the non-negligible risk of prostate cancer and high-grade disease even for low PSA values and the sharply increasing risk with increasing PSA. The risk of prostate cancer rose from 11.1% for PSA values less than 1 ng/mL to 43.3% for PSA

Table 2
Numbers (Percentages) of Prostate Cancers and High-Grade Prostate Cancers by PSA Level

| PSA level (ng/mL) | N | No. of prostate cancers (%) | No. of high-grade prostate cancers (%) |
|---|---|---|---|
| 0–1 | 1,963 | 217 (11.1) | 19 (1.0) |
| 1.1–2 | 1,640 | 337 (20.5) | 43 (2.6) |
| 2.1–3 | 775 | 205 (26.5) | 44 (5.7) |
| 3.1–4 | 510 | 153 (30.0) | 48 (9.4) |
| 4.1–6 | 481 | 234 (48.6) | 70 (14.6) |
| >6 | 150 | 65 (43.3) | 33 (22.0) |
| Total | 5,519 | 1211 (21.9) | 257 (21.2) |

values greater than 6 ng/mL and the risk of high-grade disease rose from 1.0% to 22.0% across these two PSA intervals.

Given the high-predictive power of PSA the next step in developing the PCPT risk model was to see if any other risk factors added independent prognostic information. Many factors are associated with increased risk of prostate cancer. Family history predicts prostate cancer as does an abnormal DRE. The challenge is whether or not a risk factor contributes independent prognostic prediction above that already achieved by PSA. This can only be evaluated by putting all competing risk factors into a single multivariable model and assessing the relative strengths of the risk factors that adjusts for the other factors. For the 5,519 PCPT participants the factors that contributed to independent prognostic information when evaluated in this manner were PSA (odds ratio (OR) = 2.34, 95% confidence interval (CI) = (2.13, 2.56) for unit increase in log PSA, $p$-value < 0.0001), family history (OR = 1.31, 95% CI = (1.11, 1.55), $p$-value = 0.002), DRE (OR = 2.47, 95% CI=(2.03, 3.01), $p$-value < 0.0001), and history of prior biopsy (OR = 0.64, 95% CI=(0.53,0.78), $p$-value < 0.0001). An increase in PSA was associated with an increase in the risk of cancer, a positive family history increased the odds by 31.0%, an abnormal DRE more than doubled the odds, and having had one or more prior biopsies decreased the odds of prostate cancer on the current biopsy. The latter effect is somewhat artificial, induced by the screening nature of the study.

There is currently increased interest in the role of PSA velocity in prostate cancer *(2)*. Although PSA velocity has been associated with risk of prostate cancer recurrence and mortality as an isolated risk factor, it is not clear that it provides independent prognostic information to PSA for biopsy-detectable prostate cancer in healthy men undergoing screening. In the screening situation, where participants essentially participate or begin follow-up with a low PSA value (less than 3 ng/mL in the case of the PCPT) PSA velocity evaluated thereafter is highly correlated with the current or last PSA value. A high-current PSA implies it must have increased from the baseline low value, or in other words, have had a change in velocity. Therefore in the screening context current PSA is confounded with PSA velocity and velocity somewhat duplicates the information contained in PSA. In the PCPT analysis, when evaluated in absence of the other risk factors, including in absence of PSA, velocity was highly associated with increased risk of prostate cancer with OR = 5.65 and 95% CI = (4.13, 7.74) ($p$-value < 0.0001). However, when the other risk factors were adjusted for in the analysis, although velocity was still associated with an increase in prostate cancer risk, it was no longer statistically significant (OR = 1.18, 95% CI = (0.82, 1.69), $p$-value = 0.38), meaning that it did not add independent prognostic value to PSA.

Similarly, age, which is also a predictor of prostate cancer in the absence of other factors, did not add independent prognostic information to PSA, DRE, family history, and prior biopsy. This may have been induced by the narrow distribution of older ages in the PCPT due to the eligibility criterion that men be over 55 years old at study entry. Finally, race also did not contribute independent prognostic information to the other risk factors, a finding most likely due, however, to lack of power based on the small number of African Americans enrolled in the PCPT.

With all of the statistically significant risk factors assembled into a single logistic regression model, the risk of prostate cancer could be computed for the individual man based on all of his risk factors. Figure 1 shows prostate cancer risk by PSA, DRE, and family history status for a man with no prior biopsy. The risk increases with PSA across all four groups determined by DRE and family history status and there is a difference in

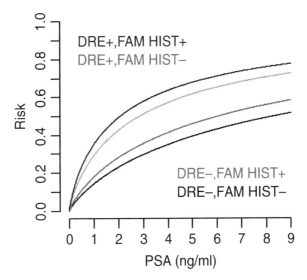

**Fig. 1.** Risk of prostate cancer by PSA for four groups of participants according to their DRE and family history status; + denotes abnormal for DRE and positive for family history, – denotes normal for DRE and negative for family history. Assumes no prior negative biopsy. (*see* Color Plate 2)

risk between the groups. Participants with the lowest risk for all levels of PSA are those with a normal DRE and no family history and participants with the highest risk are those with an abnormal DRE and positive family history. As a risk factor, DRE is more influential than family history in shifting risk. The graph provides an easy-to-read visual display understandable by both the clinician and patient. For instance, at a PSA value of 5 ng/mL, if a man has no family history and a normal DRE, the graph indicates a risk of approximately 40%, but at the same PSA value, for another patient with a positive DRE and positive family history, the graph indicates a risk of 65%. This example shows how the other risk factors add independent prognostic information to prostate cancer above that provided by PSA.

The same model-building procedure was repeated for predicting high-grade disease, defined as Gleason grade greater than or equal to 7. Similar results were obtained. PSA, DRE, and a history of a prior biopsy were independent predictors but PSA velocity was not. Family history was no longer significant but age was, indicating a minor increase in risk of high-grade disease for older age. Figure 2 and Color Plate 3 shows the graph of high-grade disease risk by PSA for groups defined by DRE status and for ages 75 versus 65, since family history was not predictive of high-grade disease. DRE remains the next strongest predictor to PSA. Risks are lower for high-grade disease since there is lower prevalence of high-grade disease than prostate cancer.

## THE PCPT RISK CALCULATOR

The PCPT risk equation is available as an online calculator, at http://www.compass. fhcrc.org/edrnnci/bin/calculator/main.asp. Figure 3 shows the entry page for the calculator. At the website the user types in the individual risk factors, presses the submit button, and gets in return an individual risk of prostate cancer and high-grade disease, both with 95% confidence intervals; sample output is shown in Fig. 4. How does a physician use

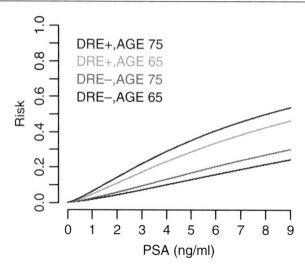

**Fig. 2.** Risk of high-grade prostate cancer by PSA for four groups of caucasian participants according to DRE age and; + abnormal DRE, − normal DRE. Assumes no prior negative biopsy. (*see* Color Plate 3)

### Predicting Likelihood Of Cancer If A Prostate Biopsy Is Performed

The fields with ✳ sign are required.

| Race: ✳ | Caucasian ▾ | |
|---|---|---|
| Age: ✳ | 65 | |
| PSA Level: ✳ | 2.5 | ng/ml |
| Family History of Prostate Cancer: ✳ | No ▾ | |
| Digital Rectal Examination Result: ✳ | Normal ▾ | |
| Prior Negative Prostate Biopsy: ✳ | No ▾ | |

Submit

**Fig. 3.** Entry webpage for the PCPT Risk of Prostate Cancer Calculator available at http://www.compass.fhcrc.org/edrnnci/bin/calculator/main.asp.

this calculator? When a physician sees a patient he assembles all risk factors and integrates them with his own experience with past patients and the literature. What the calculator is doing is quantifying this experience from a group of 5,519 men, as if providing the physician with 5,519 past patients. Although a physician may be confident in his own personal experience, it is no substitution for quantifiable evidence. The PCPT Risk Calculator brings this evidence directly to the clinic.

The PCPT Risk Calculator provides a probability or risk of prostate cancer. For the physician more comfortable or familiar with PSA rather than risk, the PCPT Risk Calculator can be inverted to provide adjusted PSA cut-offs given the set of risk factors and a desirable level of risk. For example, a physician may want to refer a man to biopsy who has no family history, a normal DRE, and no prior biopsy at a higher-PSA cut-off than a man with one or more of the other risk factors. If a 25% risk of disease is considered sufficient for referral to biopsy, then for a patient who is 65 years old, has no

## Predicting Likelihood Of Cancer If A Prostate Biopsy Is Performed

### The Result:

Based on the data provided, the person's estimated risk of biopsy-detectable cancer is **27 %** .

The **95%** Confidence Interval for this prediction is **25%** to **28%**.
More information about confidence interval ...

The person's estimated risk of biopsy-detectable <u>high grade</u> prostate cancer is **4 %** .

The **95%** Confidence Interval for this prediction is **3.5%** to **5.3%**.
More information about confidence interval ...

### The result is based on:

| | |
|---|---|
| Age: | 65 |
| Race: | Caucasian |
| PSA Level: | 2.5 ng/ml |
| Family History of Prostate Cancer: | No |
| Digital Rectal Examination Result: | Normal |
| Prior Negative Prostate Biopsy: | No |

### Predicting Likelihood Of Cancer If A Prostate Biopsy Is Performed

**The Result:**

Based on the data provided, the person's estimated risk of biopsy-detectable cancer is 27 % .

The 95% Confidence Interval for this prediction is 25% to 28%.
More information about confidence interval ...

The person's estimated risk of biopsy-detectable high grade prostate cancer is 4 % .

The 95% Confidence Interval for this prediction is 3.5% to 5.3%.
More information about confidence interval ...

**The result is based on:**

| | |
|---|---|
| Age: | 65 |
| Race: | Caucasian |
| PSA Level: | 2.5 ng/ml |
| Family History of Prostate Cancer: | No |
| Digital Rectal Examination Result: | Normal |
| Prior Negative Prostate Biopsy: | No |

**Fig. 4.** Results produced by the online PCPT Risk Calculator after submitting the risk factor input from Fig. 3.

family history and has a normal DRE, the calculator is inverted to give a PSA cut-off of 2.22 ng/mL. For another man with the same profile except who has a family history of prostate cancer, the PSA cut-off for referral to biopsy to achieve 25% risk is 1.61 ng/mL, less than the cut-off for the other patient because this man has an additional risk factor for prostate cancer. Figure 5 and Color Plate 4 shows the adjusted PSA cut-offs (*y*-axis) for varying levels of risk of prostate cancer (*x*-axis).

On the other hand, patients are more likely to understand risks rather than PSA values so may prefer monitoring risks and establishing their own subjective thresholds for referral to biopsy. For example, suppose a man has a positive family history, normal DRE, and a PSA of 1.9 ng/mL. He types in this information and gets a risk of 27.2%. Following discussions with his physician, he decides to get a biopsy and it turns out negative for prostate cancer. Suppose he returns the next year and his PSA has increased to 2 ng/mL. Now despite that his PSA has actually increased, he now has had a prior negative biopsy, a factor which decreases the risk and his risk falls to 19.9% this year. On the

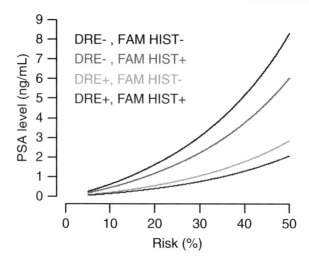

**Fig. 5.** Prostate-specific antigen levels achieving specified risks of prostate cancer adjusted for risk factors DRE and family history of prostate cancer. (*see* Color Plate 4)

basis of all of his updated information, including the fall in risk, he and his physician may decide that he does not get a biopsy this year.

## VALIDATION OF THE PCPT RISK CALCULATOR

In the report that published the PCPT Risk Calculator, Thompson and colleagues *(1)* validated it on the PCPT population of 5,519 men on which it was developed using four-fold cross-validation, where the population was split into four random sets, the model repeatedly fit to three of the four sets and then tested on the remaining one set not included in the development of the model. They reported an internally validated area underneath the receiver operating characteristic curve (AUC) of 70.2% for the prostate cancer calculator and 69.8% for the high-grade disease calculator. Internal validation, however, is known to be overly optimistic since it does not account for model selection and is on the same population as which the model was developed. Parekh and colleagues *(3)* performed the first external validation of the calculator on 446 men who received a prostate biopsy from the significantly younger and more ethnically diverse San Antonio Biomarkers Of Risk of prostate cancer (SABOR) population and obtained an only slightly diminished AUC of 65.5%. Two validations have recently been published in 2007 as American Urological Association (AUA) abstracts by Johns Hopkins University and the University of Chicago, reporting AUCs for the PCPT Risk Calculator for prostate cancer of 66% ($N = 4,672$) and 67% ($N = 1,108$) and for the high-grade risk calculator, 63% and 74%, respectively. Thompson and colleagues *(4)* recently prescribed modified use of the calculator on a population receiving the chemopreventative agent finasteride, suggesting that the PSA value be doubled for entry to the PCPT calculator since finasteride approximately halves PSA. They validated the calculator on 4,440 men on the finasteride arm of the PCPT and obtained AUCs of 76.8% for prostate cancer and 85.5% for high-grade disease. AUCs were higher on the finasteride arm than on the placebo arm of the PCPT due to the increased sensitivity of PSA on finasteride as shown by Thompson and colleagues *(5)*.

AUCs in the range of 65–70% may seem low for a risk calculator yet the Gail risk model for female breast cancer risk, first developed in 1989 and available on the Internet, has an AUC of 59.6%, and is widely used for recommendation for more invasive diagnostic testing and for enrollment in prevention trials. Nevertheless, the suboptimal operating characteristics (low sensitivity and high false positive rates) of PSA and the PCPT Risk Calculator limit its use for population screening.

## ENHANCING THE PCPT RISK CALCULATOR FOR NEW MARKERS AND RISK FACTORS

Given the limitations of PSA and the established risk factors for accurate diagnosis of prostate cancer, the search continues for new biomarkers. The Early Detection Research Network (EDRN) of the National Cancer Institute (NCI) along with other groups are dedicated to the aim of discovery of new markers for prostate cancer, through a variety of high-dimensional platforms and new targeted assays. One promising new marker is the urine marker PCA3 *(6)*. In addition there are inexpensive risk factors that can be evaluated for contribution to risk, including detailed family history and body mass index (BMI). Therefore Drs. Ankerst and Thompson are currently developing new statistical methods for expanding the PCPT Risk Calculator to incorporate new markers and risk factors by means of combining information from multiple sources, including smaller case-control studies of expensive marker panels. The methodology uses Bayes formula for updating prior odds of disease, based on the PCPT Risk Calculator, to the posterior odds of disease based on the PCPT risk factors and the new markers through use of the likelihood ratio. The likelihood ratio is the ratio of the probability of the new markers for diseased to non-diseased individuals and can be estimated by a separate case control study to the PCPT.

The PCPT Risk Calculator will expand along with the discovery of new markers and risk factors for prostate cancer, continuing to provide the most current accurate risk prediction for prostate cancer screening.

## REFERENCES

1. Thompson, I. M., Ankerst, D.P., Chi, C., Goodman, P.J., Tangen, C.M., Lucia, M.S., Feng, Z., Parnes, H.L., Coltman, C.A., Jr. (2006) Assessing prostate cancer risk: Results from the Prostate Cancer Prevention Trial *Journal of the National Cancer Institute* **98**, 529–34.
2. Etzioni, R.D., Ankerst, D.P., Thompson, I.M. (2007) Is PSA velocity useful in early detection of prostate cancer? A critical appraisal of the evidence *Journal of the National Cancer Institute* **99**, 489–90.
3. Parekh, D.J., Ankerst, D.P., Higgins, B.A., Hernandez, J., Canby-Hagino, E., Brand, T., Troyer, D., Leach, R., Thompson, I.M. (2006) External validation of the Prostate Cancer Prevention Trial risk calculator *Urology* **68**, 1152–5.
4. Thompson, I.M., Ankerst, D.P., Chi, C., Goodman, P.J., Tangen, C.M., Lippman, S.M., Lucia, M.S., Parnes, H.L., Coltman, C.A., Jr. (2007) Prediction of prostate cancer for patients receiving finasteride: results from the Prostate Cancer Prevention Trial *Journal of Clinical Oncology* **25**, 3076–81.
5. Thompson, I.M., Chi, C., Ankerst, D.P., Goodman, P., Tangen, C., Lippman, S., Lucia, M.S., Parnes, H.L., Coltman, C.A. (2006) Effect of finasteride on the sensitivity of PSA for detecting prostate cancer *Journal of the National Cancer Institute* **98**, 1128–33.
6. Marks, L.S., Fradet, Y., Deras, I.L., Blase, A., Mathis, J., Aubin, S.M.J., Cancio, A.T., Desaulniers, M., Ellis, W.J., Rittenhouse, H., Groskopf, J. (2007) PCA3 molecular urine assay for prostate cancer in men undergoing repeat biopsy *Urology* **69**, 532–5.

# 13 Integration of Risk Assessment in Prostate Cancer Screening

*Kadee E Thompson, Amanda Reed, and Dipen J Parekh*

## Contents

## Summary

While the current value of prostate cancer screening in reducing mortality is debatable, there is no doubt that screening has created overdetection of clinically insignificant cancers. An individualized risk assessment model incorporating the known risk factors associated with prostate cancer could be of potential value for predicting the risk of prostate cancer and helping individual patients make rational decisions regarding further diagnostic evaluation. Promising risk assessment tools, combining multiple established risk factors, current and newly developed markers for prostate cancer detection could impact downstream decisions, including screening options. This chapter will summarize some of the currently available risk assessment models for prostate cancer detection.

**Key Words:** Prostate cancer risk assessment, PCPT risk calculator, Age and race-specific reference ranges.

## BODY TEXT

Since the introduction of prostate-specific antigen (PSA), prostate cancer screening has witnessed a decrease in the number of detected life-threatening cancers in the USA. While the number of men diagnosed with advanced prostate cancers has dwindled, the

From: *Current Clinical Urology: Prostate Cancer Screening*, Edited by: D. P. Ankerst et al.
DOI 10.1007/978-1-60327-281-0_13 © Humana Press, a part of Springer Science+Business Media, LLC 2009

widespread use of PSA screening has invoked concern regarding overdetection of clinically insignificant disease. Traditionally, a PSA threshold value of 4.0 ng/mL with an abnormal digital rectal examination (DRE) has been considered the ideal indication for biopsy among men of all ages. Catalona et al. reported a cancer detection rate of 78% afforded by use of a total PSA threshold of 4.0 ng/mL and abnormal DRE in an early detection screening study of 6,630 men (1). Others, however, have cautioned against dichotomizing PSA results, arguing that an unacceptable number of patients with clinically significant, organ-confined cancer would be missed if a single reference range were used for all age and risk groups. As early as 1995, Gann showed that the risk of being diagnosed with an aggressive cancer increased incrementally during the 10 years following a baseline PSA measurement, even for PSA levels below 4.0 ng/mL (2). This concern was supported by the Prostate Cancer Prevention Trial (PCPT) study as well as data from the National Health and Nutrition Examination Survey 2001–2002 (NHANES 2001–2002), both studies confirming a large number of biopsy-detectable cancers in men with a "normal" PSA value (3,4). The PCPT has initiated the concept of chemoprevention for prostate cancer. The results of upcoming chemoprevention trials such as the SELECT and the REDUCE are keenly awaited and may establish the role of chemoprevention in prostate cancer.

While the current value of prostate cancer screening in reducing mortality is debatable, there is no doubt about the overdetection of clinically insignificant cancers. The questions faced by a man regarding screening for prostate cancer are multifold–What are the chances of getting diagnosed with life-threatening prostate cancer, what are the chemoprevention options available and should are they be expected to alter the risk of prostate cancer? The above questions cannot be satisfactorily answered using the current screening practices. An individualized risk assessment model incorporating the known risk factors associated with prostate cancer could be of potential value in accurately predicting a man's current risk of prostate cancer and enabling him, along with his physician, to make a rational decision while facing the above questions. Integration of risk assessment has been successfully adopted in the field of breast cancer detection and screening. Several risk assessment tools exist that provide individualized risk for breast cancer development thereby channeling women with high risk to seek appropriate chemopreventive, diagnostic, as well as therapeutic strategies (5–7). Furthermore, with the emergence of novel biomarkers, an ideal platform would integrate the existing risk factors into a user-friendly format for both patients and clinicians. Promising risk assessment tools have been recently developed for prostate cancer detection that will impact the entire decision-making process a man faces when confronted with screening options. This chapter will summarize the currently available risk assessment models for prostate cancer detection. Many of these models have been described in more detail in separate chapters devoted to them.

## PROSTATE CANCER PREVENTION TRIAL (PCPT) RISK CALCULATOR

The Prostate Cancer Prevention Trial (PCPT ) was a randomized trial that assigned 18,882 men to either finasteride or placebo for 7 years (3). Eligibility criteria included men 55 years old or older with a normal DRE and a PSA level less than or equal to 3 ng/mL. The unique feature of this trial was the requirement of all men not diagnosed with prostate cancer to undergo an end of the study biopsy regardless of the PSA level and DRE findings. The PCPT risk calculator was derived from the placebo arm of the

PCPT trial (8). A total of 5,519 subjects in the placebo group who had a PSA test and DRE within 1 year of biopsy were selected for this study. In a multivariable analysis, a statistically significant association was found between the following variables with an increased risk of prostate cancer: increasing log (PSA) (odds ratio [OR] = 2.34, P < 0.001), positive family history of prostate cancer (OR = 1.31, P = 0.002), and abnormal DRE result (OR = 2.47, P < 0.001). Previous history of one or more negative biopsies was statistically significantly associated with a decreased risk of prostate cancer (OR = 0.64, 95% CI = 0.53–0.78, P < 0.001). Statistically significant predictors of high-grade disease included the logarithm of the PSA level (OR = 3.64, P < 0.001), the DRE result (OR = 2.72, P < 0.001), and previous prostate biopsy (OR = 0.70, P = 0.04). Race was a statistically significant predictor of high-grade disease with African Americans having a higher risk of high-grade disease than non-African Americans (OR = 2.61, P < 0.001).

In collaboration with the Early Detection Research Network of the National Cancer Institute, the above-mentioned risk factors were incorporated to develop a prostate cancer risk calculator. The risk calculator is available in a user-friendly web-based format at http://www.compass.fhcrc.org/edrnnci/bin/calculator/main.asp. Values of predetermined variables can be entered to obtain percentage risks of prostate cancer as well as high-grade cancer on prostate biopsy. Further details regarding the performance characteristics of the PCPT risk calculator are covered in a separate chapter. The PCPT risk calculator enables a patient to know his risk in percentage for developing prostate cancer. Different patients will have unique perspectives and variable comfort levels while deciding a percent risk value that would then trigger a biopsy. At the present time, there are no set guidelines regarding the use of percentage risk that should prompt biopsy in men. Ideally it would be prudent not to set such guidelines that would again dichotomize the use of the risk calculator. The value of the risk calculator would be mainly in educating patients and informing them about their individualized risk for developing prostate cancer based on their own unique variables and letting them decide what would be an acceptable level of risk to trigger a biopsy. The following example, while highlighting the utility of the risk-based approach, also points out the flaws in the current screening strategies. A 60-year-old Caucasian man with a PSA of 3.0 ng/mL, normal DRE, negative family history, and no prior prostate biopsy has a 30% risk estimate of biopsy-detectable prostate cancer based on the PCPT risk calculator. On a separate note, if a 60-year-old Caucasian man has a positive family history of prostate cancer, a PSA value of 2.2 ng/mL would give him an equivalent 30% risk of prostate cancer detection. As per our current clinical practice, while the man in the first scenario would be offered a biopsy using a PSA cut-off value of 2.5 ng/mL, the man in the second scenario would not be offered a biopsy despite having the same individualized risk of prostate cancer as the man in the first scenario.

The PCPT risk calculator has been validated in a separate external cohort (9). The San Antonio Center of Biomarkers Of Risk for Prostate Cancer (SABOR) is a clinical and epidemiologic validation center of the Early Detection Research Network of the National Cancer Institute. Since 2000, SABOR has recruited 3,379 men without a diagnosis of prostate cancer into a longitudinal follow-up study. The break up of the cohort with regards to ethnicity was as follows: 1,712 (49.1%) non-Hispanic whites, 1,296 (37.2%) Hispanics, 472 (13.5%) African Americans, and 8 men of other minorities (0.2%). Study subjects were followed-up annually with PSA and DRE, with prostate biopsy offered for a PSA level of 2.5 ng/mL or more, abnormal DRE findings, or a positive family history of prostate cancer. From the above cohort, 446 participants who had undergone a prostate biopsy were selected. The risk of prostate cancer for each SABOR participant as determined by the PCPT risk calculator was calculated using the risk equation developed from the PCPT data. The PCPT risk score was highly associated with an increasing risk of prostate cancer, with 9.8% of the 41 participants with a PCPT risk of less than 15% diagnosed with cancer and increasing to 53.2% of the 47 participants with a PCPT risk greater than 50. The area underneath the receiver operating characteristic curve (AUC) for the PCPT risk score was 65.5%.

The utility of the PCPT risk calculator as an attractive screening tool was underlined recently by Reed et al. (10). In light of the discordance in recommended screening strategies for high-risk men, they evaluated the impact of age and race on the development of high-grade prostate cancer using the PCPT risk calculator. Reed et al. identified the risk of high-grade disease at which a man would be referred for biopsy using specific age and race cut-offs. Tables 1 and 2 characterize the risk of high-grade disease using the PCPT risk calculator for age and PSA values. Highlighted boxes illustrate the PSA threshold values at which a biopsy would be recommended if age-specific reference ranges were to be implemented (11,12). For instance, a 55-year-old Caucasian male would be advised to proceed with prostate biopsy when his risk of high-grade disease reached 5% (Table 1). However, a 55-year-old African American man with identical risk factors would have a 12% risk of high-grade disease at the time a biopsy would be

Table 1

Risk of Biopsy-Detected High-Grade Prostate Cancer (%). Caucasian Man, Normal Rectal Examination, No Family History of Prostate Cancer, No Previous Prostate Biopsy

| Age | PSA (ng/mL) | | | | | | | | | | | | |
|-----|-----|-----|-----|-----|-----|-----|-----|-----|-----|-----|-----|-----|-----|
|     | 0.5 | 1.0 | 1.5 | 2.0 | 2.5 | 3.0 | 3.5 | 4.0 | 4.5 | 5.0 | 5.5 | 6.0 | 6.5 |
| 55  | 0 | 1 | 2 | 2 | 3 | 4 | 5 | 6 | 7 | 8 | 9 | 10 | 11 |
| 60  | 0 | 1 | 2 | 3 | 4 | 5 | 6 | 7 | 8 | 9 | 10 | 11 | 12 |
| 65  | 1 | 1 | 2 | 3 | 4 | 6 | 7 | 8 | 9 | 10 | 11 | 13 | 14 |
| 70  | 1 | 2 | 3 | 4 | 5 | 6 | 8 | 9 | 10 | 12 | 13 | 14 | 16 |
| 75  | 1 | 2 | 3 | 5 | 6 | 7 | 9 | 10 | 12 | 13 | 15 | 16 | 18 |

Table 2

Risk of Biopsy-Detected High Grade Prostate Cancer (%). African American Man, Normal Rectal Examination, No Family History of Prostate Cancer, No Previous Prostate Biopsy

| Age | PSA (ng/mL) | | | | | | | | | | | | |
|-----|-----|-----|-----|-----|-----|-----|-----|-----|-----|-----|-----|-----|-----|
|     | 0.5 | 1.0 | 1.5 | 2.0 | 2.5 | 3.0 | 3.5 | 4.0 | 4.5 | 5.0 | 5.5 | 6.0 | 6.5 |
| 55  | 1 | 3 | 4 | 6 | 8 | 10 | 12 | 14 | 16 | 18 | 20 | 22 | 23 |
| 60  | 1 | 3 | 5 | 7 | 9 | 12 | 14 | 16 | 18 | 20 | 22 | 24 | 26 |
| 65  | 1 | 4 | 6 | 8 | 11 | 13 | 16 | 18 | 21 | 23 | 25 | 27 | 29 |
| 70  | 2 | 4 | 7 | 10 | 12 | 15 | 18 | 21 | 23 | 26 | 28 | 30 | 33 |
| 75  | 2 | 5 | 8 | 11 | 14 | 17 | 20 | 23 | 26 | 29 | 31 | 34 | 36 |

recommended. A 70-year-old Caucasian male would possess a 16% risk of high-grade disease before biopsy would be recommended while a 70-year-old African American man would reach 33% risk before biopsy was advised (Table 2).

Using these data, many men with high-grade prostate cancer might be advised that biopsy would be unnecessary if age or race-adjusted PSA cut-offs were utilized. As shown by Reed et al., the use of PCPT risk calculator obviates the deficiencies of utilizing the age and race-specific PSA reference ranges to guide decision-making regarding offering a prostate biopsy.

## NOMOGRAMS ASSESSING INDIVIDUAL RISK FOR PROSTATE CANCER

In an effort to aid patients undergoing PSA screening, a clinical nomogram was recently devised by Nam et al. to estimate individual risk for having prostate cancer using all known risk factors associated with prostate cancer *(13)*. The nomogram was based on 3,108 men who were referred between June 1999 and June 2005 to the University of Toronto network. From these, 2,700 subjects either had a PSA value $\geq$ 4.0 ng/mL or abnormal DRE. All patients underwent transrectal ultrasonography-guided needle core biopsies with a median number of 8 cores. Patients with a previous history of prostate cancer or with PSA greater than 50 ng/mL were excluded from the study. All study patients provided adequate baseline information regarding known risk factors associated with prostate cancer such as family history and ethnicity. From a separate prostate cancer screening program offered to the general public, 408 volunteers who were willing to undergo a prostate biopsy with a PSA in the range of 0–4.0 ng/mL were also included in the study. Abnormal DRE was found in 160 (39.2%) subjects. Variables evaluated included AUA Symptom Score, DRE results, serum PSA level, family history of prostate cancer information, and ethnic background. Stored serum (at −70°C) was evaluated for free:total PSA ratio measurements for each patient. Cases were defined as those with presence of prostate cancer on biopsies whereas controls had no evidence of prostate cancer on biopsy. Risk factors associated with prostate cancer such as age, family history of prostate cancer, ethnicity, the presence of lower urinary tract voiding symptoms, total PSA levels, free:total PSA ratio, and DRE findings were compared between cases and controls using unconditional logistic regression. While creating a nomogram, ordinal logistic regression was used to model the probability of having low- or high-grade cancer. From a total of 3,108 patients, two thirds were used for model building, and the remaining one third was used for model assessment. The nomogram was validated using discrimination and calibration. Of 3,108 men, 1,304 men (42%) were found to have adenocarcinoma of the prostate at biopsy (cases), and 1,804 patients (58%) had no evidence of cancer (controls). From the 408 subjects with a PSA < 4.0 ng/mL, 99 (24.3%) had cancer at biopsy. Of 1,304 patients with cancer, more than one half had a Gleason score of 7 or higher; 19 (1.5%) had a Gleason score of 4–5; 534 (40.9%) had a Gleason score of 6; 606 (46.5%) had a Gleason score of 7, and 145 (11.1%) had a Gleason score of 8–10 cancer. All the above-mentioned risk factors were found to be significantly associated with prostate cancer detection from univariate and multivariate analyses. The nomogram can predict both the presence of prostate cancer as well as high-grade cancers. The area underneath the receiver operating characteristic curve (AUC) in predicting overall prostate cancer was 0.74, while the AUC for predicting high-grade cancer was 0.77. A separate nomogram was then obtained from exactly the same dataset using the conventional screening tools such as the PSA and DRE alone. The results of the two nomograms were then compared. The total AUC for the nomogram using the conventional screening methods was significantly lower than the more comprehensive nomogram (AUC, 0.62; for any cancer; AUC, 0.69; for high-grade cancer). The authors performed further analysis to determine the importance of each individual risk factor by removing them individually from the model and then evaluating the AUC of the rest of the factors and noting the difference or drop in the prediction. The removal of PSA and DRE from the nomogram model resulted in an incremental AUC drop of 0.010 whereas the removal of all of the other risk factors resulted in an incremental AUC drop of 0.082. When compared to PSA, each of the individual risk factors performed in a similar or better fashion regarding the incremental drop in the AUC. The nomogram also performed better than the conventional screening methods in patients with PSA levels < 4.0 ng/mL. For patients with a PSA ≥ 4.0 ng/mL, the ratio of free:total PSA was the most important predictor. For prediction of high-grade cancers, age, DRE, PSA, and free:total PSA ratio were found to be statistically significant variables. The nomogram constructed by the authors is more comprehensive compared to the existing nomograms for prostate cancer risk prediction *(14,15)*.

In the future, other variables of risk such as the genetic status, body mass index, ethnicity as well as newly discovered biomarkers will be folded into the existent risk assessment tools to further increase their predictive value. Most recently, PCA3, a novel urine biomarker for prostate cancer has been added to the PCPT risk calculator and validated in an independent population (Ankerst et al, in press).

## CONCLUSIONS

The integration of risk assessment into screening for disease, though novel to the field of prostate cancer detection, has been in widespread use in other areas of clinical medicine. For example, individual cardiology decisions for preventive or therapeutic interventions are often based on the individual risk of cardiovascular disease based on the unique individual characteristics and risk factors for the individual. The cardiac event risk calculator, which was developed from the data from the Framingham study, is widely used to inform patients about their individual risk of developing a cardiac event during a 10-year period *(16)*. Based on their individual risk, patients are offered preventive interventions to potentially alter or diminish their risk of a future cardiac event. A similar paradigm of individualized risk assessment is very commonly used in breast cancer detection where patients at high-risk of being diagnosed with breast cancer are offered prophylactic options that could be highly invasive in nature *(17)*. Preventive health decisions, as in other areas of medicine and cancer, should not be forced, but preference driven. The decision to undergo a prostate biopsy is not made with an endpoint of diagnosis of prostate cancer. The diagnosis of prostate cancer is just the beginning of a phase that involves a multitude of complex therapeutic choices that confronts the patient and his family. Every treatment option currently in use for prostate cancer has a potential adverse impact on the quality of life of that individual. The final decision balancing quality versus quantity of life rests on the individual patient. Against the above-background, it is clear that the current dichotomous strategies of prostate cancer screening are flawed and do not take into account a man's unique individualized attributes that could significantly alter his own risk of developing prostate cancer. It would be erroneous to use the tools of risk assessment to simplify the clinical recommendations for biopsy by recommending a single threshold of risk. Instead, the decision to undergo a biopsy should be made on an elective basis by the patient based on the degree of concern for risk of prostate cancer along with the general health of the patient, overall life expectancy, as well as degree of aversion to potential downstream treatment related interventions.

# REFERENCES

1. Catalona WJ, Richie JP, Ahmann FR, et al. Comparison of digital rectal examination and serum prostate specific antigen in the early detection of prostate cancer: results of a multicenter clinical trial of 6,630 men. The Journal of Urology 1994;151(5):1283–90.
2. Gann PH, Hennekens CH, Stampfer MJ. A prospective evaluation of plasma prostate-specific antigen for detection of prostatic cancer. JAMA 1995;273(4):289–94.
3. Thompson IM, Goodman PJ, Tangen CM, et al. The influence of finasteride on the development of prostate cancer. The New England Journal of Medicine 2003;349(3):215–24.
4. Porter MP, Stanford JL, Lange PH. The distribution of serum prostate-specific antigen levels among American men: implications for prostate cancer prevalence and screening. The Prostate 2006;66(10):1044–51.
5. Gail MH, Costantino JP, Pee D, et al. Projecting individualized absolute invasive breast cancer risk in African American women. Journal of the National Cancer Institute 2007;99(23):1782–92.
6. Gail MH, Costantino JP. Validating and improving models for projecting the absolute risk of breast cancer. Journal of the National Cancer Institute 2001;93(5):334–5.
7. Gail MH, Anderson WF, Garcia-Closas M, Sherman ME. Absolute risk models for subtypes of breast cancer. Journal of the National Cancer Institute 2007;99(22):1657–9.
8. Thompson IM, Ankerst DP, Chi C, et al. Assessing prostate cancer risk: results from the Prostate Cancer Prevention Trial. Journal of the National Cancer Institute 2006;98(8):529–34.
9. Parekh DJ, Ankerst DP, Higgins BA, et al. External validation of the prostate cancer prevention trial risk calculator in a screened population. Urology 2006;68(6):1152–5.
10. Reed A, Ankerst DP, Pollock BH, Thompson IM, Parekh DJ. Current age and race adjusted prostate specific antigen threshold values delay diagnosis of high grade prostate cancer. The Journal of Urology 2007;178(5):1929–32; discussion 32.
11. Oesterling JE. Age-specific reference ranges for serum PSA. The New England Journal of Medicine 1996;335(5):345–6.
12. Morgan TO, Jacobsen SJ, McCarthy WF, Jacobson DJ, McLeod DG, Moul JW. Age-specific reference ranges for prostate-specific antigen in black men. The New England Journal of Medicine 1996;335(5):304–10.
13. Nam RK, Toi A, Klotz LH, et al. Assessing individual risk for prostate cancer. Journal of Clinical Oncology 2007;25(24):3582–8.
14. Finne P, Auvinen A, Aro J, et al. Estimation of prostate cancer risk on the basis of total and free prostate-specific antigen, prostate volume and digital rectal examination. European Urology 2002;41(6):619–26; discussion 26–7.
15. Karakiewicz PI, Benayoun S, Kattan MW, et al. Development and validation of a nomogram predicting the outcome of prostate biopsy based on patient age, digital rectal examination and serum prostate specific antigen. The Journal of Urology 2005;173(6):1930–4.
16. Wilson PW, D'Agostino RB, Levy D, Belanger AM, Silbershatz H, Kannel WB. Prediction of coronary heart disease using risk factor categories. Circulation 1998;97(18):1837–47.
17. Ozanne EM, Klemp JR, Esserman LJ. Breast cancer risk assessment and prevention: a framework for shared decision-making consultations. The Breast Journal 2006;12(2):103–13.

# 14 Family History of Prostate Cancer During Rapidly Increasing Incidence

## Kari Hemminki and Justo Lorenzo Bermejo

CONTENTS

## SUMMARY

The Swedish Family-Cancer Database has been used for some 12 years in the study of familial risks of cancer at all common sites. The current version VII was assembled in the year 2006 and it includes all residents in Sweden born or immigrated in 1932 and later (offspring) with their biological parents, a total of 11.5 million individuals. Cancer cases were retrieved from the Swedish Cancer Registry from years 1958 to 2004, including over 1.0 million cancers. We show applications of the Database in the study of familial risks in prostate cancer, with special reference to the modification of familial risk at the time of about 50% increase in incidence due to prostate-specific antigen (PSA) screening. The familial relative risks for prostate cancer were 1.88 for sons and 3.42 for brothers of affected patients. Familial risks were calculated for two overlapping birth cohorts, separated by 8 years. The risk for sons of affected fathers was 3.85 in the period 1961–1996 compared to 3.48 in 1969–2004. For brothers, the corresponding risks were 2.57 and 4.35. The explanations to these reverse effects were assumed to be the increasing background rate and availability of PSA testing. The consideration of the time after diagnosis of the first family member revealed that the familial risk of prostate cancer was significantly higher when the two family members were diagnosed in the same year compared to 5+ years apart. Increased surveillance and the availability of PSA screening are the likely reasons for the overestimated familial relative risk shortly after the first diagnosis. This lead time bias should be considered in clinical counseling.

From: *Current Clinical Urology: Prostate Cancer Screening*, Edited by: D. P. Ankerst et al.
DOI 10.1007/978-1-60327-281-0_14 © Humana Press, a part of Springer Science+Business Media, LLC 2009

**Key Words:** Familial cancers, Offspring, Brother, Familial risk, Genes, PSA screening, Clinical counseling.

## BODY TEXT

According to the Swedish Family-Cancer Database, 20.2% of men up to age 72 years diagnosed with prostate cancer have a paternal or fraternal family history, this being the highest familial proportion for any cancer site, followed by breast (13.6%) and colorectal (12.8%) cancers *(1)*. The proportion of familial prostate cancers has been equally high in a study from Utah *(2)*. The family history is the prime anamnestic piece of information for the clinical genetic counseling of many cancers, including breast, prostate, and colorectal cancers *(3,4)*. A confirmed family history of a disease has been the initial clue about its heritable causation and a starting point for gene identification of most hereditary diseases, with recent successes for prostate cancer *(5–7)*.

Public awareness of familial risks and the demand for counseling have increased. In USA, increasing numbers of the National Cancer Institute-designated cancer centers offer clinical genetic counseling, not only to patients and their families but also to any concerned individuals *(8)*. Awareness of familial risks and concern after diagnosis of a family member may lead to an early diagnosis of the same disease, if screening methods are available *(9)*. The usefulness of the family history is critically dependent on its accuracy. A recommendation for mutation testing for a disease gene is usually based on the family history, and incomplete/false information on family history may result in inappropriate advice. Unfortunately patients tend often to be unaware of the medical histories of their relatives. Data on the accuracy of family histories have been accumulated by comparing reported histories to those with medical documentation. Murff et al. collected literature on the accuracy of family history data for cancer *(10)*. The positive predictive value (positives of true positives) of the reported family history compared to medical diagnosis in a first-degree relative was 85% for prostate cancer when reported by cancer patients. When the family histories were reported by healthy controls, the positive predictive value was only 68%. The percentages were lower for the second-degree relatives than for the first-degree relatives. Many of the findings were similar in a Swedish study *(11)*. These data are worrisome as they are, but they may be even worse for many internal cancers, let alone for other diseases, for which the diagnostics have not been as uniform as they have been for cancer during the past half-century.

Familial clustering of cancer can be identified through a number of approaches. The clinical identification of probands and construction of pedigrees have been the classical approach into heritable diseases. Population-based datasets on familial cancer have been assembled in Utah, Iceland, UK, Denmark, Finland, and Sweden *(12–15)*. The largest dataset on familial cancer is the Swedish Family-Cancer Database, which has been updated periodically, and in the present article we use the seventh update (FCD2004), covering cancers up to year 2004. We show an application of the Database on prostate cancer, with a special reference to the familial risks during a period of an increasing incidence.

## THE FAMILY-CANCER DATABASE OF YEAR 2004

Statistics Sweden created a family database, "Second Generation Register" in 1995 *(16)*. After a few expansions, it covered offspring born after 1931 with their parents, renamed to "Multigeneration Register" to indicate that the number of generations was more than two. We have linked this Register to the Swedish Cancer Registry (1958–2004) to make the Family-Cancer Database (MigMed2) in year 2006 for the seventh time, called here FCD2004 *(17,18)*. As a novelty, FCD2004 contains data on all immigrants, whereas the previous versions only included those who had had children in Sweden. In FCD all data are organized in child–mother–father triplets; the parents have been registered at the time of birth of the child, allowing tracking of "biological" parents in spite of divorce and remarriage.

FCD2004 identified a total of 11.5 million persons, divided into parental and offspring generations. An overwhelming proportion (97.9%) of offsprings born in Sweden have information on parents, but the proportion is much smaller for offspring born outside Sweden, for obvious reasons. Even for those born in Sweden, the parental links are more numerous for living than for deceased individuals; 10.9% of offspring with cancer lack parental links. FCD2004 contains 1.2 million tumor notifications, 796,000 are first primary cancers, 85,000 are multiple primaries, and 237,000 are in situ cancers, dominated by cervical in situ cancers. The offspring generation was born after 1931 and their parents before that year. Thus the oldest age of the offspring generation was 74 years while the ages of the parents were not limited.

## INCIDENCE OF PROSTATE CANCER IN SWEDEN

The increase in the incidence of prostate cancer has been 3.4-fold in Sweden for the period 1960–2004, based on the Swedish Cancer Registry *(19)*. We surveyed the trend further and show in Fig. 1 the age-standardized incidence for years 1980–2005. The incidence in year 2005 is lower than in the previous year but it is unclear whether the decrease will continue. In the US SEER data, a joinpoint analysis showed a temporary downward reflection for period 1992–1995, followed by a slow increase again in period 1995–2002 *(20)*. In Germany, a joinpoint analysis showed a downward trend

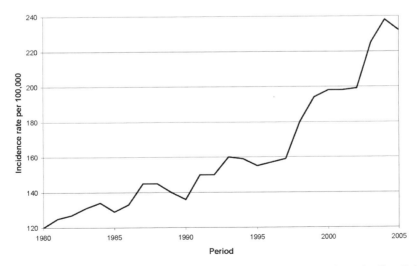

**Fig. 1.** Annual age-standardized incidence rate of prostate cancer, based on the Swedish Cancer Registry.

for the last observation period, 1994–2002 *(21)*. An introduction of a successful population screening method is initially expected to increase the incidence and subsequently decrease it. The Swedish experience is yet too recent to show any trend shifts, and like any uncontrolled introduction of a new screening tool, the results may remain impossible to interpret even in the future.

In interpreting the Swedish incidence trends two different patterns have been discerned. The first phase prevailed until about year 1995, and it was characterized by a preferential increase in incidence in those older than 70 years *(19)*. This increase coincided with a more common and intense application of prostatic biopsies and transurethral resection techniques *(22)*. In the second phase, after year 1997, the 50% increase extended preferentially to younger age groups and it coincided with a wide application of opportunistic prostate-specific antigen (PSA) testing *(23,24)*. The widespread use of PSA testing was the probable cause of the upward shift in the incidence between years 1998 and 2004. The official policy on PSA testing has been restrictive in Sweden, which probably delayed the wide-spread use of the PSA testing compared to USA, even though the test was developed in Sweden. This may be the reason for the late steep upraise and saturation of prostate cancer incidence.

Prostate cancer has been a disease of old men but the age-incidence relationships have changed drastically in the past decade and an ever larger proportion of younger men are affected *(19)*. Although we have no proof that the diagnostic procedures are the only cause of the observed changes, it appears reasonable to assume that they have contributed to the shift. A similar shift in age-incidence relationships has been observed for breast cancer in countries where mammographic screening has a high penetration *(25–27)*.

## FAMILIAL RISKS

Age-specific familial incidence rates for prostate cancer are shown in Fig. 2, based on FCD2004 (oldest age for sons being 72 years). The lowest curve shows the overall incidence in Sweden, the next higher curves show the incidence in sons of affected

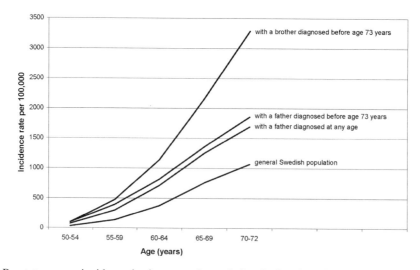

**Fig. 2.** Prostate cancer incidence in the general population in Sweden (*bottom*), in sons of affected fathers, in sons of affected fathers when fathers were diagnosed before age 73 years and in brothers of prostate cancer patients (*top*).

fathers of all ages and in those whose fathers were diagnosed before age 73 years; these two curves show the effect of proband age on familial risk. The top curve is the incidence for brothers. The differences between the familial and overall rates give the familial risks which are higher in the young ages. The familial risk, given as standardized incidence ratios (SIRs, adjusted for age, period, socioeconomic status, and region) in son–father pairs was 1.88 (2,472 affected sons) and in brothers 3.42 (859 affected brothers).

We analyze the effect of age on familial risk by contour plots for familial SIRs in son–father pairs (Fig. 3) and in brothers (Fig. 4). Figures 3a and 4a are based on the observed SIRs, which were smoothed by weighted robust linear regression in Figs. 3b and 4b. We have no direct interpretation for the irregularities of the "crude" contours but

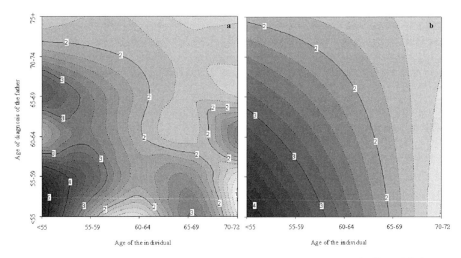

**Fig. 3.** Contour plots of familial relative risks for prostate cancer in sons of affected fathers according to age, (**A**) plots based on raw familial risks, (**B**) plots smoothened by weighted robust linear regression.

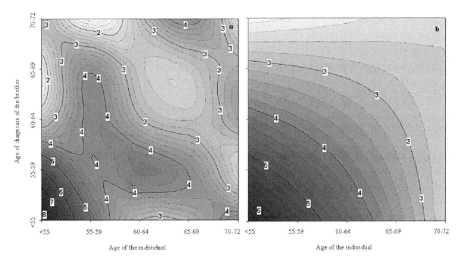

**Fig. 4.** Contour plots of familial relative risks for prostate cancer in brothers of patients according to age, (**A**) plots based on raw familial risks, (**B**) plots smoothened by weighted robust linear regression.

## Table 1
### Age-Specific Incidence Rates Per 100,000 Person-Years and Incidence Ratios of Prostate Cancer According to Family History and Diagnostic Period

| Age (years) | General Swedish population | | With affected father* | | | | With affected brother* | | | |
|---|---|---|---|---|---|---|---|---|---|---|
| | 1961–1996 | 1969–2004 | 1961–1996 | | 1969–2004 | | 1961–1996 | | 1969–2004 | |
| | IR | IR | IR | N, SIR (95%CI) | IR | N, SIR (95%CI) | IR | N, SIR (95%CI) | IR | N, SIR (95%CI) |
| 45–49 | 2.8 | 5.4 | 28.7 | 2, 10.4 (2.58–42.3) | 26.6 | 3, 4.96 (1.59–15.5) | 6.0 | 2, 2.20 (0.31–15.7) | 41.6 | 8, 7.76 (2.89–20.8) |
| 50–54 | 16.6 | 40.4 | 111.8 | 4, 6.75 (2.52–18.1) | 200.5 | 15, 4.96 (2.98–8.25) | 30.4 | 7, 1.83 (0.64–5.25) | 177.4 | 29, 4.39 (2.62–7.37) |
| 55–59 | 68.4 | 172.5 | 300.1 | 4, 4.38 (1.64–11.7) | 621.7 | 25, 3.60 (2.43–5.34) | 228.4 | 27, 3.34 (1.95–5.72) | 792.8 | 84, 4.60 (3.39–6.23) |
| 60–64 | 186.2 | 478.9 | – | – | 1208.2 | 13, 2.52 (1.46–4.35) | 388.1 | 12, 2.08 (0.93–4.66) | 1791.9 | 57, 3.74 (2.59–5.41) |
| 45–64 | 24.4 | 74.3 | 94.1 | 10, 3.85 (2.07–7.17) | 258.9 | 56, 3.48 (2.68–4.53) | 62.7 | 48, 2.57 (1.72–3.84) | 323.2 | 178, 4.35 (3.53–5.36) |

*Both the father and the brother were diagnosed before age 65 years.

these are likely to be related to the large changes in incidence, which we address below. The smoothened contours show clearly the higher familial risks for brothers compared to sons of affected prostate cancer patients.

In order to assess the effect of increasing incidence on familial risks, we derived familial risks for two overlapping birth cohorts. Individuals born after 1931 were followed-up from 1961 to year 1996, individuals born after 1939 were followed-up from 1969 to 2004; thus the birth cohorts were shifted by 8 years (Table 1). The age of diagnosis of the fathers was also restricted to 64 years. Unfortunately, the numbers of cases were limited because the highest age of cases was 64 years. The overall relative risk (SIRs adjusted for age) for sons of affected fathers was 3.85 in the early period compared to 3.48 in the later period. For brothers, the risks were 2.57 and 4.35, respectively. It is notable that the largest difference for brothers in the early and in the late periods was in the youngest age group, 45–49 years, with SIRs of 2.20 and 7.76 and in the next youngest group, 50–54 years, with SIRs 1.83 and 4.39. The small number of cases in the early period guards against definite conclusions, but in every age group the SIRs for sons of affected fathers were higher in the earlier periods, while the opposite was observed for brothers. We hypothesize that the reasons for these reverse effects rest on the increasing background rates and the availability of PSA testing. The increasing rate of prostate cancer in the general population would drop in both paternal and fraternal familial relative risks, but PSA testing would have a stronger effect for brothers (fathers would have been tested rarely compared to their sons) and this would result in an overall higher SIR for brothers of prostate cancer patients, as discussed below.

## FAMILIAL CONCERNS FOR PROSTATE CANCER

The diagnosis of cancer in a family member raises concerns about the risks among the remaining members. The concern is greater if the cancer is diagnosed in a sibling, particularly at early age. The likely consequence is to seek medical advice, which in the case of prostate cancer leads to an examination and a probable PSA testing and a possible detection of a tumor. As practically all prostate cancers are histologically verified in the Swedish Cancer Registry, a false diagnosis is unlikely. Instead, the consequence is an early detection (lead time bias) or the detection of asymptomatic tumors that would have remained latent during the person's life time. The lead time may be substantial, 5–7 years, in prostate cancer *(28)*. For the familial risk, the consequence would be a decrease because of the increasing background rate (for sons of affected fathers, assuming that fathers have not undergone PSA testing), or an elevation if family members will be tested preferentially, a most likely scenario for brothers. We have some previous evidence for increasing risks of cancer shortly after a family member has been diagnosed for prostate; similar data were found also for some other cancers for which screening methods are available *(9,19,26)*.

We assessed familial risk (analyzed as relative risks, RR, adjusted for age and current calendar year) for prostate cancer in father–son pairs and brothers according to the time since the first family member was diagnosed (Fig. 5). The risk for sons was highest during the year of father's diagnosis; the risk difference between the same year (RR 3.37, $N = 31$, 95%CI 2.34–4.86) and the reference, 5+ years (RR 2.10, $N = 2,504$, 95%CIs 2.01–2.19) was significant with a $p = 0.011$. However, the only difference was noted when father and son were diagnosed in the same year. The analysis for brothers showed a somewhat different result, as the RRs decreased systematically according to the time

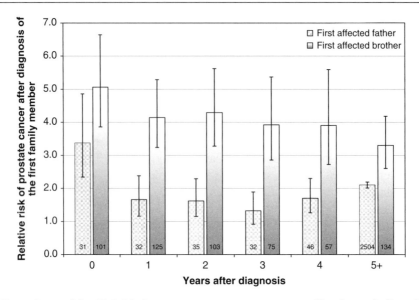

**Fig. 5.** Dependence of familial risk for prostate cancer among sons and brothers of affected patients on the time since first diagnosis.

after first diagnosis. The difference between the same and 5+ years remained. In the same year the RR was 5.06 ($N = 101$, 95%CIs 3.86–6.64) compared to 3.30 ($N = 134$, 95%CIs 2.60–4.18) in 5+ years, $p = 0.019$.

## CONCLUSIONS

Empirical risk estimates from epidemiological studies have been useful in clinical genetic counseling for prostate cancers (3,29). According to the present data from the Swedish Family-Cancer Database, the familial risk for prostate cancer in son–father pairs was 1.88 and in brothers it was 3.42. The age of the second generation was less than 73 years. The difference between the SIR for sons of affected fathers and brothers was highly significant (30). The effects through different probands could be interpreted genetically, if environmental factors have been excluded, as discussed (30). The father history could be due to dominant heritable effects and brother history (without an affected father) due to recessive or X-chromosome linked effects. However, with the present findings on the apparent bias due to screening, conclusions on higher risks among brothers than among sons of affected individuals should be drawn with caution. Patient recruitment schemes for genetic studies on prostate cancer need to consider the possibility of bias, because recruitment through health campaigns and advertisements are likely to select health conscious individuals whose familial risk may not always signal a heritable predisposition. Twin studies, which have been an important argument for the large heritable component in prostate cancer, would also be vulnerable to this type of bias, and monozygotic twins may be affected more than dizygotic twins. In the Nordic twin study, most cases of prostate cancer were diagnosed before PSA assays became commonplace (31); however, screening bias may also be caused by other diagnostic methods, such as digital rectal examination. The identification of heritable prostate cancer susceptibility genes has turned out to be cumbersome (22), and the accuracy of defining familial cases, as illustrated in the present analysis, may be one of the contributing problems which is not easy to avoid or correct. So far no evidence on recessive susceptibility for prostate cancer has been found. The newly detected prostate cancer loci on chromosome 8 are relatively common variants with genotype relative risks (risks of variant homozygotes) varying from 2.6 to 4.4; the effects of the genotypes are multiplicative *(5–7,32)*. Interestingly, this locus is also associated with the risk of colorectal cancer *(7,33,34)*. The risk is only about 1.2, which is probably the reason for the lack of familial association between prostate and colorectal cancers *(35)*.

Increased surveillance and the availability of screening methods may result in over-estimated familial relative risks shortly after the first diagnosis. We show here increased risks for prostate cancer both for father–son pairs and for brothers in the year of the first family member's diagnosis, consistent with the previous data *(9,19,26)*. However, even though the overall effect of this bias on familial risks is small, it calls for consideration in clinical counseling of individuals from families in which synchronous cancers were diagnosed. The lead time bias should not misguide the doctor, who should instead explain the possibility of overdiagnosis to the patients and their family members in order to comfort their anxiety.

## REFERENCES

1. Hemminki K., Sundquist J., Lorenzo Bermejo J. (2007) How common is familial cancer *Ann Oncol* **19,** 163–7.
2. Goldgar D.E., Easton D.F., Cannon-Albright L.A., Skolnick M.H. (1994) Systematic population-based assessment of cancer risk in first-degree relatives of cancer probands *J Natl Cancer Inst* **86,** 1600–7.
3. ASCO (2003) American Society for Clinical Oncology policy statement update: Genetic testing for cancer susceptibility *J Clin Oncol* **21,** 2397–406.
4. Hampel H., Sweet K., Westman J., Offit K., Eng C. (2004) Referral for cancer genetics consultation: a review and compilation of risk assessment criteria *J Med Genet* **41,** 81–91.
5. Amundadottir L.T., Sulem P., Gudmundsson J., et al. (2006) A common variant associated with prostate cancer in European and African populations *Nat Genet* **38,** 652–8.
6. Gudmundsson J., Sulem P., Manolescu A., et al. (2007) Genome-wide association study identifies a second prostate cancer susceptibility variant at 8q24 *Nat Genet* **39,** 631–7.
7. Haiman C.A., Patterson N., Freedman M.L., et al. (2007) Multiple regions within 8q24 independently affect risk for prostate cancer *Nat Genet* **39,** 638–44.
8. Epplein M., Koon K.P., Ramsey S.D., Potter J.D. (2005) Genetic services for familial cancer patients: a follow-up survey of National Cancer Institute Cancer Centers *J Clin Oncol* **23,** 4713–8.
9. Lorenzo Bermejo J., Hemminki K. (2005) Familial risk of cancer shortly after diagnosis of the first familial tumor *J Natl Cancer Inst* **97,** 1575–9.
10. Murff H.J., Spigel D.R., Syngal S. (2004) Does this patient have a family history of cancer? An evidence-based analysis of the accuracy of family cancer history *Jama* **292,** 1480–9.
11. Chang E., Ekström Smedby K., Hjalgrim H., Glimelius B., Adami H.O. (2006) Reliability of self-reported family history of cancer in a large case-control study of lymphoma *J Natl Cancer Inst* **98,** 61–8.
12. Amundadottir L.T., Thorvaldsson S., Gudbjartsson D.F., et al. (2004) Cancer as a complex phenotype: Pattern of cancer distribution within and beyond the Nuclear Family *PLoS Med* **1,** e65.
13. Kerber R.A., O'Brien E. (2005) A cohort study of cancer risk in relation to family histories of cancer in the Utah population database *Cancer* **103,** 1906–15.
14. Peto J., Easton D., Matthews F., Ford D., Swerdlow A. (1996) Cancer mortality in relatives of women with breast cancer: the OPCS study *Int J Cancer* **65,** 275–83.
15. Matikainen M., Pukkala E., Schleutker J., et al. (2001) Relatives of prostate cancer patients have an increased risk of prostate and stomach cancers: a population-based, cancer registry study in Finland *Cancer Causes Control* **12,** 223–30.
16. Hemminki K., Vaittinen P. (1997) Familial cancer in Sweden: population-based study *Int J Oncol* **11,** 273–80.

17. Hemminki K., Li X., Plna K., Granström C., Vaittinen P. (2001) The nation-wide Swedish Family-Cancer Database: updated structure and familial rates *Acta Oncol* **40,** 772–7.
18. Hemminki K., Granstrom C., Chen B. (2005) The Swedish Family-Cancer: update, application to colorectal cancer and clinical relevance *Heredit Cancer Clin Pract* **3,** 7–18.
19. Hemminki K., Rawal R., Lorenzo Bermejo J. (2005) Prostate cancer screening, changing age-specific incidence trends and implications on familial risk *Int J Cancer* **113,** 312–5.
20. Edwards B.K., Brown M.L., Wingo P.A., et al. (2005) Annual report to the nation on the status of cancer, 1975–2002, featuring population-based trends in cancer treatment *J Natl Cancer Inst* **97,** 1407–27.
21. Becker N., Altenburg H.P., Stegmaier C., Ziegler H. (2007) Report on trends of incidence (1970–2002) of and mortality (1952–2002) from cancer in Germany *J Cancer Res Clin Oncol* **133,** 23–35.
22. Gronberg H. (2003) Prostate cancer epidemiology *Lancet* **361,** 859–64.
23. Pilebro B., Johansson R., Damber L., Damber J.E., Stattin P. (2003) Population-based study of prostate-specific antigen testing and prostate cancer detection in clinical practice in northern Sweden *Scand J Urol Nephrol* **37,** 210–2.
24. Stattin P., Johansson R., Damber J.E., et al. (2003) Non-systematic screening for prostate cancer in Sweden – survey from the national prostate cancer registry *Scand J Urol Nephrol* **37,** 461–5.
25. Zahl P.H., Strand B.H., Maehlen J. (2004) Incidence of breast cancer in Norway and Sweden during introduction of nationwide screening: prospective cohort study *Bmj* **328,** 921–4.
26. Hemminki K., Lorenzo Bermejo J. (2005) Effects of screening for breast cancer on its age-incidence relationships and familial risk *Int J Cancer* **117,** 145–9.
27. Moller B., Weedon-Fekjaer H., Hakulinen T., et al. (2005) The influence of mammographic screening on national trends in breast cancer incidence *Eur J Cancer Prev* **14,** 117–28.
28. Auvinen A., Maattanen L., Stenman U.H., et al. (2002) Lead-time in prostate cancer screening (Finland) *Cancer Causes Control* **13,** 279–85.
29. Hemminki K., Eng C. (2004) Clinical genetic counseling for familial cancers requires reliable data on familial cancer risks and general action plans *J Med Genet* **41,** 801–7.
30. Hemminki K., Li X. (2004) Familial risks of cancer as a guide to gene identification and mode of inheritance *Int J Cancer* **110,** 291–4.
31. Lichtenstein P., Holm N., Verkasalo P., et al. (2000) Environmental and heritable factors in the causation of cancer *N Engl J Med* **343,** 78–85.
32. Yeager M., Orr N., Hayes R.B., et al. (2007) Genome-wide association study of prostate cancer identifies a second risk locus at 8q24 *Nat Genet* **39,** 645–9.
33. Zanke B.W., Greenwood C.M., Rangrej J., et al. (2007) Genome-wide association scan identifies a colorectal cancer susceptibility locus on chromosome 8q24 *Nat Genet* **39,** 989–94.
34. Tomlinson I., Webb E.L., Carvajal-Carmona L., et al. (2007) A genome-wide association scan of tag SNPs identifies a susceptibility variant for colorectal cancer at 8q24.21 *Nat Genet* **39,** 984–8.
35. Hemminki K., Chen B. (2005) Familial association of prostate cancer with other cancers in the Swedish-Family-Cancer Database *Prostate* **65,** 188–94.

# IV RECENT BIOMARKERS FOR PROSTATE CANCER

# 15 PSA Isoforms: [−2]proPSA Significant Adjunct to Free PSA

*Jeffrey E. Tam*

## Contents

## Summary

Prostate-Specific Antigen (PSA) is a widely used serum marker to aid in the diagnosis of prostate cancer and monitor its treatment. PSA by itself has limited specificity, and cannot distinguish between early stage prostate cancer and benign prostatic hyperplasia (BPH), resulting in many unnecessary biopsies. The specificity of PSA for prostate cancer was improved when it was discovered that complex and free forms of PSA existed in serum and the ratio of free to complexed PSA (%free PSA) correlated to prostate cancer. It is now known that the free form of PSA is actually composed of several proenzyme forms and enzymatically nicked PSA. The major nicked form is common to benign hyperplasia and is referred to as Benign PSA (BPSA). The proenzyme forms of PSA are collectively called proPSA and are associated with prostate cancer. There are three recognized proPSA isoforms ([−5/−7]proPSA, [−4]proPSA, and [−2]proPSA) that increase the utility of PSA in prostate cancer diagnosis.

**Key Words:** Prostate, Cancer, PSA, proPSA, Immunoassay, Diagnosis, Markers.

The concentration of prostate-specific antigen (PSA) in serum is commonly used to screen prostate cancer (PCa), despite the fact that PSA levels cannot differentiate early stage PCa from benign prostatic hyperplasia (BPH) when serum levels are between 4 and 10 ng/mL. In these cases, biopsy of the prostate is indicated to detect PCa. The specificity of PSA to detect early stages of PCa is improved when total PSA and the free proportion of PSA in serum (%free PSA) are combined. Over the last 10 years investigators have discovered that at least five PSA isoforms comprise free PSA in serum *(1)*. The concentration of one isoform versus another is often associated with certain pathologies such as PCa or BPH. The hallmark of these PSA isoforms is that they do not exhibit enzymatic activity, nor do they readily form complexes with $\alpha$-1-antichymotrypsin

From: *Current Clinical Urology: Prostate Cancer Screening*, Edited by: D. P. Ankerst et al.
DOI 10.1007/978-1-60327-281-0_15 © Humana Press, a part of Springer Science+Business Media, LLC 2009

(ACT; 2, 3). Four isoforms of free PSA have been extensively characterized. Benign PSA (BPSA) is a nicked form of PSA and is more associated with BPH. The proenzyme forms of PSA (proPSA) are isoforms which have retained all or part of the 7-amino acid leader sequence. Three proPSA isoforms are associated with PCa and are considered to have potential as tumor markers, [−5/−7]proPSA, [−4]proPSA, and [−2]proPSA isoforms.

This chapter will focus on proPSA isoforms as tumor markers, and especially on the potential utility of [−2]proPSA. The biology of PSA isoforms has been reviewed in the literature many times since 2000 and the reader is directed to these excellent and comprehensive reviews for background (1–6). Nonetheless, there are some milestones in proPSA research that deserve highlighting. Perhaps the most significant milestone was the cloning of pre-proPSA into the mammalian cell line AV12-664, and demonstration that proPSA was produced by the cell line and could be purified in quantity (7). Mikolajczyk et al. (2) later showed that recombinant cell line-produced proPSA digested with human kallikrein-2 produced PSA. The significance of this recombinant cell line was that a ready supply of proPSA analyte was now available.

Concomitant with the cloning of proPSA was the generation of monoclonal antibodies specific to the N-terminus of [−5/−7]proPSA, [−4]proPSA and [−2]proPSA. For each of the proPSA isoforms, mice were immunized with peptides representing the leader sequence of the particular PSA isoform plus the first 7 amino acids of the mature PSA molecule. The resultant monoclonal antibodies (mAbs) were reactive to the recombinant proPSA isoforms, but not to PSA. More importantly, these mAbs were reactive to proPSA in PCa serum samples (2). These data confirmed that proPSA was indeed present in serum. Further confirmation that serum contained proPSA isoforms was made by Peter et al. (8) who collected PSA from PCa patients' sera and, using mass spectrometry, identified the proPSA isoforms. These results, using non-related technology, verified Mikolajczyk's hypothesis that PSA isoforms were in the sera of PCa patients.

Further proof of the relationship between proPSA isoforms and PCa came from immunohistological staining of prostate tissue. Prostate tissue from PCa patients stained positive for [−2]proPSA, and the heaviest staining was localized to the transition zone of the prostate. Benign tissue demonstrated no significant staining (8,9).

With a ready source of recombinant [−5/−7]proPSA, [−4]proPSA, and [−2]proPSA, and monoclonal antibodies to these analytes, investigators began to quantify serum levels of these proPSA isoforms and assess their utility in differentiating PCa from BPH. Mikolajczyk et al. (10), employing the monoclonal antibodies specific for the proPSA isoforms, developed a microplate enzyme immunoassay (EIA) specific for the [−5/−7]proPSA, [−4]proPSA, and [−2]proPSA isoforms. Briefly, proPSA isoforms were captured by an anti-PSA monoclonal antibody, PSM773. The captured, or bound, proPSA was detected using [−5/−7]proPSA-, [−4]proPSA-, and [−2]proPSA-specific monoclonal antibodies labeled with europium. The assays were calibrated using recombinant [−5/−7]proPSA, [−4]proPSA, or [−2]proPSA purified from AV12-664 cells. The mass of calibrator proPSA in each was determined by a free PSA immunoassay. Table 1 shows the minimal detectable concentration and approximate precision of each of the assays.

Several investigators have used these assays to assess the clinical utility of proPSA isoforms in the detection of PCa in men with PSA levels < 10 ng/mL. Table 2 summarizes the results of these studies. All studies used retrospective samples for which disease outcome was known. Generally, it was found that none of the proPSA isoforms alone

Table 1
Assay Parameters of proPSA Microplate EIA and Access p2PSA

| Analyte | Minimum detectable concentration (pg/mL) | Imprecision (CV%) |
|---|---|---|
| [−2]proPSA | 15 | 9–14 |
| [−4]proPSA | 25 | 6–18 |
| [−5/−7]proPSA | 25 | 4–11 |
| p2PSA | <2.3 | <8% |

out-performed total PSA or %free PSA in detecting PCa. However, a ratio of proPSA (all isoforms) to free PSA (%proPSA) did give an improvement in PCa detection – as indicated by an increase in the area under the curve (AUC) of a receiver operator characteristic curve (ROC). The improvement in specificity of PCa detection cannot be overstated. For example, Sokoll et al. *(12)* found that among men with PSA levels of 2.5–4 ng/mL, 75% of the cancers would have been detected and 59% of unnecessary biopsies avoided. Using %free PSA, only 33% of the unnecessary biopsies would have been avoided. In general, Table 2 shows that the greatest benefit from proPSA is realized with serum PSA levels between 2 and 10 ng/mL.

In PCa, high-Gleason scores are equated with tumor aggressiveness and adverse prognosis. Studies attempting to relate serum PSA, free PSA, or complexed PSA concentrations to tumor aggressiveness have resulted in mixed results *(14)*. The reported association between proPSA and aggressive prostate tumors *(1)* raises the possibility that PCa aggressiveness can be predicted by %proPSA. Catalona et al. *(14)* studied the ability of %proPSA to detect PCa. Using retrospective samples from patients with Gleason scores of 7 or greater and PSA levels 2.5–4 ng/mL these investigators showed that %[−2]proPSA was indeed a better predictor of tumor aggression than either PSA or %free PSA. Paradoxically, this was not true when serum PSA was between 4 and 10 ng/mL.

While the studies cited above provided strong and consistent evidence of the clinical utility of [−2]proPSA, they carried the proviso that verification with larger and more comprehensive studies that include prospective samples was needed. To assist in this goal an automated version of the [−2]proPSA enzyme immunoassay described by Mikolajczyk et al. is under development for the Access® Immmunoassay System, called the p2PSA assay. While the Access p2PSA assay shares many of the original design attributes of the microplate EIA, the automated version has improved precision and sensitivity (Table 1). To assess the performance of this assay on patient samples, 177 serum samples from biopsied men were run on the Access Hybritech PSA, free PSA, and p2PSA assays. The median PSA concentration was 4.65 ng/mL with a range of 0.8–19 ng/mL. The median [−2]proPSA concentration was 8.3 pg/mL with a range of 2.8–119 pg/mL (Table 3). From these data, testing men with PSA levels between 4 and 10 ng/mL should have [−2]proPSA levels between 3 and 119 pg/mL *(15)*.

The Access p2PSA assay was independently evaluated by the National Cancer Institute's (NCI) Early Detection Research Network (EDRN) as a blinded study of 123 retrospective samples, collected from roughly equal numbers of PCa and non-PCa patients *(16)*. The analysis of all patients showed that the ratio of the [−2]proPSA isoform to all free forms of PSA (%[−2]proPSA) was slightly more specific for cancer

Table 2
Summary of Studies Using proPSA EIA

| Study size (N) | PSA range (ng/mL) | ROC results (AUC) | Ref |
|---|---|---|---|
| 43 | 0.4–12 | • %freePSA 0.620<br>• [−2]proPSA/(free PSA−proPSA) 0.768<br>• [−2]proPSA/(free PSA−BPSA) 0.714<br>• [−2]proPSA/(free PSA−BPSA) 0.714<br>• [−2]proPSA/(free PSA) 0.644 | (11) |
| 308 | 4–10 | • %free PSA 0.627<br>• proPSA/free PSA (%) 0.689<br>• [−2]proPSA/free PSA (%) 0.635<br><br>**When %free PSA > 25%**<br><br>• %free PSA 0.527<br>• proPSA/free PSA (%) 0.694<br>• [−2]proPSA/free PSA (%) 0.770 | (10) |
| 119 | 2.5–4 | • %free PSA 0.527<br>• pPSA/free PSA (%) 0.688 | (12) |
| 1091 | 2–10 | **PSA 2–6 ng/mL**<br><br>• %free PSA 0.568<br>• proPSA/free PSA (%) 0.623<br>• [−2]proPSA (%) 0.624<br><br>**PSA 2–6 ng/mL**<br><br>• %free PSA 0.586<br>• proPSA/free PSA (%) 0.656<br>• [−2]proPSA (%) 0.633<br><br>**PSA 4–10 ng/mL**<br><br>• %free PSA 0.633<br>• proPSA/free PSA (%) 0.683<br>• [−2]proPSA (%) 0.655<br><br>**PSA 2–10 ng/mL**<br><br>• %free PSA 0.602<br>• proPSA/free PSA (%) 0.650<br>• [−2]proPSA (%) 0.638 | (13) |

than the ratio of all free forms of PSA to total PSA (%free PSA) with ROC AUC of 0.69 (95% CI 0.60–0.79) and 0.61 (95% CI 0.51–0.71), respectively. However, when patients with PSA levels 2–10 ng/mL were considered ($N = 89$) %[−2] proPSA was clearly different from %free PSA with ROC AUC of 0.73 (95% CI 0.63–0.84) versus 0.53 (95% CI 0.41–0.65). The reported results were similar to those seen with the earlier [−2]proPSA microplate assay.

Table 3
Median [−2]proPSA Concentrations for 177 Serum Samples Taken from Men
with and Without Cancer (Biopsy Confirmed)

| Assay | Median concentration | Median concentration 95% CI | Range |
|-------|----------------------|-----------------------------|-------|
| Access p2PSA | 8.30 pg/mL | 7.43–8.91 pg/mL | 2.8–119.9 pg/mL |
| Access Hybritech® PSA | 4.65 ng/mL | 4.42–4.89 ng/mL | 0.8–19 ng/mL |
| Access Hybritech® free PSA | 0.48 ng/mL | 0.57–0.70 ng/mL | 0.2–3.8 ng/mL |

Stephan et al. *(17)* screened 475 sera with PSA levels 2–10 ng/mL with the Access Hybritech PSA, free PSA, and p2PSA assays. Their results were also similar to those reported previously for the microplate assay. The AUC for %[−2]proPSA (0.78) was the highest of the assays followed by %free PSA (0.77) and PSA (0.56). In addition, this study employed an artificial neural network (ANN) that incorporated all three PSA markers. The AUC for the ANN was 0.85, with a specificity of 40.9% at 95% sensitivity. This is compared to <30% specificity for any of three markers by themselves. These results clearly need further validation, but they do demonstrate the potential of multivariate models or algorithms that incorporate PSA results. The same investigators also suggested that [−2]proPSA could differentiate pT2 PCa from pT3 PCa, and Gleason scores 7, and greater, from Gleason scores less than 7. The latter is consistent with the observation that proPSA microplate assays can detect more aggressive PCa. Finally, Jensen et al. (manuscript in preparation) tested the utility of the Access p2PSA assay to predict the recurrence of PCa after prostatectomy. In this study serum samples from 135 PCa patients who had undergone a radical prostatectomy were tested. Approximately 30% of the patients had recurrence of cancer in less than 5 years post-prostatectomy. These investigators noted a relationship between recurrence of cancer and pre-surgery [−2]proPSA levels. In this case, [−2]proPSA serum concentration and prostate volume were statistically significant in predicting post-prostatectomy cancer recurrence, implicating [−2]proPSA as a predictor of PCa aggression.

In addition to the Access p2PSA assay, an automated [−5/−7] proPSA assay was recently developed (Roche Research Laboratories; Penzberg, Germany). This assay was evaluated in two large retrospective studies. In the first study, 2,055 patients with PSA concentrations between 0.28 and 81 ng/mL were tested. In this study, [−5/−7]proPSA/free PSA was no better than total PSA in the 2–10 ng/mL range. However, [−5/−7]proPSA/free PSA performed marginally better than total PSA in the 4–10 ng/mL range. But in this PSA range it performed no better than free PSA/total PSA *(18)*. In the second study, 898 patients with PSA between 1 and 10 ng/mL were tested. This study showed similar results: [−5/−7] proPSA by itself or as a ratio with free PSA did not outperform either total PSA or free PSA/total PSA. *(19)*. These data are consistent with the immunohistological results of Chan et al. *(9)* who reported that tissue stained with [−5/−7]proPSA mAbs appeared to be similar in both PCa and BPH, and that [−5/−7]proPSA lacked specificity for PCa.

As stated at the beginning of this chapter, PSA isoforms have been studied for over 10 years yet very little is known about their roles and functions. In the case of proPSA, the data show that these isoforms can be utilized to aid in diagnosing PCa. Recent studies have shown that [−2]proPSA has the greatest potential of all the proPSA isoforms for improving the role of PSA in detecting PCa. The data also show that the greater sensitivity and specificity in PCa diagnosis probably does not reside in a single new tumor marker, but rather in the generation of algorithms that incorporate many tumor markers – old and new. Given the data seen thus far, we expect that [−2]proPSA will play a major role in the future of PCa diagnosis, and perhaps treatment.

# REFERENCES

1. Mikolajczyk, S.D. and Rittenhouse, H.G. (2003) Pro PSA: a more cancer specific form of prostate specific antigen for the early detection of prostate cancer *Keio J Med* **52**, 86–91.
2. Mikolajczyk, S.D., Marker, K.M., Millar, L.S., Kumar, A., Saedi, M.S., Payne, J.K., Evans, C.L., Gasior, C.L., Linton, H.J., Carpenter, P., and Rittenhouse, H.G. (2001) A truncated precursor form of prostate-specific antigen is a more specific serum marker of prostate cancer *Cancer Res* **61**, 6958–6963.
3. Mikolajczyk, S.D., Marks, L.S., Partin, A.W., and Rittenhouse, H.G. (2002) Free Prostate-specific Antigen in serum is becoming more complex U*rology* **50**, 797–802.
4. Mikolajczyk, S.D., Song,Y., Wong, J.R., Matson, R.S., and Rittenhouse, H.G. (2004) Are multiple markers the future of prostate cancer diagnostics? *Clin Biochem* **37**, 519–528.
5. Balk, S.P. Ko, Y-J., and Bubley, G.J. (2003) Biology of Prostate-specific Antigen *J Clin Oncol* **21**, 383–391.
6. Haese, A., Graefen, M., Huland, H., and Lilja, H. (2004) Prostate-specific Antigen and related isoforms in the diagnosis and management of prostate cancer *Curr Urol Reports* **5**, 231–240.
7. Kumar, A., Mikolajczyk, S.D., Goel, AS, Millar, L.S., and Saedi, M.S. (1997) Expression of pro forms of Prostate-specific Antigen by mammalian cells and its conversion to mature, active form by Human Kallikrein2 *Cancer Res* **57**, 3111–3114.
8. Peter, J., Unverzagt, C., Krogh, T.N., Vorm, O., and Hoesel, W. (2001) Identification of precursor forms of free Prostate-specific Antigen in serum of prostate cancer patients by immunosorption and mass spectrometry *Cancer Res* **61**, 957–962.
9. Chan, T.Y., Mikolajczyk, S.D., Lecksell, K., Shue, M.J., Rittenhouse, H.G., Partin, A.W., and Epstein, J.I. (2003) Immunohistochemical staining of prostate cancer with monoclonal antibodies to the precursor of Prostate-specific Antigen *Urology* **62**, 177–181.
10. Mikolajczyk, S.D., Catalona, W.J., Evans, C.L. Linton, H.J., Millar, L.S. Marker, K.M, Katir, D., Amirkhan, A., and Rittenhouse, H.G. (2004) Proenzyme forms of Prostate-specific Antigen in serum improve the detection of prostate cancer Clin Chem **50**, 1017–1025.
11. Naya, Y., Fritsche, H.A., Bhadkamkar, V.A., Mikolajczyk, S.D., Rittenhouse, H.G., and Babaian, R.J. (2005) Evaluation of precursor prostate-specific antigen isoform ratios in the detection of prostate cancer *Urol Oncol* **23**, 16–21
12. Sokoll, L.J., Chan, D.W., Mikolajczyk, S.D., Rittenhouse, H.G., Evans, C.L., Linton, H.J., Mangold, L.A., Mohr, P., Bartsch, G., Klocker, H., Horninger, W., and Partin, A. (2003) Proenzyme PSA for the early detection of prostate cancer in the 2.5–4.0 ng/mL total PSA range: Primary analysis *Urology* **61**, 274–276.
13. Catalona, W.J., Bartsch, G., Rittenhouse, H.G., Evans, C.L., Linton, H.J., Amirkhan, A., Horninger, W., Klocker, H., and Mikolajczyk, S.D. (2003) Serum pro prostate specific antigen improves cancer detection compared to free and complexed prostate specific antigen in men with prostate specific antigen 2 to 4 ng/mL *J Urol* **170**, 2181–2185.
14. Catalona, W.J., Bartsch, G., Rittenhouse, H.G., Evans, C.L., Linton, H.J., Horninger, W., Klocker, H., and Mikolajczyk, S.D. (2004) Serum pro-prostate specific antigen preferentially detects aggressive prostate cancers in men with 2 to 4 ng/mL prostate specific antigen *J Urol* **171**, 2239–2244.
15. Weinzierl, C.F, Su, S.X., Pierson, T.B., Arockiasamy, D.A., Mizrahi, I.A., Broyles, D. L, and Tam, J.E., (2007) (C-38) Measuring [−2]proPSA in serum: Analytical performance of the Access p2PSA assay from Beckman Coulter. Annual Meeting of the American Association for Clinical Chemistry. *Abstract No. C-38.*
16. Sokoll, L.J., Wang, Y., Feng, Z., Kagan, J., Partin, A.W., Sanda, M.G., Thompson, I.M., and Chan, D.W., (2008) [-2]proPSA for prostate cancer detection: an NCI Early Detection Research Network validation study *J Urol* **180**, 539–543.

17. Stephan, C., Cammann, H., Jung, K., and Lein, M. (2008) –2proPSA enhanced prostate cancer detection at tPSA 2–10 µg/l within multivariate models and detects aggressive Pca The 2nd World Congress on Controversies in Urology, *Abstract No. 457762.*

18. Lein, M., Semjonow, A., Graefen, M., Kwiatkowski, M., Abramjuk, C., Stephan, C. et al. (2005) A multicenter clinical trial on the use of (−5, −7) pro prostate specific antigen *J Urol* **174**, 2150–2153.

19. Stephan, C., Meyer, H.A., Kwiatkowski, M., Recker, F. Camman, H. Loening, S. A. et al. (2006) A (−5, −7) proPSA based artificial neural network to detect prostate cancer *Eur Urol* **50**, 1014–1020.

# 16  PCA3

## Jack Groskopf, Jack Schalken, and Harry Rittenhouse

**CONTENTS**

## INTRODUCTION

The current standard for early detection of prostate cancer (PCa) consists of a digital rectal exam (DRE) and a serum test for prostate-specific antigen (PSA). Serum PSA levels have been widely used for diagnostic purposes for more than 25 years, but falsely positive and negative results are commonplace *(1)*. Thompson and colleagues have concluded that no certain PSA level can accurately separate men with cancer from men with only benign prostatic hyperplasia *(2)*. In addition, a large population of men with chronically elevated serum PSA and one or more negative prostate biopsies has now emerged. These men are at risk of developing clinically significant prostate cancer as they age, but serum PSA and its derivative assays may not allow effective management of these patients. Consequently, many men with negative biopsies undergo repeat biopsies to rule out cancer. While prostate biopsy remains the gold standard for PCa diagnosis, this method has its own limitations and associated co-morbidities. More accurate diagnostic tests are needed to help guide decisions to biopsy the prostate.

The paradigm of direct detection of cancer cells in biological fluids is attractive due to the expected improvement in specificity compared to the measurement of surrogate protein markers in blood. In addition, since these two mechanisms of detection are completely independent of one another, gene-based assays for cancer cell detection should

From: *Current Clinical Urology: Prostate Cancer Screening*, Edited by: D. P. Ankerst et al.
DOI 10.1007/978-1-60327-281-0_16 © Humana Press, a part of Springer Science+Business Media, LLC 2009

be synergistic with immunoassays for blood antigens such as serum PSA. A number of molecular markers with the potential to improve PCa diagnosis have been identified *(3,4)*. PCA3 is the first non-invasive molecular test for the diagnosis of PCa, and therefore provides a case study for the successful translation of a molecular marker from the research laboratory to clinical practice.

In this chapter we describe the PCA3 story, from discovery and characterization of its expression in prostate tissue to the evolution of PCA3-based molecular urine tests and their application for predicting prostate biopsy outcome. We also review the most recent data demonstrating the potential diagnostic and prognostic utilities of PCA3, either alone or as part of algorithm including serum PSA and other clinical information.

**Key Words:** PCA3, DD3, Prostate cancer, PSA.

## PCA3: DISCOVERY AND EARLY CHARACTERIZATION

Prostate cancer gene 3 (*PCA3*), also referred to in the literature as *PCA3*[DD3] or DD3[*PCA3*], was first described in 1999 by Bussemakers and colleagues *(5)*. Researchers in the Isaacs laboratory at Johns Hopkins University used differential display analysis to compare mRNA expression patterns in benign vs. malignant prostate tissue, with the goal of identifying unknown genes involved in prostate tumorigenesis. One of the clones, DD3 (*d*ifferential *d*isplay-3), was chosen as the primary candidate for further characterization based on the high level of expression in prostate tumors and apparent absence of expression in benign tissue. The gene was subsequently re-named *PCA3*.

Further analyses using sensitive RT-PCR methodology demonstrated low but quantifiable PCA3 mRNA expression in benign prostate tissue, but undetectable levels in normal and malignant tissue from other organs *(6)*. Over 90% of prostate tumors examined showed over-expression of PCA3 mRNA, with a median 66-fold up-regulation in PCa relative to benign tissue *(7)*. Moreover, a median 11-fold up-regulation was found in prostate tissue samples containing <10% PCa cells *(7)*. Receiver-operating characteristic (ROC) curve analysis was employed and measurement of PCA3 yielded an area under the curve (AUC) of 0.98, indicating a very high sensitivity and specificity for prostate cancer when isolated prostate tissues are directly examined *(6)*. These studies demonstrated the prostate cancer specificity of PCA3 in tissue, and the potential for non-invasive clinical application using bodily fluids as the specimen.

The gene for PCA3 was mapped to chromosome 9q21–22 but extensive characterization of the transcription unit yielded no indication of function. In fact, the presence of alternative splicing and polyadenylation sites and a lack of any extensive open reading frame indicated that PCA3 is a non-coding RNA (ncRNA). Although the function of PCA3 is not yet known, this is an area of active research *(8)* and there is evidence that another prostate-specific ncRNA, PCGEM-1, might be involved in regulating apoptosis *(9)*.

## FEASIBILITY OF A PCA3-BASED URINE TEST

Based on the results from prostate tissue, researchers in the Schalken laboratory at Radboud University determined the feasibility of a non-invasive PCA3-based test for predicting biopsy outcome. It was hypothesized that manipulation of the prostate would release cells into the urethra, so sediments from urine collected following a DRE were utilized. This represents a unique specimen type, and a mechanism for detection that is completely distinct from current blood-based immunoassays. This difference is illustrated in Fig. 1 and Color Plate 5, which depicts the release of prostate cells into urine (Fig. 1a) compared to the barriers that PSA protein must cross to enter the bloodstream (Fig. 1b, *(10)*). The leakage of PSA protein into the bloodstream due to damage or disease of the prostate is analogous to the release of Troponin I into blood following

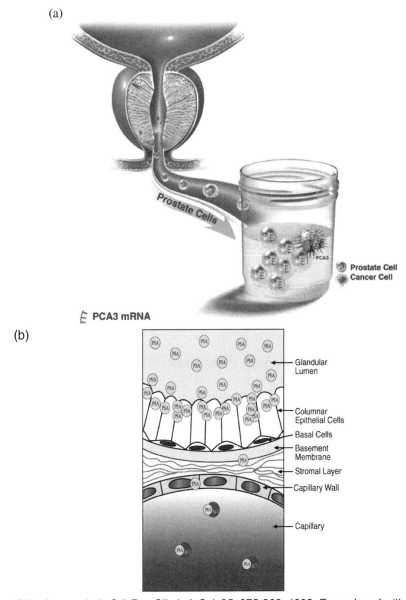

*Rittenhouse et al., Crit.Rev.Clin.Lab Sci, 35, 275-368, 1998. Reproduced with permission of the publisher (Taylor and Francis, Ltd, http://www.tandf.co.uk/journals)*

**Fig. 1.** Release of prostate cells into the urethra following DRE (**a**) vs. release of PSA protein into the bloodstream (**b**). (*see* Color Plate 5)

a myocardial infarction. Elevation of PSA is a very good indicator of damage to the integrity of the prostate gland; however, both benign conditions (e.g., BPH) and cancer can cause PSA leakage, which severely limits the specificity of PSA for cancer detection.

Although PCA3 mRNA is highly expressed in PCa, it is also present at low levels in benign prostate cells. To detect PCA3 up-regulation in cancer cells against the background of normal prostate cells, it was therefore necessary to normalize PCA3 levels to the amount of prostate RNA recovered from the post-DRE urine. *KLK3*, the gene encoding PSA, is prostate-specific and has been shown not to be up-regulated in PCa *(11)*; PSA mRNA was thus selected as the normalizing factor (note: PSA mRNA levels in prostate cells released into urine are completely unrelated to PSA protein levels in blood, i.e., serum PSA). PCA3 and PSA mRNA levels were quantified, with the latter functioning as a housekeeping gene to which the PCA3 mRNA levels were normalized. The final output of the test was ratio of PCA3/PSA mRNA (multiplied by 1,000); this measure of the degree of PCA3 over-expression in urine is referred to as the "PCA3 Score".

Hessels et al. used a time-resolved fluorescence (TRF) RT-PCR method to measure PCA3 and PSA mRNA levels in urine sediments collected following DRE *(7)*. The study population consisted of 108 men admitted to the hospital for prostate biopsy due to serum PSA levels $\geq 3$ ng/mL, of whom 24 were subsequently found to be biopsy positive for PCa. Applying biopsy as the reference standard, ROC analysis yielded an AUC of 0.72 (95% confidence interval 0.58–0.85). A PCA3 Score cutpoint corresponding to the greatest diagnostic accuracy yielded sensitivity of 67% and specificity of 83%; for comparison, serum PSA assay specificity (cutoff of 3 ng/mL) was 22%. This study was the first to demonstrate the potential of a quantitative urinary PCA3 test to aid in the prediction of biopsy outcome. The clinical performance of the TRF RT-PCR method was verified in a recent European multi-center study *(12)* that included 583 men with serum PSA between 3 and 15 ng/mL (the so-called PSA gray zone). The AUC for PCA3 was 0.66 compared to 0.57 for serum PSA. At a sensitivity of 65%, the specificities for PCA3 and serum PSA were 66 and 47%, respectively.

Fradet and co-workers at DiagnoCure Incorporated developed the first commercially available PCA3 urine test, uPM3. This qualitative assay utilized post-DRE urine sediments and nucleic acid sequence-based amplification technology, and two independent studies confirmed the results obtained with the quantitative TRF assay *(13,14)*.

## TRANSCRIPTION-MEDIATED AMPLIFICATION ASSAY FOR PCA3

Gen-Probe Incorporated developed a quantitative PCA3-based urine test with the potential for widespread implementation in clinical laboratories *(15)*. Whole urine (instead of sediments) is collected following a DRE consisting of 3 strokes per prostate lobe. The urine is then mixed with an equal volume of detergent-based stabilization buffer, which lyses the cells and stabilizes the RNA; the processed urine sample can then be shipped overnight to testing labs or stored frozen for longer time periods. PCA3 and PSA mRNAs are quantified utilizing like protocols and reagents with components specific for the two analytes. The target RNAs are purified via capture onto magnetic particles coated with target-specific oligonucleotides, amplified using transcription-mediated amplification (TMA), and the amplification products detected with chemiluminescent DNA probes using a hybridization protection assay. All assay steps occur in a single tube, and the assay is performed with instrumentation currently utilized in several FDA-approved products.

In 2006, Groskopf et al. applied the TMA method to urine specimens collected following DRE from 52 healthy men with no known risk factors, 70 men scheduled for prostate biopsy based on existing risk factors ($n$ = 16 positive for PCa) and 21 men who had previously undergone radical prostatectomy *(15)*. Mean PCA3 Scores were highest in biopsy positive patients, and mean values were significantly different between biopsy positive, biopsy negative, and normal patient groups ($p$ <0.01). ROC analysis for the pre-biopsy group yielded an AUC of 0.746; at the optimal cutpoint, sensitivity was 69% and specificity 79%. For the post-radical prostatectomy group, 20/21 of these specimens yielded PCA3 and PSA assay signals at or near background levels, and mRNA copy levels below the amount required for analysis. The remaining post-prostatectomy specimen yielded a PCA3 Score of 55; follow-up indicated that, during the 4 months between the radical prostatectomy and collection of urine for PCA3 testing, the subject had a local recurrence and became biopsy positive. Importantly, TMA PCA3 assay diagnostic accuracy was equivalent to the TRF RT-PCR method, demonstrating the utility of a quantitative PCA3-based urine test using two different technologies.

The analytical performance of the TMA PCA3 assay has been extensively characterized. The specimen informative rate (i.e., the fraction of specimens that yield sufficient RNA levels for analysis) has been >95% across several studies *(15–17)*. This improvement relative to earlier PCA3-based urine tests (~80%) was a significant advance in terms of implementation into clinical practice; non-informative specimens require a return visit to the physician's office, a clear inconvenience to the patient and to the healthcare system. The improved informative rate of the TMA assay was likely due to the simplified specimen processing procedure utilizing whole urine instead of sediments, as well as the analytical sensitivity of the assay.

In the initial study *(15)*, the TMA method demonstrated good reproducibility for PCA3 and PSA mRNA quantitation, with intra- and inter-assay CVs of <13% and <12%, respectively, and total variation of <20%. The inter-run CV for the PCA3 Score [(PCA3 c/mL)/(PSA c/mL) × 1000] was 15–24%. This analytical performance has been confirmed in a recent multi-center evaluation *(18)*; the observed intra- and inter-assay CVs were <14% and <10%, respectively, and the inter-site CV was <9%. This study by Sokoll et al. also assessed the pre-analytical effects of specimen collection type and DRE procedure. In the absence of prostate manipulation, informative rates were relatively low (~80%). However, what might be considered merely a "good urologic DRE" of 3 strokes per prostate lobe provided an informative rate of >95%, and was equivalent to a more aggressive procedure incorporating 8 strokes per prostate lobe. Furthermore, the resulting PCA3 Scores of informative samples were equivalent irrespective of specimen type or DRE procedure, indicating the substantial insensitivity of the method to pre-analytical effects.

## APPLICATION OF THE TMA PCA3 ASSAY IN CLINICAL STUDIES

In a 2007 study *(16)* by Marks et al. of 233 men with serum PSA levels persistently above 2.5 ng/mL but with previous negative biopsies, the TMA PCA3 method yielded an AUC of 0.68 (95% CI 0.60–0.76), a finding that was superior to the AUC of 0.52 (95% CI 0.44–0.61) for serum PSA in the same cohort ($p$ = 0.008). At a PCA3 Score cutoff of 35, sensitivity was 58% and specificity 72%. Another important conclusion from this study was that the quantitative PCA3 Score correlated with the probability of a positive biopsy.

In a more recent study including 570 North American men scheduled for prostate biopsy *(17)*, PCA3 Score was correlated with prostate volume, serum PSA, and biopsy outcome. The ability of the PCA3 Score to synergize with other patient information to predict biopsy outcome was also examined.

The correlation between PCA3 Score and the probability of a positive biopsy is shown in Fig. 2. For this subject population (34% biopsy positive for PCa), men with a PCA3 Score less than 5 showed a positive biopsy rate of 14%, whereas 69% of men with a PCA3 Score of greater than 100 were biopsy positive. The probability of a positive biopsy for prostate cancer increased continuously as the PCA3 Score increased. The performance of the PCA3 assay was equivalent in men undergoing first biopsy (AUC = 0.70, $n$ = 277) and men with one or more previous negative biopsies (AUC = 0.68, $n$ = 280).

In contrast to serum PSA, the PCA3 Score did not correlate with prostate size determined by trans-rectal ultrasound. This result highlights the difference between direct detection of PCA3 RNA from cancer cells vs. use of the surrogate marker serum PSA. PCA3 assay performance was also found to be independent of serum PSA level; subjects with serum PSA <4, 4–10 and >10 ng/mL yielded equivalent sensitivity and specificity.

To determine if PCA3 could improve diagnostic accuracy when combined with other clinical information, logistic regression (LR) models were developed using the following independent variables: PCA3 Score, serum PSA, suspicious vs. normal DRE, age, and prostate gland volume. First, the complete dataset of 553 subjects with no missing values for the 5 independent variables was randomly divided into 4 groups of equal size and equal prevalence using a block randomization scheme. Three of the four groups were then used as a training set to develop the LR model; the trained model was subsequently applied to the remaining group, which acted as the test set. Permutations were made four times to obtain prediction results for all four groups, and the prediction results of the cross-validated LR model were assessed using ROC analysis. The best model

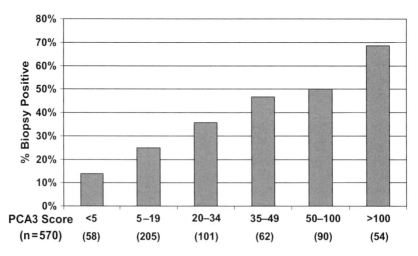

**Fig. 2.** Percent of men with positive biopsy vs. PCA3 Score range. The number of men in each group is shown at bottom in parentheses.

included PCA3 Score, serum PSA, DRE result, and prostate volume. The AUCs for serum PSA alone, PCA3 alone, and the LR model were 0.55, 0.69, and 0.75, respectively (Fig. 3 and Color Plate 6). At a sensitivity of 70%, specificities were 35% (serum PSA), 56% (PCA3 Score), and 67% (LR). The increase in the AUC by the LR model was strongly significant ($p = 0.0002$); if PCA3 Score was omitted from the model the AUC decreased from 0.75 to 0.67. These data indicated that PCA3 has the potential to add diagnostic accuracy when used in conjunction with other patient information.

The PCA3 Score is dependent on the fraction of PCa vs. benign cells released into the urethra following DRE. Larger, more aggressive tumors might shed cells more easily than smaller, less invasive tumors, resulting in higher PCA3 Scores. Nakanishi et al. tested this hypothesis in a study in which PCA3 Scores were determined for 96 men scheduled for radical prostatectomy, then correlated with tumor volume and other pathologic features of the radical prostatectomy specimens *(19)*. The PCA3 Score was significantly correlated with total tumor volume in prostatectomy specimens ($R = 0.269$, $p = 0.008$), and was also associated with prostatectomy Gleason score (6 vs. 7 or greater, $p = 0.005$) but not with other clinical and pathological features or tumor location (peripheral vs. transition zone). Furthermore, the PCA3 score was significantly lower when comparing low-volume/low-grade cancer (dominant tumor volume <0.5 cc, Gleason score 6) and "significant" cancer ($p = 0.004$, Fig. 4 and Color Plate 7). These results have been confirmed in a more recent study of 72 pre-prostatectomy subjects *(20)*. PCA3 Score correlated with tumor volume and stage (pT3 >pT2), and the combination of PCA3 and serum PSA improved accuracy for predicting extracapsular extension. While preliminary, these data suggest that the PCA3 Score may have prognostic value, and could therefore assist in identifying which cancers require more aggressive treatment.

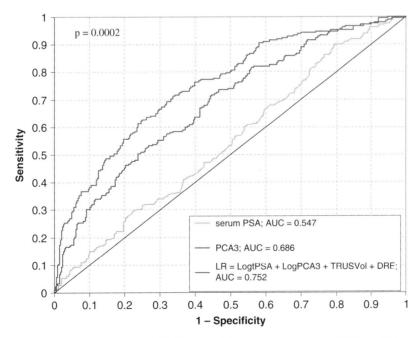

**Fig. 3.** ROC curves for serum PSA, PCA3 Score, and the logistic regression (LR) model incorporating serum PSA, PCA3 Score, diagnostic DRE result, and prostate gland volume. (*see* Color Plate 6)

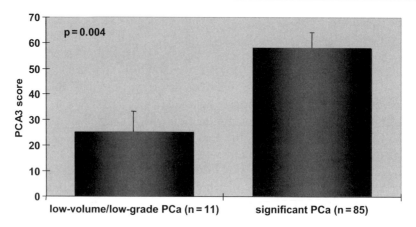

**Fig. 4.** Mean PCA3 Scores for men with low-volume / low-grade PCa (<0.5 cc, Gleason 6) vs. "significant" PCa (>0.5 cc, Gleason ≥7). Error bars represent the standard error of the mean. (*see* Color Plate 7)

## SUMMARY AND FUTURE DIRECTIONS

The Gen-Probe PCA3 assay is commercially available in several reference laboratories in the United States featuring their own laboratory-developed assays with ASRs (analyte-specific reagents). These laboratories have independently validated the PCA3 assay with results remarkably similar to previous research studies. The CE-marked version of the product was launched in Europe in late 2006 and is commercially available under the brand name PROGENSA™ PCA3.

The PCA3 assay provides a novel method to assist in PCa diagnosis. In contrast to surrogate markers such as serum PSA, the assay directly detects cancer cells released into the urine following DRE. PCA3 is not affected by prostate size but does correlate with tumor burden, and functions similarly at all serum PSA levels. The equivalent PCA3 sensitivity and specificity at all serum PSA levels are especially important in clinical testing today. As the average PSA levels have decreased over the last 15 years, the PSA range of 2.5–4 ng/mL has become more relevant for biopsy decisions.

Multiple independent studies (using different technologies) have confirmed the diagnostic accuracy of the PCA3 assay for predicting biopsy outcome. PCA3 may have the most immediate utility for men with serum PSA that is chronically elevated for non-cancer reasons, although the equivalent performance in men undergoing first biopsy indicates that PCA3 could have utility in this setting as well. Importantly, the quantitative PCA3 Score correlates with the probability of positive biopsy; PCA3 can therefore be used to stratify patients who are at risk of PCa. Using an LR model approach, we have demonstrated that the PCA3 Score has potential to add value when incorporated into existing nomograms to further improve the accuracy of PCa diagnosis. It will be important to verify this result, and to include other markers such as PSA isoforms and free PSA.

Perhaps the greatest unmet need in PCa diagnostics is the discrimination of "indolent" vs. "significant" cancers. Preliminary data suggest that PCA3 Scores are higher in patients with larger, more invasive tumors; PCA3 may therefore assist in determining whether patients require aggressive treatment/follow-up or might be considered as candidates for active surveillance. Studies are ongoing to validate the correlation of PCA3

Score with tumor volume, and to assess the potential of nomograms to increase tumor volume predictive value.

Efforts to further validate and expand the clinical utility of the PCA3 assay continue. Potential applications include use of PCA3 testing prior to first biopsy, detecting recurrence following radical prostatectomy or radiation therapy, or monitoring patients receiving drug therapies that affect serum PSA levels (e.g., 5α-reductase inhibitors).

The PCA3 test is emerging as the first fully translated molecular diagnostic assay for prostate cancer cells in biological fluids, and holds promise as a valuable tool for aiding in the diagnosis of PCa.

# REFERENCES

1. Freedland SJ, Partin AW. Prostate-specific antigen: update 2006. Urology 2006;67:458–60.
2. Thompson IM, Ankerst DP, Chi C, et al. Operating characteristics of prostate-specific antigen in men with an initial PSA level of 3.0 ng/mL or lower. JAMA 2005;294:66–70.
3. Reynolds MA, Kastury K, Groskopf J, Schalken JA, Rittenhouse H. Molecular markers for prostate cancer. Cancer Lett 2007;249:5–13.
4. Hessels D, Verhaegh GW, Schalken JA, Witjes JA. Applicability of biomarkers in the early diagnosis of prostate cancer. Expert Rev Mol Diagn 2004;4:513–26.
5. Bussemakers MJ, van Bokhoven A, Verhaegh GW, et al. DD3: a new prostate-specific gene, highly overexpressed in prostate cancer. Cancer Res 1999;59:5975–9.
6. de Kok JB, Verhaegh GW, Roelofs RW, et al. DD3(PCA3), a very sensitive and specific marker to detect prostate tumors. Cancer Res 2002;62:2695–8.
7. Hessels D, Klein Gunnewiek JM, van Oort I, et al. DD3(PCA3)-based molecular urine analysis for the diagnosis of prostate cancer. Eur Urol 2003;44:8,15; discussion 15–6.
8. Mattick JS, Makunin IV. Non-coding RNA. Hum Mol Genet 2006;15 Spec No 1:R17–29.
9. Fu X, Ravindranath L, Tran N, Petrovics G, Srivastava S. Regulation of apoptosis by a prostate-specific and prostate cancer-associated noncoding gene, PCGEM1. DNA Cell Biol 2006;25:135–41.
10. Rittenhouse HG, Finlay JA, Mikolajczyk SD, Partin AW. Human Kallikrein 2 (hK2) and prostate-specific antigen (PSA): two closely related, but distinct, kallikreins in the prostate. Crit Rev Clin Lab Sci 1998;35:275–368.
11. Meng FJ, Shan A, Jin L, Young CY. The expression of a variant prostate-specific antigen in human prostate. Cancer Epidemiol Biomarkers Prev 2002;11:305–9.
12. van Gils MP, Hessels D, van Hooij O, et al. The time-resolved fluorescence-based PCA3 test on urinary sediments after digital rectal examination; a Dutch multicenter validation of the diagnostic performance. Clin Cancer Res 2007;13:939–43.
13. Fradet Y, Saad F, Aprikian A, et al. uPM3, a new molecular urine test for the detection of prostate cancer. Urology 2004;64:311,5; discussion 315–6.
14. Tinzl M, Marberger M, Horvath S, Chypre C. DD3PCA3 RNA analysis in urine – a new perspective for detecting prostate cancer. Eur Urol 2004;46:182,6; discussion 187.
15. Groskopf J, Aubin SM, Deras IL, et al. Aptima PCA3 Molecular Urine Test: Development of a Method to Aid in the Diagnosis of Prostate Cancer. Clin Chem 2006;52:1089.
16. Marks LS, Fradet Y, Deras IL, et al. PCA3 molecular urine assay for prostate cancer in men undergoing repeat biopsy. Urology 2007;69:532–5.
17. Deras IL, Aubin SMJ, Blase A, et al. PCA3 – a molecular urine assay for predicting biopsy outcome. J Urol 2008;179:1587–92.
18. Sokoll LJ, Ellis WJ, Lange PH, et al. A multicenter evaluation of the PCA3 molecular urine test: preanalytical effects, analytical performance and diagnostic accuracy. Clinica Chimica Acta 2008; 389:1–6.
19. Nakanishi H, Groskopf J, Fritsche HA, et al. PCA3 molecular urine assay correlates with prostate cancer tumor volume; implication in selecting candidates for active surveillance. J Urol 2008;179:1804–1810.
20. Whitman EJ, Groskopf J, Ali A, et al. PCA3 Score Before Radical Prostatectomy Predicts Extracapsular Extension and Tumor Volume. J Urol 2008;180:1975–8.

# 17 Transcriptional Profiling of Prostate Cancer: Biomarker Identification and Clinical Applications

*Nigel Clegg and Peter S. Nelson*

## Contents

## Summary

Cancer of the prostate is nearly universal with advanced age. However, the propensity for a given prostate cancer to cause morbidity or influence survival varies tremendously. New biomarkers are needed with higher specificity and sensitivity to accurately diagnose prostate cancer, to predict outcomes, and ultimately to categorize prostate cancers into subtypes for personalized treatment. Taking full advantage of the information encoded in the genomes and proteomes of cancer cells and their attendant micro- and macro-environments has provided new opportunities for identifying biomarkers capable of defining the presence of disease and stratifying tumor phenotypes with distinct behaviors. This review provides an overview of the basic technologies associated with gene expression profiling, describes recent advances in the transcript-based search for prostate cancer biomarkers, and discusses future applications of these strategies in the context of prostate cancer diagnosis and treatment stratification.

**Key Words:** Gene expression, Profiles, Biomarker, Prediction, Outcome, Microarray.

From: *Current Clinical Urology: Prostate Cancer Screening*, Edited by: D. P. Ankerst et al.
DOI 10.1007/978-1-60327-281-0_17 © Humana Press, a part of Springer Science+Business Media, LLC 2009

# INTRODUCTION

Cancer of the prostate may be unique among malignancies affecting man in that the prevalence of the disease is nearly universal with advanced age. Detailed autopsy studies of men dying of causes unrelated to prostatic disease have identified foci of prostate cancer in 2, 32, and 64%, of men aged 30, 50, and 70, respectively *(1)*. The overall numbers of prevalent biopsy-detectable prostate cancers in the US population exceed 3 million men *(2)*. In contrast, a relatively smaller, yet substantial number of prostate cancer cases are diagnosed clinically, approximately 220,000 new cases yearly *(3)*. Considerable debate continues to center on what type of treatment, if any, is optimal for these men, and a major component of these deliberations centers on defining features of prostate cancers that reflect indolent versus aggressive behavior. Evidence for the importance of this topic is provided by the tremendous morbidity and mortality attributed to prostate cancers that were not identified at a disease stage amenable to localized therapy.

As reviewed elsewhere, prostate-specific antigen (PSA), the most widely used blood-based screening test for any malignancy, has limited prognostic ability. Further, the sensitivity and specificity of PSA for prostate cancer are suboptimal, with many aggressive cancers missed at any PSA threshold *(4)*, resulting in many needless biopsy procedures due to the influence of benign disease on serum PSA concentrations. New biomarkers are needed with higher specificity and sensitivity to accurately diagnose prostate cancer, to predict outcomes, and ultimately to stratify prostate cancers into subtypes for personalized treatment. In identifying such markers, it is likely that significant insights into the biology of prostate cancer will be gained, although this is not a prerequisite for a useful marker.

The sheer magnitude of the task of biomarker discovery is arguably best suited for high-throughput technologies. Thousands of features (genes, transcripts, or proteins) can be queried simultaneously, in a relatively unbiased fashion, to identify individual or multi-featured marker panels that associate with the presence of disease or with particular disease phenotypes. In this context, tools and methods developed for comprehensive studies of the human genome; *genomics,* and proteome; *proteomics,* represent attractive approaches to the problem. The information presented in this review is restricted to a subfield of functional genomics that involves the comprehensive assessment of gene expression measured at the level of transcription. Transcript-based searches for biomarkers are aided by the fact that RNA can be isolated and stored and, unlike proteins, amplified and labeled with relative ease using standard molecular biology techniques. Further, methods such as high-density microarrays have been developed for the simultaneous quantitation of tens of thousands of transcripts. Here, we describe the basic technologies associated with gene expression profiling, review recent advances in the transcript-based search for prostate cancer biomarkers, and discuss future applications of these strategies for the diagnostic and prognostic determination of prostate carcinoma.

# TECHNIQUES

## *Expressed Sequence Tags (ESTs) and Serial Analysis of Gene Expression (SAGE)*

Expressed sequence tags (ESTs) are gene specific tags determined by sequencing 200–800 bp stretches of clones randomly picked from a cDNA library that represents that component of the genome actively utilized by a given cell, tissue, or organism *(5)*. ESTs represent that component of the genome that is used or *expressed* as messenger RNA (mRNA) (subsequently converted to cDNA in the laboratory); each EST is a particular *sequence* of DNA bases that identifies a specific gene as the source of the mRNA, but represents only a portion or *tag* of the entire cloned cDNA fragment. If a large number of individual clones are sequenced and assigned to specific genes, then the frequency of a specific set of ESTs in the library should be proportional to the actual expression level – corresponding to the number of transcripts or mRNAs – of the gene in the tissue of interest. Serial Analysis of Gene Expression (SAGE) is similar to EST creation, except that even shorter fragments or tags of cDNAs are isolated for each mRNA molecule. The short fragments are ligated together and subsequently inserted into a cloning vector. The result is a series of short concatenated 9–14 bp gene-specific tags that can be used to infer the level of expression of each gene represented by a tag *(6)*. The basic method for exploiting ESTs and SAGE tags centers on quantitating tag counts between different cell or tissue phenotypes such as benign versus cancer epithelium to determine those genes with differential expression patterns.

## *Differential Display*

Differential display identifies differences in gene expression based on the controlled amplification of randomly chosen transcripts in target and reference samples *(7)*. First, cDNA is synthesized from an RNA sample using a fixed 3'-oligonucleotide. This cDNA is then amplified with the fixed primer and a small set of oligonucleotides that are mathematically predicted to hybridize to 50–100 genes. The resultant PCR products for the target and reference samples are compared side-by-side using gel electrophoresis to visualize products that are present in one sample and absent, or of lower abundance in the other.

## *Microarray Expression Profiling*

Microarrays are composed of a series of DNA molecules spotted in a stereotyped grid pattern on a solid support such as a glass slide, silicon wafer, or nylon membrane (a "chip"). The microarray spots serve as hybridization targets for cDNA or amplified RNA that is enzymatically synthesized in vitro from endogenous RNA isolated from a tissue source of interest (amplified RNA is frequently used if the amount of tissue is limiting, such as in core needle biopsies). In a typical experiment, a test sample and a reference sample are differentially labeled with fluorophores capable of emitting different light wavelengths, then combined and hybridized to the DNA chip. After stringent washing, the target molecules bind exclusively to spots with a complementary sequence. The level of gene expression for any given gene (represented by the spotted or affixed DNA segment) is expressed as the ratio of intensities of the two different fluorophores.

Microarrays have been developed in several different formats. Early versions were primarily constructed by spotting aliquots of cDNA clones (cDNA arrays) onto a solid support. Subsequent methods have involved spotting or chemically synthesizing short (25 nucleotides) or long (70 nucleotides) sequences on a solid support. Multiple different oligonucleotides may be synthesized for each gene. Other approaches have been developed that include the use of digital tags and bead-anchored oligonucleotides *(8)*. A variety of commercially available platforms have been reviewed by Hardiman *(9,10)*.

## TRANSCRIPTIONAL ANALYSES OF PROSTATE CANCER

### Transcript Alterations Distinguishing Cancer from Benign Prostate Tissue

EST and SAGE methods have been used to identify specific genes with altered expression in cancer compared to benign tissue (see Table 1). Of particular interest are data mining approaches that utilized large public databases such as Unigene, dbEST, and SAGEMap because they deeply sample the transcriptomes of benign and neoplastic cells. Asmann et al. *(11)* used a novel search algorithm (the Binary Indexing Search Algorithm) to interrogate approximately 130,000 prostate ESTs in the dbEST database. They identified nine genes with statistically significant differential expression in cancer versus normal tissue. One of the genes that was verified to be up-regulated in cancer, CRISP-3, is currently being investigated as a cancer biomarker *(12)*. Data mining of public databases has also shown HOXB13, AMACR, and ALCAM to have altered expression in cancer (Table 1).

Prostate Cancer Gene 3 (PCA3) is one of several potential prostate cancer markers identified by differential display (Table 1). PCA3 is overexpressed in more than 95% of primary prostate cancers and metastases. Its clinical relevance is described in more detail elsewhere in this volume. In a recent study of 106 samples, Schmidt et al. *(13)* found that while quantitative real-time PCR of PCA3 was a powerful predictor of primary prostate cancer, even more diagnostic power was possible if EZH2, SLC45A3, and TRPM8 expression levels were also considered. Promising efforts are underway to develop a urine-based PCA3 assay as a diagnostic test for the presence of prostate carcinoma *(14,15)*.

Several microarray-based expression profiling studies have identified substantial alterations in the transcript levels of individual genes between normal prostate tissue, BPH, and prostate cancer. The number of observed differentially regulated genes in these studies depends on the diversity of genes represented on the array platform, the number of samples evaluated, and the statistical methods used to analyze the data, but most studies have identified more than 50 significant cancer-associated alterations. Table 1 lists some potential prostate cancer markers that were highlighted in published microarray studies. Many genes have been observed repeatedly *(16)*, but most have not been investigated further because they are abundant in multiple other human tissues and thus may lack the specificity required for a prostate cancer biomarker. One frequently identified gene, $\alpha$-methylacyl-CoA racemase (AMACR), is highly expressed in up to 90% of prostate tumors and is used clinically for confirming a histological diagnosis of prostate cancer. Additional genes of interest are the proto-oncogene PIM1 and hepsin (HPN), which have increased expression in cancer, and CDH1, which has decreased expression. Other markers such as IGFBP5, FAT, RAB5A, and MTA1 are primarily altered in metastases *(17,18)*.

### TMPRSS2-ETS Family Gene Rearrangements and ERG Expression

Microarray-based profiling of prostate cancers identified overexpression of the ETS-oncogene family member *ERG* in the vast majority of human prostate cancers *(19)*. However, the relative overexpression of ERG varied substantially across prostate cancer samples. Using a bioinformatics approach termed Cancer Outlier Profile Analysis (COPA) to search microarray data for genes with marked overexpression in subsets

Table 1
Selected Examples of Genes Differentially Expressed in Prostate Cancer Versus Benign Prostate Tissue Identified Using Genomics Approaches

| Method | No. of genes studied | Benign | PIN or cancer | Examples | Reference |
|---|---|---|---|---|---|
| Differential display | – | 7 | 7 | TRPM8, ADAMTS9 | Bai et al. (57) |
| Differential display | – | 3 | 3 | ENPP1 | Konishi et al. (58) |
| Differential display | – | – | – | PTOV1 | Benedit et al. (59) |
| Differential display | – | – | – | PBOV1 | An et al. (60) |
| Differential display | – | – | – | PCGEM1 | Srikantan et al. (61) |
| Differential display | – | – | – | PCA3 | Bussemakers et al. (62) |
| SAGE | ~6,500 | 1 | 1 | FASN | Cho-Vega et al. (63) |
| SAGE (db mining) | – | – | – | HOXB13 | Edwards et al. (64) |
| SAGE (db mining) | – | – | – | AMACR | Zhou et al. (65) |
| SAGE | 19,287 | – | – | DAXX, E2F4 | Waghray et al. (66) |
| ESTs | 8,794 | – | – | ALCAM | Clegg et al. (67) |
| ESTs | – | – | – | CRISP3, DAN | Asmann et al. [11] |
| ESTs | – | – | – | GDEP | Olsson et al. (68) |
| ESTs | – | – | – | PSGR | Xu et al. (69) |
| cDNA microarray | 36,864 | – | 35 | ANLN, SNRPE | Tamura et al. (70) |
| Short-oligo microarray | 18,400 | 7 | 13 | SPRY1, SPRY2 | Fritzsche et al. (71) |
| Short-oligo microarray | 44,928 | 8 | 32 | FABP5, SOX4 | Vanaja et al. (72) |
| Bead microarray | 1,532 | – | – | AMACR, CACNAID | Li et al. (73) |
| cDNA microarray | 5,760 | 10 | 11 | HOXB13 | Edwards et al. (64) |
| cDNA microarray | 40,000 | 48 | 23 | HPN, AMACR | Halvorsen et al. (74) |
| Short-oligo microarray | 3,950 | 42 | 42 | ALCAM, CD24 | Kristiansen et al. (75) |
| cDNA microarray | 23,040 | – | 26 | PCOTH, MICAL2 | Ashida et al. (76) |
| cDNA microarray | ~43,500 | 41 | 62 | MUC1, AZGP1 | Lapointe et al. (29) |
| Short-oligo microarray | 12,625 | 50 | 38 | HPN, AMACR | Stuart et al. (77) |
| cDNA microarray | 6,400 | Pool | 13 | HPN, PVRL3 | Best et al. (78) |
| cDNA microarray | 46,000 | – | 72 | TRPM8, DHCR24 | Henshall et al. (35) |

Table 1
[Continued]

| | | | | |
|---|---|---|---|---|
| Short-oligo microarray | 12,600 | 8 | 32 | HPN, AMACR | Vanaja et al. (79) |
| cDNA microarray | 12,600 | 9 | 17 | HPN, AMACR | Ernest et al. (80) |
| Short-oligo microarray | 12,626 | 3 | 41 | STK15, STK11 | LaTulippe et al. (81) |
| cDNA microarray | ~6,112 | 9 | 16 | HPN | Luo et al. (82) |
| Short-oligo microarray | ~35,000 | 15 | 15 | HPN, AMACR | Luo et al. (83) |
| Short-oligo microarray | 12,600 | 50 | 52 | HPN, TSPN1 | Singh et al. (27) |
| cDNA microarray | 588 | 1 | 1 | VEGF | Chaib et al. (84) |
| cDNA microarray | 588 | 1 | 1 | GSTM1 | Chetcuti et al. (85) |
| cDNA microarray | ~9,980 | Pool | 56 | HPN, PIM1 | Dhanasekaran et al. (18) |
| Short-oligo microarray | ~4,712 | 4 | 14 | HPN | Magee et al. (86) |
| Short-oligo microarray | ~6,800 | 8 | 9 | HPN, PSMA | Stamey et al. (87) |
| short-oligo microarray | 12,626 | 9 | 24 | HPN, MIC1, FASN | Welsh et al. (88) |

Table 2

Predictive Profiles Derived from Microarray Expression Signatures

| Predictor type | Prostate-specific | No. of genes | Accuracy | No. of samples[1] | No. of data sets[2] | Reference |
|---|---|---|---|---|---|---|
| Cancer versus normal[3] | Yes | 128 | 0.92 | 38 | 1[4] | Zhang et al.(89) |
| Cancer versus normal | Yes | 32 | 0.87 | 38 | 1[4] | Zhang et al. (89) |
| Cancer versus normal | No | 67 | – | – | 39 | Rhodes et al. (90) |
| Cancer versus normal | Yes | 16 | 0.86 | 35 | 2 | Singh et al. (27) |
| Gleason pattern 3 versus 4 and 5 | Yes | 86 | 0.76 | 30 | 2 | True et al. (31) |
| Recurrence | Yes | 16 | – | 71 | – | Bibikova et al. (30) |
| Recurrence | Yes | 5–8 | 0.75 | 79 | 1[4] | Stephenson et al. (37) |
| Recurrence | No | 14[5] | 0.82 | 79 | 2 | Glinksy et al. (36) |
| Recurrence | Yes | 5 | 0.9 | 29 | 1[4] | Singh et al. (27) |
| Invasiveness/ survival | No | 186 | – | 295 | 2 | Liu et al. (42) |
| Death-from-cancer | No | 11 | – | – | >10 | Glinsky et al. (34) |
| Serum response signature | No | 512 | – | – | 4 | Chang et al. (41) |
| Tumor aggressiveness | Yes | 70 | 0.78 | 23 | 1 | Yu et al. (25) |
| Metastasis and poor outcome | No | 17 | – | 21 | 3 | Ramaswamy et al. (33) |
| PTEN/PI3K pathway | No | ~246 | – | 105 | 3 | Saal et al. (43) |

[1]Data set used to calculate accuracy.
[2]Independent data sets used to validate the predictor including[1].
[3]Using transcript splice forms.
[4]Leave-one-out cross-validation.
[5]Three small signatures used in a single algorithm.

of tumors, two members of the ETS family, ERG and ETV1, were found to be up-regulated in a distinct group of prostate cancers *(20)*. Further analyses of these cancers revealed chromosomal rearrangements fusing parts of the coding region of ERG, ETV1, and subsequently, ETV4, to the 5'-untranslated region of the androgen-regulated gene *TMPRSS2 (20)*. Fluorescent in situ hybridization and quantitative real-time PCR analysis confirmed that TMPRSS2 is frequently fused with ERG in prostate carcinoma and high-grade PIN *(21,22)*, and rarely fused with *ETV1* and *ETV4 (20,23)*. The high frequency of TMPRSS2–ERG fusions makes this one of the most common genetic aberrations in human malignancies. It is also highly specific since both the DNA rearrangement and TMPRSS2–ERG fusion transcripts are detectable only in high-grade PIN and prostate cancer. Additional incentive for the continued development of a TMPRSS2–ERG cancer marker is the presence of fusion transcripts in the urine of prostate cancer patients, raising the possibility of a relatively non-invasive assay for prostate cancer *(24)*.

## Prostate Cancer Field Effect

When expression profiles of benign prostate tissues acquired from glands with no evidence of cancer were compared with profiles derived from prostate cancers or from histologically benign tissue adjacent to neoplastic glandular epithelium, the cancer tissue and the cancer-adjacent tissue were found to have substantial overlap in the subset of genes that distinguished them from benign samples *(25,26)*. Yu et al. *(25)* hypothesized that histologically benign tissues adjacent to cancer may have undergone genetic changes similar to prostate cancer. Though provocative, it remains unclear whether changes in benign-appearing epithelium associated with cancer precede or follow the histological appearance of the adjacent tumor. Nor is it clear if transcriptional changes need involve genetic alterations. The field effect may represent a paracrine phenomenon or a consequence of underlying genetic alterations in regions of the prostate, or both. Follow-up studies may determine if these molecular alterations could be used as biomarker predictors of the subsequent development of prostate cancers in the setting of biopsy screening where no malignancy was initially identified.

## Gene Expression Signatures of Prostate Neoplasia

In addition to identifying individual genes that may serve as cancer markers, expression profiling allows the construction of expression signatures: collections of genes whose expression states, when considered together, can classify samples into distinct groups. Expression signatures increase the search-space for markers, as the incremental contribution of multiple genes can classify samples where no single gene has sufficient power to do so.

Two categories of expression signatures have been described that differentiate benign prostate tissue from prostate cancer: those applicable to multiple types of cancer, and those that are prostate-specific. In the former category, Rhodes et al. *(16)* compared the expression signatures from 12 different tissue types (including prostate) and constructed a 67-gene meta-signature of neoplastic transformation. This signature likely represents transcriptional features of cancer that are independent of tissue of origin or initial transformation mechanism. Several prostate-specific cancer gene expression signatures have been described, but most have not been validated on independent data sets. However,

Singh et al. *(27)* described a 16-gene class predictor capable of classifying samples with 86% accuracy in an independent data set. While unlikely to replace standard methodologies for cancer determination such as histology, the 16-gene classifier might complement other approaches, or represent a basis for non-invasive biomarker development.

## *Molecular Correlates of Gleason Grade*

Histological grade is one of the key parameters taken into account when assessing prostate cancer prognosis and choice of therapy. The grading system developed by Gleason describes microscopic tumor architecture and consists of five categories, ranging from well differentiated (pattern 1) to poorly differentiated features (pattern 5) *(28)*. Two numbers are reported, one for the most prevalent pattern and one for the second-most prevalent pattern. Of greatest clinical significance are Gleason patterns 4 and 5: the amount of pattern 4 and the presence of any pattern 5 is highly correlated with probability of cancer dissemination, response to therapy, and disease outcome. Given the clinical significance of Gleason scores, molecular correlates of the Gleason grading system have been sought both to complement pathologist's determinations and to elucidate the molecular mechanisms of cancer progression.

Several expression profiling studies used the Gleason-sum score to find expression correlates of histological patterns. Singh et al. *(27)* and Lapointe et al. *(29)* identified 29 and 41 genes, respectively that associated with Gleason-sum scores; but only three genes were found in common between the analyses. Bibikova et al. *(30)* screened 512 candidate genes chosen from the literature and identified 16 different genes that associated with Gleason scores. One possible reason for the low concordance between studies is the use of whole tissue which, while enriched for tumor, also contains other cell and tissue types such as stroma and benign glands. In contrast to previous studies, True et al. *(31)* used laser capture microscopy to specifically isolate tissue from Gleason patterns 3, 4, and 5 tumors. Following expression profiling, a supervised learning approach was used to generate an 86-gene model that could distinguish Gleason pattern 3 from patterns 4 and 5. In an independent set of 30 prostate biopsies the model had an overall 76% correct classification rate. No classifier could be found that distinguished Gleason pattern 4 from pattern 5, suggesting that they are relatively similar with respect to gene expression.

## *Prediction of Tumor Behavior*

Despite advances in therapies for advanced prostate cancer, the cure rates remain low *(32)*. To optimize opportunities for long-term survival, prostate cancer must be diagnosed early while the tumor is confined to the prostate, at which point it can be surgically removed or destroyed by radiation. However, approximately one third of patients with presumed organ-confined cancers undergoing radical prostatectomy will experience disease recurrence, indicating that many tumors disseminate early in the disease course. Thus, biomarkers correlating with cancer behavior, such as the propensity for invasive growth and metastasis, may enhance the ability to predict prostate cancer recurrence, stratify patients for additional therapies, and potentially define specific molecular mechanisms that could be targeted.

Gene expression signatures have been described with prognostic value for multiple types of cancer. Ramaswamy et al. *(33)* analyzed the gene expression profiles of distant metastases originating from 5 different organs (including prostate) and identified a 17-gene signature associated with metastasis. Patients with primary tumors bearing the signature were more likely to develop distant metastases than those lacking the signature; they also had significantly shorter survival times. Interestingly, this study found that several genes in the gene-expression signature appeared to be derived from non-epithelial components of the tumor: an observation consistent with the fact that epithelial–stromal interactions influence tumor behavior. These data also suggest that different (or overlapping) outcome predictors could be identified if the stromal and epithelial compartments were separated.

Using a mouse/human translational comparative genomics approach Glinsky et al. *(34)* identified an 11-gene expression signature that predicted outcome in patients with 11 distinct types of cancer, including prostate cancer. The authors intersected gene expression signatures for mouse neural stem cell renewal with a metastasis signature identified in a transgenic mouse model (TRAMP). The resulting stem cell-like expression signature was then used to interrogate expression patterns of human cancers. Across multiple data sets (and 1,153 cancer patients), the presence of a stem cell-like expression profile in primary cancer was a good predictor of a short interval to disease recurrence, distant metastasis, and death after therapy. Since the treatments for the different cancer types are varied, it seems likely that the 11-gene signature truly represents a marker for prognosis rather than response to therapy.

Expression profiling has also revealed potential prostate-specific single gene markers and gene expression signatures for predicting relapse following prostatectomy *(17,18,25,27,29,30,35–38)*. RNA or protein expression levels of TRPM8, DHCR24, PIM1, MUC1, AZGP1, and EZH2 have all been reported to associate with recurrence. EZH2 protein expression was found to be a better predictor for clinical progression than surgical margin status, maximum tumor dimension, Gleason score, or preoperative PSA *(17)*. However, EZH2 protein is only expressed in a subset of prostate cells and at a relatively low levels, so it (along with most other single gene markers) is likely to be used as part of a prognostic panel in conjunction with other genes. In an immunohistochemical study of more than 2,000 tumor samples, Rhodes et al. *(39)* found that moderate or strong expression of EZH2 coupled with moderate expression of E-cadherin (CDH1) was strongly associated with the recurrence of prostate cancer. Bismar et al. *(40)* evaluated transcript and protein expression data and developed a 12-gene model predictive of prostate cancer progression postradical prostatectomy. A unique feature of this study involved the use of immunohistochemical quantitation of gene expression at the protein level such that this signature of outcome could be generated using procedures commonly used by practicing pathologists.

Amongst prostate-specific gene expression signatures, those described by Glinsky et al. *(36)* are novel in the use of multiple human data sets to create a predictor of prognosis. The authors analyzed postoperative radical prostatectomy samples to define a large set of genes (218) whose expression was differentially regulated in tumors from patients with recurrent versus non-recurrent cancer. Subsequently, expression profiles from prostate cancer xenografts were used to identify members of the larger gene set that were concordantly regulated across multiple data sets. With these data a recurrence predictor algorithm was created that correctly identified 88% of patients with recurrent disease and 92% of patients with non-recurrent disease. In an independent set of 79 clinical samples, patient groups were separated by clinical criteria (Gleason score, PSA level, and tumor stage) and the recurrence predictor was used to discriminate outcome. For each clinical criterion, the recurrence algorithm provided additional predictive value (measured using Kaplan–Meier analysis), suggesting it may be suitable for stratification of prostate cancer patients into subgroups with distinct survival probability after therapy.

## INSIGHTS FROM EXPRESSION PROFILING OF OTHER TUMOR TYPES

### *Outcome Prediction*

For other malignancies, gene signatures and class predictors have been created using biological characteristics of tumors rather than clinical outcomes. Subsequently, these signatures have been shown to also associate with disease outcome. Such signatures are of special interest as they provide more readily identifiable biological insights into the cancers, both for diagnosis and treatment. Based on gene expression profiles of fibroblasts from 10 different anatomic locations, Chang et al. *(41)* defined a 512-gene activated serum-response (and cell cycle independent) signature, also called the "wound response" signature. Breast cancer patients whose tumors expressed wound response signature were more likely to progress to metastasis and death in a 5-year follow-up period. The prognostic value of the wound response signature was also demonstrated for lung adenocarcinomas and gastric carcinomas, though it was found to have limited utility in predicting prostate cancer recurrence, as only a small sample of prostate cancers expressed the genes comprising this phenotype.

Biological characteristics of tumor invasiveness have also been used to identify molecular features that could be used as prognostic markers. A small population of breast cancer cells characterized by CD44 expression, but negligible levels of CD24 (CD44+CD24−/low) were found to produce a high incidence of tumor formation when injected into immunodeficient mice *(42)*. In contrast, other breast cancer cells do not. A 186-gene invasiveness gene signature (IGS) was identified by comparing the gene expression profiles of CD44+CD24−/low tumorigenic breast cancer cells with those of normal breast epithelium. Amongst 295 patients, there was a significant association between the IGS and metastasis-free survival. Patients identified as having high-risk early breast cancer using clinical criteria were further divided by the IGS into good and poor prognosis categories: the 10-year rate of metastasis-free survival was 81% in the former category, and 57% in the latter category. The prognostic power of the IGS signature was increased when the wound-healing signature was considered simultaneously, demonstrating the potential power of a "multiplex" approach. The IGS was also prognostic for survival in a sample of 21 prostate cancer patients *(42)*.

Another approach to using expression profiling for marker discovery has been to target specific biochemical or signaling pathways. In this context, a 246-gene PTEN/PI3K expression signature was found in stage 2 breast cancer samples that could classify tumors based on the presence or absence of defects in the PTEN/PI3K signaling pathway *(43)*. Patients with a PTEN/PI3K expression signature similar to that associated with loss of PTEN gene activity had a significantly higher proportion of distant metastases. The PTEN/PI3K expression signature was also able to stratify outcomes for patients with prostate and bladder cancers. The identification of gene expression signatures for signaling pathways may ultimately lead to the identification of customized patient therapies.

## Predicting Response to Therapy

Breast cancer studies, such as those involving tamoxifen, demonstrate the potential of using gene expression signatures as biomarkers to predict response to specific chemotherapeutic regimens. Estrogen receptor-positive breast cancer is frequently treated with tamoxifen, yet up to 40% of patients do not respond, or develop resistance to this treatment, leading to incurable metastatic disease (44). Using a 44-gene signature, Jansen et al. were able to correctly predict the outcome for 66 patients in response to tamoxifen treatment with 77% specificity and 48% sensitivity (45). Other expression signatures with prognostic value for response to tamoxifen have been identified (46–48). The usefulness of expression signatures to predict response to therapeutic agents remains to be demonstrated for prostate cancer.

## Integration of Expression Profiles and Biomarkers in Clinical Trials

The utility of expression profiles as prognostic tools is being tested in two clinical trials involving breast cancer. The MINDACT (Microarray In Node negative Disease may Avoid ChemoTherapy) trial, is a multi-center prospective, phase 3 randomized study designed to compare a 70-gene-based expression signature with the prognostic tool "Adjuvant Online!" in selecting node-negative patients for adjuvant therapy. Nine thousand people are being recruited for the trial. In the original study leading to the trial, the 70-gene model predicted poor prognosis (defined as occurrence of distant metastases within 5 years) with an accuracy of 83% in node-negative patients under 55 years of age. This trial will test both the utility of the expression signature and the feasibility of using small custom microarrays in a clinical setting. The US Food and Drug Administration recently (Spring, 2007) approved a commercial version of the 70-gene test, Agendia's MammaPrint breast cancer prognosis test. A similar product has been offered in the Netherlands since 2005.

A second study, TAILORx (Trial Assigning IndividuaLized Options for Treatment(Rx)), was designed to validate the usefulness of a 21-gene quantitative RT-PCR expression assay (Oncotype DX, created by Genomic Health) as a predictor of response to tamoxifen for patients with ER positive, node negative breast cancer. Oncotype DX was developed by integrating information from a variety of sources, including microarray expression profiling studies; and it has already performed successfully in a retrospective study of 668 tamoxifen-treated, hormone receptor positive patients (49). PCR-based expression profiling may prove easier to implement in a controlled clinical setting than a more technically demanding microarray method.

## EXPRESSION PROFILING CAVEATS

Microarray-based clinical research has grown explosively in the past decade, but both the validity and reproducibility of findings have been questioned (50). One major area of contention is the technical reproducibility of data between labs, especially where different microarray platforms are used. However, recent studies suggest that a key factor in multi-lab and multi-platform reproducibility is RNA quality *(51)*. Also, rapid changes in gene expression can also occur as a result of tissue handling and iatrogenic ischemia *(52,53)*. Thus, one major technical hurdle involves standardizing tissue collection and extraction protocols.

Problems associated with data reporting and data analysis have also cast a shadow on the reproducibility of microarray data. This subject has been critically reviewed elsewhere *(54–56)*. Two points stand out: (1) virtually all studies fail to address key statistical parameters such as sample size and power and (2) the inappropriate use of statistical methodologies is widespread. Additional concerns about study design such as the use of heterogeneous groups of patients, tumors, and treatment regimens; and the lack of external validation are common to all biomarker studies. Clearly, these issues mandate a highly critical case-by-case assessment of published results. Fortunately, the recent advent of public repositories for formatted raw and processed microarray data (such as GEO, ArrayExpress, and CIBEX) make it possible for researchers to verify published results. Many journals now demand that authors deposit microarray data in public repositories as a prerequisite to publication.

## SUMMARY AND FUTURE DIRECTIONS

The information encoded in the genomes and proteomes of cancer cells and their attendant micro- and macro-environments has provided new opportunities for identifying biomarkers capable of defining the presence of disease and stratifying tumor phenotypes with distinct behaviors. We now recognize that prostate cancers exhibit substantial molecular diversity. Recent technological advances in microarray construction now allow for queries of the entire genome including alternatively spliced forms of genes and microRNAs, further adding to the information detailing and defining characteristics of tumor behavior. The greatest potential for genomics and proteomics to impact the care of cancer patients may ultimately involve the personalization of diagnosis and treatment through phenotype-defining markers. To validate the promising results of completed studies, it will be critical to compile and analyze related data sets to create a consensus gene expression prognosis predictor that can be validated in large adequately powered prospective cohorts. To this end, standards should be implemented to ensure recruitment of patients who have undergone similar treatments. Ideally molecular correlates would be incorporated as integral components into clinical trial design such that tumor and host biomarkers are able to stratify risk, forecast responses to chemoprevention, specify effective drug dosing, and predict treatment outcomes.

## REFERENCES

1. Sakr WA, Grignon DJ, Crissman JD, et al. High grade prostatic intraepithelial neoplasia (HGPIN) and prostatic adenocarcinoma between the ages of 20–69: an autopsy study of 249 cases. In-vivo 1994;8(3):439–43.
2. Porter MP, Stanford JL, Lange PH. The distribution of serum prostate-specific antigen levels among American men: implications for prostate cancer prevalence and screening. Prostate 2006;66(10):1044–51.
3. Jemal A, Siegel R, Ward E, Murray T, Xu J, Thun MJ. Cancer statistics, 2007. CA Cancer J Clin 2007;57(1):43–66.

4. Thompson IM, Pauler DK, Goodman PJ, et al. Prevalence of prostate cancer among men with a prostate-specific antigen level < or =4.0 ng per milliliter. N Engl J Med 2004;350(22):2239–46.

5. Nagaraj SH, Gasser RB, Ranganathan S. A hitchhiker's guide to expressed sequence tag (EST) analysis. Brief Bioinform 2007;8(1):6–21.

6. Porter D, Yao J, Polyak K. SAGE and related approaches for cancer target identification. Drug Discov Today 2006;11(3–4):110–8.

7. Liang P, Pardee AB. Analysing differential gene expression in cancer. Nat Rev Cancer 2003;3(11):869–76.

8. Fan JB, Yeakley JM, Bibikova M, et al. A versatile assay for high-throughput gene expression profiling on universal array matrices. Genome Res 2004;14(5):878–85.

9. Hardiman G. Microarray platforms – comparisons and contrasts. Pharmacogenomics 2004;5(5):487–502.

10. Hardiman G. Microarrays Technologies 2006: an overview. Pharmacogenomics 2006;7(8):1153–8.

11. Asmann YW, Kosari F, Wang K, Cheville JC, Vasmatzis G. Identification of differentially expressed genes in normal and malignant prostate by electronic profiling of expressed sequence tags. Cancer Res 2002;62(11):3308–14.

12. Bjartell A, Johansson R, Bjork T, et al. Immunohistochemical detection of cysteine-rich secretory protein 3 in tissue and in serum from men with cancer or benign enlargement of the prostate gland. Prostate 2006;66(6):591–603.

13. Schmidt U, Fuessel S, Koch R, et al. Quantitative multi-gene expression profiling of primary prostate cancer. Prostate 2006;66(14):1521–34.

14. Tinzl M, Marberger M, Horvath S, Chypre C. DD3PCA3 RNA analysis in urine – a new perspective for detecting prostate cancer. Eur Urol 2004;46(2):182–6; discussion 7.

15. Marks LS, Fradet Y, Deras IL, et al. PCA3 molecular urine assay for prostate cancer in men undergoing repeat biopsy. Urology 2007;69(3):532–5.

16. Rhodes DR, Barrette TR, Rubin MA, Ghosh D, Chinnaiyan AM. Meta-analysis of microarrays: inter-study validation of gene expression profiles reveals pathway dysregulation in prostate cancer. Cancer Res 2002;62(15):4427–33.

17. Varambally S, Dhanasekaran SM, Zhou M, et al. The polycomb group protein EZH2 is involved in progression of prostate cancer. Nature 2002;419(6907):624–9.

18. Dhanasekaran SM, Barrette TR, Ghosh D, et al. Delineation of prognostic biomarkers in prostate cancer. Nature 2001;412(6849):822–6.

19. Petrovics G, Liu A, Shaheduzzaman S, et al. Frequent overexpression of ETS-related gene-1 (ERG1) in prostate cancer transcriptome. Oncogene 2005;24(23):3847–52.

20. Tomlins SA, Rhodes DR, Perner S, et al. Recurrent fusion of TMPRSS2 and ETS transcription factor genes in prostate cancer. Science 2005;310(5748):644–8.

21. Demichelis F, Fall K, Perner S, et al. TMPRSS2:ERG gene fusion associated with lethal prostate cancer in a watchful waiting cohort. Oncogene 2007;26(31):4596–9.

22. Soller MJ, Isaksson M, Elfving P, Soller W, Lundgren R, Panagopoulos I. Confirmation of the high frequency of the TMPRSS2/ERG fusion gene in prostate cancer. Genes Chromosomes Cancer 2006;45(7):717–9.

23. Perner S, Demichelis F, Beroukhim R, et al. TMPRSS2:ERG Fusion-Associated Deletions Provide Insight into the Heterogeneity of Prostate Cancer. Cancer Res 2006;66(17):8337–41.

24. Laxman B, Tomlins SA, Mehra R, et al. Noninvasive detection of TMPRSS2:ERG fusion transcripts in the urine of men with prostate cancer. Neoplasia 2006;8(10):885–8.

25. Yu YP, Landsittel D, Jing L, et al. Gene expression alterations in prostate cancer predicting tumor aggression and preceding development of malignancy. J Clin Oncol 2004;22(14):2790–9.

26. Chandran UR, Dhir R, Ma C, Michalopoulos G, Becich M, Gilbertson J. Differences in gene expression in prostate cancer, normal appearing prostate tissue adjacent to cancer and prostate tissue from cancer free organ donors. BMC Cancer 2005;5(1):45.

27. Singh D, Febbo PG, Ross K, et al. Gene expression correlates of clinical prostate cancer behavior. Cancer Cell 2002;1(2):203–9.

28. Gleason DF. Histologic grading of prostate cancer: a perspective. Hum Pathol 1992;23(3):273–9.

29. Lapointe J, Li C, Higgins JP, et al. Gene expression profiling identifies clinically relevant subtypes of prostate cancer. Proc Natl Acad Sci USA 2004;101(3):811–6.

30. Bibikova M, Chudin E, Arsanjani A, et al. Expression signatures that correlated with Gleason score and relapse in prostate cancer. Genomics 2007;89(6):666–72.

31. True L, Coleman I, Hawley S, et al. A molecular correlate to the Gleason grading system for prostate adenocarcinoma. Proc Natl Acad Sci USA 2006;103(29):10991–6.

32. Petrylak D, Tangen C, Hussain M, et al. SWOG 99-16: Randomized phase III trial of docetaxel/estramustine versus mitoxantrone/prednisone in men with androgen-independent prostate cancer. Proc Amer Soc Clin Onc 2004;Abstract 3.

33. Ramaswamy S, Ross KN, Lander ES, Golub TR. A molecular signature of metastasis in primary solid tumors. Nat Genet 2003;33(1):49–54.

34. Glinsky GV, Berezovska O, Glinskii AB. Microarray analysis identifies a death-from-cancer signature predicting therapy failure in patients with multiple types of cancer. J Clin Invest 2005;115(6):1503–21.

35. Henshall SM, Afar DE, Hiller J, et al. Survival analysis of genome-wide gene expression profiles of prostate cancers identifies new prognostic targets of disease relapse. Cancer Res 2003;63(14):4196–203.

36. Glinsky GV, Glinskii AB, Stephenson AJ, Hoffman RM, Gerald WL. Gene expression profiling predicts clinical outcome of prostate cancer. J Clin Invest 2004;113(6):913–23.

37. Stephenson AJ, Smith A, Kattan MW, et al. Integration of gene expression profiling and clinical variables to predict prostate carcinoma recurrence after radical prostatectomy. Cancer 2005;104(2):290–8.

38. Varambally S, Yu J, Laxman B, et al. Integrative genomic and proteomic analysis of prostate cancer reveals signatures of metastatic progression. Cancer Cell 2005;8(5):393–406.

39. Rhodes DR, Sanda MG, Otte AP, Chinnaiyan AM, Rubin MA. Multiplex biomarker approach for determining risk of prostate-specific antigen-defined recurrence of prostate cancer. J Natl Cancer Inst 2003;95(9):661–8.

40. Bismar TA, Demichelis F, Riva A, et al. Defining aggressive prostate cancer using a 12-gene model. Neoplasia 2006;8(1):59–68.

41. Chang HY, Sneddon JB, Alizadeh AA, et al. Gene expression signature of fibroblast serum response predicts human cancer progression: similarities between tumors and wounds. PLoS Biol 2004;2(2):E7.

42. Liu R, Wang X, Chen GY, et al. The prognostic role of a gene signature from tumorigenic breast-cancer cells. N Engl J Med 2007;356(3):217–26.

43. Saal LH, Johansson P, Holm K, et al. Poor prognosis in carcinoma is associated with a gene expression signature of aberrant PTEN tumor suppressor pathway activity. Proc Natl Acad Sci USA 2007;104(18):7564–9.

44. Clarke R, Liu MC, Bouker KB, et al. Antiestrogen resistance in breast cancer and the role of estrogen receptor signaling. Oncogene 2003;22(47):7316–39.

45. Jansen MP, Foekens JA, van Staveren IL, et al. Molecular classification of tamoxifen-resistant breast carcinomas by gene expression profiling. J Clin Oncol 2005;23(4):732–40.

46. Jansen MP, Sieuwerts AM, Look MP, et al. HOXB13-to-IL17BR expression ratio is related with tumor aggressiveness and response to tamoxifen of recurrent breast cancer: a retrospective study. J Clin Oncol 2007;25(6):662–8.

47. Ma XJ, Wang Z, Ryan PD, et al. A two-gene expression ratio predicts clinical outcome in breast cancer patients treated with tamoxifen. Cancer Cell 2004;5(6):607–16.

48. Loi S, Haibe-Kains B, Desmedt C, et al. Definition of clinically distinct molecular subtypes in estrogen receptor-positive breast carcinomas through genomic grade. J Clin Oncol 2007;25(10):1239–46.

49. Paik S, Shak S, Tang G, et al. A multigene assay to predict recurrence of tamoxifen-treated, node-negative breast cancer. N Engl J Med 2004;351(27):2817–26.

50. Shi L, Reid LH, Jones WD, et al. The MicroArray Quality Control (MAQC) project shows inter- and intraplatform reproducibility of gene expression measurements. Nat Biotechnol 2006;24(9):1151–61.

51. Stafford P, Brun M. Three methods for optimization of cross-laboratory and cross-platform microarray expression data. Nucleic Acids Res 2007;35(10):e72.

52. Dash A, Maine IP, Varambally S, Shen R, Chinnaiyan AM, Rubin MA. Changes in differential gene expression because of warm ischemia time of radical prostatectomy specimens. Am J Pathol 2002;161(5):1743–8.

53. Lin DW, Coleman IM, Hawley S, et al. Influence of surgical manipulation on prostate gene expression: implications for molecular correlates of treatment effects and disease prognosis. J Clin Oncol 2006;24(23):3763–70. Epub 2006 Jul 5.

54. Ahmed AA, Brenton JD. Microarrays and breast cancer clinical studies: forgetting what we have not yet learnt. Breast Cancer Res 2005;7(3):96–9.

55. Dupuy A, Simon RM. Critical review of published microarray studies for cancer outcome and guidelines on statistical analysis and reporting. J Natl Cancer Inst 2007;99(2):147–57.

56. Jafari P, Azuaje F. An assessment of recently published gene expression data analyses: reporting experimental design and statistical factors. BMC Med Inform Decis Mak 2006;6:27.

57. Bai VU, Kaseb A, Tejwani S, et al. Identification of prostate cancer mRNA markers by averaged differential expression and their detection in biopsies, blood, and urine. Proc Natl Acad Sci USA 2007;104(7):2343–8.

58. Konishi N, Nakamura M, Ishida E, et al. High expression of a new marker PCA-1 in human prostate carcinoma. Clin Cancer Res 2005;11(14):5090–7.

59. Benedit P, Paciucci R, Thomson TM, et al. PTOV1, a novel protein overexpressed in prostate cancer containing a new class of protein homology blocks. Oncogene 2001;20(12):1455–64.

60. An G, Ng AY, Meka CS, et al. Cloning and characterization of UROC28, a novel gene overexpressed in prostate, breast, and bladder cancers. Cancer Res 2000;60(24):7014–20.

61. Srikantan V, Zou Z, Petrovics G, et al. PCGEM1, a prostate-specific gene, is overexpressed in prostate cancer. Proc Natl Acad Sci USA 2000;97(22):12216–21.

62. Bussemakers MJ, van Bokhoven A, Verhaegh GW, et al. DD3: a new prostate-specific gene, highly overexpressed in prostate cancer. Cancer Res 1999;59(23):5975–9.

63. Cho-Vega JH, Troncoso P, Do KA, et al. Combined laser capture microdissection and serial analysis of gene expression from human tissue samples. Mod Pathol 2005;18(4):577–84.

64. Edwards S, Campbell C, Flohr P, et al. Expression analysis onto microarrays of randomly selected cDNA clones highlights HOXB13 as a marker of human prostate cancer. Br J Cancer 2005;92(2):376–81.

65. Zhou M, Chinnaiyan AM, Kleer CG, Lucas PC, Rubin MA. Alpha-Methylacyl-CoA racemase: a novel tumor marker over-expressed in several human cancers and their precursor lesions. Am J Surg Pathol 2002;26(7):926–31.

66. Waghray A, Schober M, Feroze F, Yao F, Virgin J, Chen YQ. Identification of differentially expressed genes by serial analysis of gene expression in human prostate cancer. Cancer Res 2001;61(10): 4283–6.

67. Clegg N, Abbott D, Ferguson C, Coleman R, Nelson PS. Characterization and comparative analyses of transcriptomes from the normal and neoplastic human prostate. Prostate 2004;60(3):227–39.

68. Olsson P, Bera TK, Essand M, et al. GDEP, a new gene differentially expressed in normal prostate and prostate cancer. Prostate 2001;48(4):231–41.

69. Xu LL, Stackhouse BG, Florence K, et al. PSGR, a novel prostate-specific gene with homology to a G protein-coupled receptor, is overexpressed in prostate cancer. Cancer Res 2000;60(23):6568–72.

70. Tamura K, Furihata M, Tsunoda T, et al. Molecular features of hormone-refractory prostate cancer cells by genome-wide gene expression profiles. Cancer Res 2007;67(11):5117–25.

71. Fritzsche S, Kenzelmann M, Hoffmann MJ, et al. Concomitant down-regulation of SPRY1 and SPRY2 in prostate carcinoma. Endocr Relat Cancer 2006;13(3):839–49.

72. Vanaja DK, Ballman KV, Morlan BW, et al. PDLIM4 repression by hypermethylation as a potential biomarker for prostate cancer. Clin Cancer Res 2006;12(4):1128–36.

73. Li HR, Wang-Rodriguez J, Nair TM, et al. Two-dimensional transcriptome profiling: identification of messenger RNA isoform signatures in prostate cancer from archived paraffin-embedded cancer specimens. Cancer Res 2006;66(8):4079–88.

74. Halvorsen OJ, Oyan AM, Bo TH, et al. Gene expression profiles in prostate cancer: association with patient subgroups and tumour differentiation. Int J Oncol 2005;26(2):329–36.

75. Kristiansen G, Pilarsky C, Wissmann C, et al. Expression profiling of microdissected matched prostate cancer samples reveals CD166/MEMD and CD24 as new prognostic markers for patient survival. J Pathol 2005;205(3):359–76.

76. Ashida S, Nakagawa H, Katagiri T, et al. Molecular features of the transition from prostatic intraepithelial neoplasia (PIN) to prostate cancer: genome-wide gene-expression profiles of prostate cancers and PINs. Cancer Res 2004;64(17):5963–72.

77. Stuart RO, Wachsman W, Berry CC, et al. In silico dissection of cell-type-associated patterns of gene expression in prostate cancer. Proc Natl Acad Sci USA 2004;101(2):615–20.

78. Best CJ, Leiva IM, Chuaqui RF, et al. Molecular differentiation of high- and moderate-grade human prostate cancer by cDNA microarray analysis. Diagn Mol Pathol 2003;12(2):63–70.

79. Vanaja DK, Cheville JC, Iturria SJ, Young CY. Transcriptional silencing of zinc finger protein 185 identified by expression profiling is associated with prostate cancer progression. Cancer Res 2003;63(14):3877–82.

80. Ernst T, Hergenhahn M, Kenzelmann M, et al. Decrease and gain of gene expression are equally discriminatory markers for prostate carcinoma: a gene expression analysis on total and microdissected prostate tissue. Am J Pathol 2002;160(6):2169–80.

81. LaTulippe E, Satagopan J, Smith A, et al. Comprehensive gene expression analysis of prostate cancer reveals distinct transcriptional programs associated with metastatic disease. Cancer Res 2002;62(15):4499–506.

82. Luo JH, Yu YP, Cieply K, et al. Gene expression analysis of prostate cancers. Mol Carcinog 2002;33(1):25–35.

83. Luo J, Zha S, Gage WR, et al. Alpha-methylacyl-CoA racemase: a new molecular marker for prostate cancer. Cancer Res 2002;62(8):2220–6.

84. Chaib H, Cockrell EK, Rubin MA, Macoska JA. Profiling and verification of gene expression patterns in normal and malignant human prostate tissues by cDNA microarray analysis. Neoplasia 2001;3(1):43–52.

85. Chetcuti A, Margan S, Mann S, et al. Identification of differentially expressed genes in organ-confined prostate cancer by gene expression array. Prostate 2001;47(2):132–40.

86. Magee JA, Araki T, Patil S, et al. Expression profiling reveals hepsin overexpression in prostate cancer. Cancer Res 2001;61(15):5692–6.

87. Stamey TA, Warrington JA, Caldwell MC, et al. Molecular genetic profiling of Gleason grade 4/5 prostate cancers compared to benign prostatic hyperplasia. J Urol 2001;166(6):2171–7.

88. Welsh JB, Sapinoso LM, Su AI, et al. Analysis of gene expression identifies candidate markers and pharmacological targets in prostate cancer. Cancer Res 2001;61(16):5974–8.

89. Zhang C, Li HR, Fan JB, et al. Profiling alternatively spliced mRNA isoforms for prostate cancer classification. BMC Bioinformatics 2006;7:202.

90. Rhodes DR, Yu J, Shanker K, et al. Large-scale meta-analysis of cancer microarray data identifies common transcriptional profiles of neoplastic transformation and progression. Proc Natl Acad Sci USA 2004;101(25):9309–14.

# 18 Biomarkers for Prostate Cancer Detection: Family-Based Linkage Analysis and Case–Control Association Studies

*Joke Beuten and Teresa L Johnson-Pais*

## Contents

## Summary

For decades, it has been well-recognized that genetics plays a critical role in the development of prostate cancer. Numerous epidemiological and molecular biological studies have shown evidence for a significant but heterogeneous hereditary component in prostate cancer susceptibility. Linkage analysis in twin and family-based study designs provided targeted candidate regions for prostate cancer risk and cancer aggressiveness. Subsequent mapping efforts and mutation screening yielded several strong candidate genes. More recent tools allow investigation of gene–gene and gene–environment interactions in population-based designs, such as case–control or cohort studies. These analyses have identified associations between single nucleotide polymorphisms within candidate genes and prostate cancer susceptibility. Understanding the role of these genes may help in defining heterogeneity in prostate cancer etiology and eventually lead to better detection, treatment, and, ultimately, prevention of prostate cancer.

**Key Words:** Candidate gene, Prostate cancer risk, Association, Linkage, Single nucleotide polymorphism (SNP), Disease aggressiveness.

From: *Current Clinical Urology: Prostate Cancer Screening*, Edited by: D. P. Ankerst et al.
DOI 10.1007/978-1-60327-281-0_18 © Humana Press, a part of Springer Science+Business Media, LLC 2009

## HEREDITARY COMPONENT OF PROSTATE CANCER ETIOLOGY

The underlying etiology of prostate cancer (PCa) remains poorly understood, with both genetic predisposition and environmental factors likely to play a role. Studies published in the *New England Journal of Medicine* attempted to determine the role of hereditary factors in common cancers *(1)*. Using a large cohort of twins (*n* = 77,788) from Sweden, Denmark, and Finland, the heritable factors for several cancers including stomach, colorectal, lung, breast, and prostate were estimated. The proportion of prostate cancer risk accounted for by inheritable factors was estimated to be 42%, providing substantial evidence for a genetic component in the susceptibility to PCa. Heritable risk factors can involve highly penetrant susceptibility genes with low frequencies and/or low penetrant genes with higher frequencies in the population. Several studies suggest that the disease is more likely due to the contributions of multiple prostate cancer susceptibility genes rather than a single gene, corroborating hypotheses that the majority of prostate cancer cases involve more common, low- to moderate-penetrant alleles in genes that are components of pathways that influence prostate function, rather than mutations in high-penetrant susceptibility genes (reviewed in *(2,3)*).

Despite this strong evidence for a genetic component in prostate cancer, little progress has been made to identify a major gene or genes *(4)*. For more than 10 years, investigators have attempted to identify genes for prostate cancer using large-scale mapping methods that proved successful for breast and colon cancers. There is an increased impetus for better understanding of the molecular processes involved in prostate carcinogenesis with the ultimate goal of discovering new biomarkers, which may be beneficial in the detection, prevention, and/or treatment of this disease.

## FAMILY HISTORY

As with breast and colon cancers, familial clustering of prostate cancer has been reported frequently *(5–8)*. Familial prostate cancer represents families in which there are two first-degree or one first-degree and two or more second-degree relatives with prostate cancer. Familial prostate cancer is estimated to account for 10–20% of all cases of prostate cancer (reviewed in *(2,3)*). Genome-wide linkage analyses, using genetic markers (usually short tandem repeats) to search for regions that show excessive sharing of inherited alleles among affected men, are used to identify susceptibility genes in familial prostate cancer. To date, at least 15 genome-wide scans for prostate cancer susceptibility loci have been reported *(2–9)*. Thirteen candidate gene loci have been identified and three strong candidate genes that are involved in pathways critical to DNA damage response (*ELAC2*), apoptosis (*RNASEL*), and innate immunity (*MSR1* and *RNASEL*) were determined from these linkage findings (Table 1). The linkage findings for prostate cancer have given high hopes, but the lack of replicating promising regions of linkage showed that finding prostate cancer genes is not as "easy" as finding genes for breast cancer and colon cancer susceptibilities. Likely explanations for this failure of replication include the high prevalence of the disease, a large environmental component, the presence of weakly penetrant alleles that cause the disease, as well as the fact that non-gene carriers with prostate cancer are present in the pedigrees. Also with a late onset disease, such as prostate cancer, members of pedigree may not show the disease yet at the time of screening.

Table 1
Putative Hereditary Prostate Cancer Susceptibility Loci

| Reference | Linked locus | Gene | Location |
|---|---|---|---|
| Smith et al. 1996 (10) | HPC1 | RNASEL | 1q24–25 |
| Xu et al. 1998 (11) | HPCX | | Xq27–q28 |
| Tavtigian et al. 2001 (12) | HPC2 | ELAC2 | 17p11 |
| Berry et al. 2000 (13) | HPC3 | | 20q13 |
| Friedrichsen et al. 2004 (14) | HPC4 | | 7p11–q21 |
| Rokman et al. 2005 (15) | HPC5 | | 3p26 |
| Xu et al. 2005 (9) | HPC6 | | 22q12 |
| Lange et al. 2006 (16) | HPC7 | | 15q12 |
| Berthon et al. 1998 (17) | HPC8 | | 1q42.2–q43 |
| Gibbs et al. 1999 (18) | CAPB | | 1p36 |
| Xu et al. 2003 (19) | MSR1 | MSR1 | 8p22–p23 |
| Lange et al. 2003 (20) | HPC9 | | 17q21–q22 |
| Amundadottir et al. 2006 (21) | HPC10 | | 8q24 |

To better account for the genetic heterogeneity, linkage analyses are being conducted using clinical information related to cancer aggressiveness as an endpoint. Linkage analyses using prostate tumor Gleason score as a quantitative trait showed suggestive linkage with 19q and 5q (22–25). It is widely accepted that genetic alterations within multiple genes are responsible for the development and progression of prostate cancer, even though these genes have yet to be identified. These types of studies will provide chromosomal regions that should be further investigated in the search for prostate cancer genes.

One advantage of linkage studies is that the entire genome can be screened in an efficient manner. However, it is often difficult to collect DNA samples from multiple generations of affected men and, as a result, inheritance content is reduced. Another limitation of linkage studies is their weak power to find susceptibility genes of small-to-moderate effects. An alternative are case–control association studies which do not require family members and also tend to have greater power to detect genes of small risk.

## CASE–CONTROL STUDIES ON CANDIDATE GENES

A commonly used method to determine possible roles of genes in the susceptibility of prostate cancer is to perform a case–control study on candidate genes. After the diagnostic criteria and definition of the disease are clearly established, selection of cases (disease) and controls (no disease) is made based on disease status. Odds ratios (ORs), which measure the odds of exposure for cases compared to controls, are estimated to determine how the exposure to a particular variant influences the risk of the disease. An OR < 1 indicates that the odds of exposure for cases are less than the odds of exposure for controls and the exposure reduces the disease risk (protective factor). On the other hand, an OR > 1 implies that the odds of exposure for cases are greater than the odds of exposure for controls and thus the exposure increases the disease risk (risk factor). An OR of 1, for which the odds of exposure are equal among cases and controls, indicates that the particular exposure is not a risk factor. The main advantage of the case–control study is that it enables us to study rare health outcomes without having to follow thousands of people, and is therefore generally quicker, cheaper, and easier to conduct than the cohort study.

Critical in the case–control analysis is determining what type of exposure (which variants) will be investigated and compared between cases and controls. Single nucleotide polymorphisms (SNPs) are the most commonly analyzed variants in case–control association studies. SNPs are sites in the human genome where individuals differ in their DNA sequence by a single base. Such slight variations in DNA sequences, in particular when they are likely to be functional (e.g., result in amino acid changes), can have a major impact on the development of a disease and on particular responses to environmental insults.

The TaqMan assay (Applied Biosystems, Foster City, CA, USA), is a commonly used method for discriminating between specific alleles of an SNP and as such allows the genotyping of individuals for specific alleles. The TaqMan assay for allelic discrimination consists of sequence-specific forward and reverse primers to amplify the polymorphic sequence of interest and two different TaqMan probes, each uniquely labeled and binding preferentially to one of the alleles. A reporter dye is linked to the 5′-end and a non-fluorescent quencher attached to the 3′-end of each probe. TaqMan probes also contain a minor groove binding protein, which enhances the discrimination between match and mismatch by allowing the use of shorter probes. During polymerase chain reaction (PCR), each probe anneals specifically to complementary sequences between the forward and reverse primer sites. The exonuclease activity of AmpliTaq-Gold DNA polymerase will result in the cleavage of only the probes that hybridize to the target sequence. Cleavage of the probe separates the reporter dye from the quencher dye, which results in increased fluorescence by the reporter dye. Thus, the fluorescence signals generated by PCR amplification indicate the sequences that are present in the sample.

A finding of no association of multiple SNPs within a candidate gene does not necessarily rule the gene out, because there could still be other unmeasured variants within the gene that increase the risk for prostate cancer. Therefore, shared haplotypes are screened to obtain genomic information in the form of haplotype blocks (chromosomal regions with relatively little recombination). If all alleles within a haplotype block are highly correlated among themselves, then the block should capture the necessary information on a particular region of the candidate gene, to allow one to rule out the role of that region if no significant association is detected.

## CANDIDATE GENES

The most likely prostate cancer candidate genes that have been studied are the androgen receptor gene, genes involved in the metabolism of testosterone and other androgens, DNA repair genes, genes involved in the metabolism of environmental carcinogens, and tumor suppressor genes (summarized in Table 2).

### *Polymorphisms of Genes Involved in the Androgen-Signaling Cascade*

Androgens play an important role in both normal and abnormal prostate development (reviewed by *(26)*) and therapies designed at removing androgens from prostate cancer patients were proposed more than 60 years ago *(27)*.

Table 2

**Candidate Genes Associated with Risk for Prostate Cancer**

| | |
|---|---|
| **Genes involved in the androgen-signaling cascade** | |
| Androgen receptor gene | *AR* |
| 3β-Hydroxysteroid dehydrogenase type II gene | *HSD3B2* |
| 5α-Reductase type II gene | *SRD5A2* |
| Cytochrome P450 17 | *CYP17* |
| Cytochrome P450 19 | *CYP19* |
| **Other prostate cancer-related genes** | |
| Prostate-specific antigen | *PSA-KLK3* |
| Cytochrome P450 1B1 | *CYP1B1* |
| Cytochrome P450 3A4 | *CYP3A4* |
| Oxoguanine glycosylase 1 | *OGG1* |
| p53 tumor suppressor gene | *TP53* |
| 2′-5′-Oligoadenylate (2-5A)-dependent RNASEL | *RNASEL* |
| *N*-Acetyltransferases 1 and 2 | *NAT1, NAT2* |
| Vitamin D receptor | *VDR* |

## ANDROGEN RECEPTOR GENE

The gene that has been the focus of the most intense molecular studies is the androgen receptor *(AR)*, which binds both testosterone and dihydrotestosterone (DHT) and transactivates the genes with androgen response elements *(28)*. The androgen receptor is localized on the X chromosome and mutations in this gene result in Kennedy's disease, an adult onset disorder in which the patients have low virilization, decreased sperm production, testicular atrophy, and reduced fertility. The androgen receptor has several polymorphisms, most of which lie in the first of its eight exons *(28)*. There are two length polymorphisms, $(CAG)_n$ and $(GGC)_n$, and an SNP, G1733A, which alters an *Stu*I restriction site. Several reports demonstrated that short GGC repeats ($\leq 16$) alone or in combination with short CAG repeats are significantly associated with increased ORs for incidence of prostate cancer *(6,29–31)*. Crocitto and colleagues evaluated the *Stu*I SNP in African American prostate cancer cases and controls, and found association with a 3-fold increase in prostate cancer in men under the age of 65 years. Unfortunately, their results were only referred to in a publication by Ross et al. *(32)* and there is limited information about their data or analysis. One additional polymorphism in the androgen receptor gene has been evaluated in the Finnish population. Mononen et al. *(33)* identified a missense mutation in codon 726 in exon 5 which resulted in an arginine to leucine substitution. Although the polymorphism was rare (less than 1%), it was associated with an increased OR of 5.8.

## 3β-HYDROXYSTEROID DEHYDROGENASE TYPE II GENE

The *HSD3B2* gene codes for the 3β-hydroxysteroid dehydrogenase enzyme. This enzyme has a role in both the synthesis and the degradation of DHT, the most active form of testosterone. It is involved in the synthesis of androstenedione in the adrenal gland, which is converted into DHT in the prostate. Furthermore, it is one of the two enzymes which irreversibly inactivate DHT in the prostate. Mutations in the *HSD3B2* gene cause male pseudohermaphroditism with congenital adrenal hyperplasia *(34)*. The gene contains a complex dinucleotide repeat length polymorphism in the third intron. Some of the alleles in this locus have been implicated in increasing prostate cancer risk *(35)*.

## 5α-REDUCTASE TYPE II GENE

Steroid 5α-reductase is an enzyme that catalyzes the conversion of testosterone to dihydrotestosterone. There are two isozymes, which are coded by *SRD5A1* and *SRD5A2* genes. *SRD5A2* is primarily expressed in the genital skin and the prostate gland while *SRD5A1* is present in newborn scalp, skin, and liver *(36)*. Mutations in the *SRD5A2* gene result in recessive male pseudohermaphroditism *(37)*, in which the prostate remains undeveloped, and neither benign prostatic hyperplasia nor prostate cancer develop in these men. There are strong biochemical data supporting the role of *SRD5A2* polymorphisms in prostate cancer risk. The biochemical studies of Makridakis et al. *(38)* explored the role of ten missense single substitutions and three double mutants. Nine of these 13 mutations reduced enzyme activity by 20% or more, 3 increased activity by more than 15%, and one had no effect on enzyme activity. The V89L polymorphism, which replaces valine at codon 89 for leucine, reduces enzyme activity both *in vitro* and *in vivo* *(39)*. Significant associations with prostate cancer have been reported for the V89L polymorphism and another missense variant, suggesting a potential role of *SRD5A2* in the risk of prostate cancer *(31,40,41)*.

## CYTOCHROME P450 17 AND 19 ENZYMES

The *CYP17* gene codes for the enzyme cytochrome P450 17 and catalyzes two sequential steps in the biosynthesis of testosterone. The first step is the conversion of pregnenolone to 17-hydroxypregnenolone, the second, the conversion of 17-hydroxypregnenolone to C-19 steroid dehydroepiandrosterone *(42,43)*. The *CYP17* gene has a polymorphism in the 5′-untranslated region in a putative Sp1 binding site (designated CYP17*A1 and CYP17*A2). It is feasible that the polymorphism affects transcription of the *CYP17* gene. The majority of studies have supported the hypothesis that the CYP17*A2 allele predisposes men to prostate cancer through increasing testosterone biosynthesis *(44–47)*. Odds ratios varied from 1.23 to 2.8 in these studies, with only two studies demonstrating statistically significant findings. However, one study by Habuchi et al. *(48)* found an increase in prostate cancer risk associated with the CYP17*A1 allele.

The *CYP19* gene codes for aromatase cytochrome P450 19. The product of *CYP19* is primarily expressed in the ovary and the placenta, and it converts androgen to estrogen. In addition to being extensively studied as a risk factor for breast cancer, the *CYP19* variants have also been evaluated as a risk factor for prostate cancer *(49)*. Latil *et al.* found that individuals who were heterozygous for a length polymorphism (171 and 187 alleles) within the gene had a 3.73-fold increased risk.

## *Other Prostate Cancer-Related Genes*

Another class of genes that has been implicated for increasing prostate cancer risk is the prostate-related genes.

## PROSTATE-SPECIFIC ANTIGEN

Human prostate-specific antigen (*PSA*) is a kallikrein-like protease present in seminal plasma. *PSA* has been implicated not only as a marker for prostate cancer but may also be involved in the disease process. The *PSA* promoter has eight androgen response elements *(50,51)* and three different polymorphisms in the *PSA* promoter have been studied. Significant association with increased risk for advanced disease was reported in men with the *PSA* GG genotype of the A→G polymorphism in an androgen response element *(52)*. However, Lai and colleagues recently published a report that the presence of the A allele, rather than the GG genotype, increased the risk for prostate cancer *(53)*.

## CYTOCHROME P450 ENZYMES

The cytochromes P450 (P450) are a very large gene family of constitutive and inducible enzymes with a major role in the oxidative activation and/or deactivation of a wide range of xenobiotics including many potential carcinogens and several anticancer drugs *(54)*. Besides the previously discussed *CYP17* and *CYP19* genes, another member of the CYP1 gene family, cytochrome P450 1B1 (*CYP1B1*), is a likely candidate gene that plays a role in the susceptibility of prostate cancer. *CYP1B1* is one of the major enzymes involved in the hydroxylation of estrogens, a reaction of key relevance in hormonal carcinogenesis *(55)*. *CYP1B1* catalyzes the hydroxylation of 17B-oestradiol (E2) at the $C_4$ position *(56,57)* and testosterone at the $C_{6\beta}$ and $C_{12\alpha}$ positions *(58)*. The importance of *CYP1B1* in chemical carcinogens is well illustrated in animal models, in which metabolites of *CYP1B1* have been shown to induce prostate cancer *(59,60)*. Several polymorphisms in the *CYP1B1* gene have been described, of which four result in amino acid substitutions, including the common SNPs +142C/G (R48G), +355G/T (A119S), +4326C/G (L432V), and +4390A/G (N453S). Functional studies suggest that these non-synonymous SNPs may alter enzymatic activity and catalytic specificity of *CYP1B1*. Different allelic variants of *CYP1B1* have been shown to have different catalytic activities and specificities to a variety of procarcinogens (reviewed by *(61)*). Several studies have evaluated the relationship between *CYP1B1* polymorphisms and risk of prostate cancer, with significant associations for the L432V and/or A119S variants reported for different ethnicities *(62–65)*. Furthermore, a common haplotype within *CYP1B1* was associated with an increased risk for prostate cancer *(65,66)*.

*CYP3A4* is the most abundant cytochrome P450 in human liver *(67)*. Two studies have evaluated the A→G polymorphism in the 5′-regulatory region of the *CYP3A4* gene. Individuals carrying the G allele had a higher grade and stage than those who were homozygous for AA *(68)*. Walker et al. *(69)* observed a higher frequency of the G allele in African Americans compared to US Caucasians and Taiwanese.

## OXOGUANINE GLYCOSYLASE 1

The oxoguanine glycosylase 1 (*OGG1*) gene encodes a DNA glycosylase/apuric-apyrimidinic lyase that catalyzes the removal of 8-OH-G from damaged DNA *(70)*. Although the mechanisms of carcinogenesis are not clearly understood, they have been proposed to involve repeated tissue damage by highly reactive species *(71)*. One of the most deleterious products of reactive oxygen species (ROS) damage is 8-hydroxyguanine (8-OH-G). When left unrepaired, 8-OH-G can cause GC to TA transversions, which have frequently been observed in several oncogenes and tumor suppressor genes *(72)*. Several SNPs within *OGG1* have been identified *(73)* and numerous studies report on the association between *OGG1* SNPs and prostate cancer susceptibility, in particular, the C to G change at position 6,803, which results in an amino acid change of serine to cysteine at codon 326 *(73–75)*. In addition to the Ser326Cys SNP, Xu et al. *(73)* also identified another 17 SNPs at the *OGG1* locus. Of these, two intronic SNPs, 7143A/G and 11657A/G, were found to be associated with increased prostate cancer risk *(73)*.

## P53 TUMOR SUPPRESSOR GENE

The p53 tumor suppressor gene *(TP53)* encodes a protein that is important in cell-cycle control, apoptosis, and DNA repair. Its germline mutations play a crucial role in the development of the Li-Fraumeni familial cancer syndrome *(76)*. Germline and somatic alterations of *TP53* are frequently found in individuals with prostate cancer *(77,78)*. A common polymorphism of *TP53* within exon 4 codon 72 results in a G to C change leading to an arginine to proline substitution (Arg72Pro). The Arg72Pro polymorphism occurs within a proline-rich domain of *TP53*, which is necessary for the protein to fully induce apoptosis. Dumont et al. *(79)* reported that Arg72 induces apoptosis more efficiently than does the Pro72 variant. A meta-analysis of the published literature demonstrated that carriers of the Pro/Pro genotype have an increased cancer risk compared to Arg/Arg carriers and suggested that human p53 regulates the mammalian aging process independent of its role in suppressing cancers *(80)*.

## 2′-5′-OLIGOADENYLATE (2-5A)-DEPENDENT RNASEL

An important gene involved in innate immunity and apoptosis is the gene encoding 2′-5′-oligoadenylate (2-5A)-dependent *RNASEL*. *RNASEL* regulates cell proliferation and apoptosis through the interferon-regulated 2-5A pathway *(81,82)* that mediates antiviral and antiproliferative activities *(83,84)*. It has been suggested to be a candidate tumor suppressor gene. A previous study indicated that germline mutations in the *RNASEL* gene segregate in prostate cancer families that demonstrate linkage to the HPC1 region *(85)*. The study also reported on a truncating mutation (E265X) and an initiation-codon mutation (M1I) segregating with the disease in two HPC1-linked families. Functional studies show that both mutations were associated with a reduction in *RNASEL* activity *(85)*. Furthermore, loss of the wild-type *RNASEL* allele was found in tumor tissue from an affected patient in a family with the E265X mutation, accompanied by absent protein expression. This E265X mutation was also associated with HPC in Finnish patients *(86)*. There are numerous nucleotide variants identified in the *RNASEL* gene, with seven of them resulting in protein sequence changes *(86)*. Six variants cause missense alterations and one rare variant creates a nonsense mutation. The two most commonly found variants are the non-synonymous SNPs: Arg462Gln (G→A) and Asp541Glu (T→G). The Arg462Gln variant reduces the cell's ability to cause apoptosis in response to activation by 2–5 (A) and also has three-times less enzymatic activity than normal *(87)*, whereas the Asp541Glu variant has no known effect on *RNASEL* protein function *(88)*. The Arg462Gln AA genotype has been associated with both increased prostrate cancer risk in US Caucasian sample groups *(87,88)* as well as decreased prostrate cancer risk in Caucasian and Japanese sample groups *(89,90)*.

## *N*-ACETYLTRANSFERASES 1 AND 2

*N*-Acetyltransferase genes 1 and 2 (*NAT1* and *NAT2*) catalyze the metabolic activation of aromatic amines and heterocyclic amine carcinogens such as 4-aminobiphenyl. The enzymes also deactivate, or detoxify, these compounds. Thus, genetic polymorphisms in *NAT1* and/or *NAT2* may modify the cancer risk related to exposures to these carcinogens *(91)*. Numerous genetic variants of *NAT1* and *NAT2*, which result in alterations of acetylator phenotype, have been identified *(92)*. Fukutome et al. *(93)* examined associations between *NAT1* polymorphisms and prostate cancer and found that homozygosity for the NAT1*10 allele, a variant associated with the rapid acetylator phenotype, was associated with higher risk.

## VITAMIN D RECEPTOR GENE

Vitamin D seems to play an important role in the development and progression of prostate cancer *(94)*. The active hormonal form of vitamin D, 1,25-dihydroxyvitamin D (1,25-D), influences prostate cell division through the vitamin D receptor (*VDR*) *(30)*. In prostate cancer cell lines, 1,25-D has been shown to induce cell differentiation and inhibit proliferation *(95)*, and in some epidemiologic studies, a relationship has been observed between higher serum levels of 1,25-D and lower risk of prostate cancer *(96–98)*. Overall little evidence supports an association between *VDR* polymorphisms and prostate cancer risk (reviewed in *(99)*). A recent study, however, suggests that the vitamin D status interacts with the *VDR* FokI polymorphism, modifying prostate cancer risk *(100)*. Moreover, the findings of Cicek and colleagues support a role for *VDR* variants in prostate cancer risk based on the significant association with haplotypes within the gene, in particular in men with more advanced disease status *(100)*.

The polymorphisms in these candidate genes have been the focus of many molecular epidemiological studies and have provided a biological foundation for future research. It is clear that some investigators have implicated these genes as biomarkers for prostate cancer risk. Further studies will help elucidate the role of these genes in the development of prostate cancer.

# GENOME-WIDE ASSOCIATION STUDIES

Genome-wide association studies (GWAS) are a relatively new way for scientists to identify genes involved in human disease. This method involves scanning thousands of samples, either as case–control cohorts or in family trios, utilizing hundreds of thousands of SNP markers, located throughout the human genome and available as SNP chips. Because GWAS examine SNPs across the genome, they represent a promising way to study complex, common diseases in which many genetic variations contribute to an individual's risk. While a powerful approach, GWAS are not without challenges. Critical to success is the development of robust study designs to ensure high power to detect genes of modest risk while minimizing the potential of false association signals due to testing large numbers of markers. Key components include sufficient sample sizes, well-defined phenotypes, comprehensive maps, accurate high-throughput genotyping technologies, sophisticated IT infrastructure, rapid algorithms for data analysis, and rigorous assessment of genome-wide signatures. This approach has already identified SNPs related to several complex conditions including breast cancer, colorectal cancer, diabetes type 2, and prostate cancer.

GWAS have identified variants in five chromosomal regions that are significantly associated with a risk of prostate cancer *(101–103)*. These variants occur in three independent regions at 8q24, at 17q12, and at 17q24. The specific genes in these regions have yet to be identified. Zheng et al. *(104)* assessed a joint analysis of the associated SNPs. They found that the effects of the 8q24 loci interact with the effects of the two loci on 17q and that the SNPs in the five chromosomal regions plus a family history of prostate cancer have a cumulative and significant association with prostate cancer. This interplay underscores the complex and multifactorial influences on the pathogenesis of prostate cancer.

More recent, GWAS have also led to the discovery of susceptibility loci MSMB (10q11), TCF2 (17q21), LMTK2 (7q21–q22), SLC22A3 (6q27), JAZF1 (7p15), and CTBP2 (21q21) implicated in the risk for prostate cancer *(102,105,106)* and DAB2IP (9q33), and EHBP1 (2p15) associated with the risk of developing aggressive prostate cancer *(107,108)*. It has yet to be determined whether the findings based on GWAS can provide easily applicable tests that will assist in the identification of men who are at high risk for prostate cancer. However, the ultimate goal of SNP-based studies is the development of clinically useful molecular genetic biomarkers that can be used in conjunction with standard clinical testing to permit the practice of individualized medicine, which would include cancer diagnosis, classification, intervention, and response to therapeutics.

## CONCLUSION

The development of novel and clinically relevant markers for prostate cancer diagnosis, prognosis, and prediction is essential for optimal identification and treatment of this disease. Linkage and association studies have identified several candidate genes likely involved in the pathogenesis of prostate cancer. However, to date no single biomarker has the desired level of diagnostic accuracy and the appropriate degree of certainty to predict the course of prostate cancer. Future studies should help to answer the unsolved etiology of prostate cancer and eventually lead to the identification of clinically relevant prostate cancer markers.

## REFERENCES

1. Lichtenstein, P., Holm, N. V., Verkasalo, P. K., Iliadou, A., Kaprio, J., Koskenvuo, M., Pukkala, E., Skytthe, A. and Hemminki, K. (2000) Environmental and heritable factors in the causation of cancer – analyses of cohorts of twins from Sweden, Denmark, and Finland. *N Engl J Med* **343**, 78–85.
2. Ostrander, E. A., Markianos, K. and Stanford, J. L. (2004) Finding prostate cancer susceptibility genes. *Annu Rev Genomics Hum Genet* **5**, 151–75.
3. Schaid, D. J. (2004) The complex genetic epidemiology of prostate cancer. *Hum Mol Genet* **13 Spec No 1**, R103–21.
4. Ostrander, E. A. and Stanford, J. L. (2000) Genetics of prostate cancer: too many loci, too few genes. *Am J Hum Genet* **67**, 1367–75.
5. Ghadirian, P., Howe, G. R., Hislop, T. G. and Maisonneuve, P. (1997) Family history of prostate cancer: a multi-center case-control study in Canada. *Int J Cancer* **70**, 679–81.
6. Stanford, J. L. and Ostrander, E. A. (2001) Familial prostate cancer. *Epidemiol Rev* **23**, 19–23.
7. Steinberg, G. D., Carter, B. S., Beaty, T. H., Childs, B. and Walsh, P. C. (1990) Family history and the risk of prostate cancer. *Prostate* **17**, 337–47.
8. Carter, B. S., Beaty, T. H., Steinberg, G. D., Childs, B. and Walsh, P. C. (1992) Mendelian inheritance of familial prostate cancer. *Proc Natl Acad Sci USA* **89**, 3367–71.
9. Xu, J., Dimitrov, L., Chang, B. L., Adams, T. S., Turner, A. R., Meyers, D. A., Eeles, R. A., Easton, D. F., Foulkes, W. D., Simard, J., Giles, G. G., Hopper, J. L., Mahle, L., Moller, P., Bishop, T., Evans, C.,

Edwards, S., Meitz, J., Bullock, S., Hope, Q., Hsieh, C. L., Halpern, J., Balise, R. N., Oakley-Girvan, I., Whittemore, A. S., Ewing, C. M., Gielzak, M., Isaacs, S. D., Walsh, P. C., Wiley, K. E., Isaacs, W. B., Thibodeau, S. N., McDonnell, S. K., Cunningham, J. M., Zarfas, K. E., Hebbring, S., Schaid, D. J., Friedrichsen, D. M., Deutsch, K., Kolb, S., Badzioch, M., Jarvik, G. P., Janer, M., Hood, L., Ostrander, E. A., Stanford, J. L., Lange, E. M., Beebe-Dimmer, J. L., Mohai, C. E., Cooney, K. A., Ikonen, T., Baffoe-Bonnie, A., Fredriksson, H., Matikainen, M. P., Tammela, T., Bailey-Wilson, J., Schleutker, J., Maier, C., Herkommer, K., Hoegel, J. J., Vogel, W., Paiss, T., Wiklund, F., Emanuelsson, M., Stenman, E., Jonsson, B. A., Gronberg, H., Camp, N. J., Farnham, J., Cannon-Albright, L. A. and Seminara, D. (2005) A combined genomewide linkage scan of 1,233 families for prostate cancer-susceptibility genes conducted by the international consortium for prostate cancer genetics. *Am J Hum Genet* **77**, 219–29.

10. Smith, J. R., Freije, D., Carpten, J. D., Gronberg, H., Xu, J., Isaacs, S. D., Brownstein, M. J., Bova, G. S., Guo, H., Bujnovszky, P., Nusskern, D. R., Damber, J. E., Bergh, A., Emanuelsson, M., Kallioniemi, O. P., Walker-Daniels, J., Bailey-Wilson, J. E., Beaty, T. H., Meyers, D. A., Walsh, P. C., Collins, F. S., Trent, J. M. and Isaacs, W. B. (1996) Major susceptibility locus for prostate cancer on chromosome 1 suggested by a genome-wide search. *Science* **274**, 1371–4.

11. Xu, J., Meyers, D., Freije, D., Isaacs, S., Wiley, K., Nusskern, D., Ewing, C., Wilkens, E., Bujnovszky, P., Bova, G. S., Walsh, P., Isaacs, W., Schleutker, J., Matikainen, M., Tammela, T., Visakorpi, T., Kallioniemi, O. P., Berry, R., Schaid, D., French, A., McDonnell, S., Schroeder, J., Blute, M., Thibodeau, S., Gronberg, H., Emanuelsson, M., Damber, J. E., Bergh, A., Jonsson, B. A., Smith, J., Bailey-Wilson, J., Carpten, J., Stephan, D., Gillanders, E., Amundson, I., Kainu, T., Freas-Lutz, D., Baffoe-Bonnie, A., Van Aucken, A., Sood, R., Collins, F., Brownstein, M. and Trent, J. (1998) Evidence for a prostate cancer susceptibility locus on the X chromosome. *Nat Genet* **20**, 175–9.

12. Tavtigian, S. V., Simard, J., Teng, D. H., Abtin, V., Baumgard, M., Beck, A., Camp, N. J., Carillo, A. R., Chen, Y., Dayananth, P., Desrochers, M., Dumont, M., Farnham, J. M., Frank, D., Frye, C., Ghaffari, S., Gupte, J. S., Hu, R., Iliev, D., Janecki, T., Kort, E. N., Laity, K. E., Leavitt, A., Leblanc, G., McArthur-Morrison, J., Pederson, A., Penn, B., Peterson, K. T., Reid, J. E., Richards, S., Schroeder, M., Smith, R., Snyder, S. C., Swedlund, B., Swensen, J., Thomas, A., Tranchant, M., Woodland, A. M., Labrie, F., Skolnick, M. H., Neuhausen, S., Rommens, J. and Cannon-Albright, L. A. (2001) A candidate prostate cancer susceptibility gene at chromosome 17p. *Nat Genet* **27**, 172–80.

13. Berry, R., Schroeder, J. J., French, A. J., McDonnell, S. K., Peterson, B. J., Cunningham, J. M., Thibodeau, S. N. and Schaid, D. J. (2000) Evidence for a prostate cancer-susceptibility locus on chromosome 20. *Am J Hum Genet* **67**, 82–91.

14. Friedrichsen, D. M., Stanford, J. L., Isaacs, S. D., Janer, M., Chang, B. L., Deutsch, K., Gillanders, E., Kolb, S., Wiley, K. E., Badzioch, M. D., Zheng, S. L., Walsh, P. C., Jarvik, G. P., Hood, L., Trent, J. M., Isaacs, W. B., Ostrander, E. A. and Xu, J. (2004) Identification of a prostate cancer susceptibility locus on chromosome 7q11–21 in Jewish families. *Proc Natl Acad Sci USA* **101**, 1939–44.

15. Rokman, A., Baffoe-Bonnie, A. B., Gillanders, E., Fredriksson, H., Autio, V., Ikonen, T., Gibbs, K. D., Jr., Jones, M., Gildea, D., Freas-Lutz, D., Markey, C., Matikainen, M. P., Koivisto, P. A., Tammela, T. L., Kallioniemi, O. P., Trent, J., Bailey-Wilson, J. E. and Schleutker, J. (2005) Hereditary prostate cancer in Finland: fine-mapping validates 3p26 as a major predisposition locus. *Hum Genet* **116**, 43–50.

16. Lange, E. M., Ho, L. A., Beebe-Dimmer, J. L., Wang, Y., Gillanders, E. M., Trent, J. M., Lange, L. A., Wood, D. P. and Cooney, K. A. (2006) Genome-wide linkage scan for prostate cancer susceptibility genes in men with aggressive disease: significant evidence for linkage at chromosome 15q12. *Hum Genet* **119**, 400–7.

17. Berthon, P., Valeri, A., Cohen-Akenine, A., Drelon, E., Paiss, T., Wohr, G., Latil, A., Millasseau, P., Mellah, I., Cohen, N., Blanche, H., Bellane-Chantelot, C., Demenais, F., Teillac, P., Le Duc, A., de Petriconi, R., Hautmann, R., Chumakov, I., Bachner, L., Maitland, N. J., Lidereau, R., Vogel, W., Fournier, G., Mangin, P., Cussenot, O. and et al. (1998) Predisposing gene for early-onset prostate cancer, localized on chromosome 1q42.2–43. *Am J Hum Genet* **62**, 1416–24.

18. Gibbs, M., Stanford, J. L., McIndoe, R. A., Jarvik, G. P., Kolb, S., Goode, E. L., Chakrabarti, L., Schuster, E. F., Buckley, V. A., Miller, E. L., Brandzel, S., Li, S., Hood, L. and Ostrander, E. A. (1999) Evidence for a rare prostate cancer-susceptibility locus at chromosome 1p36. *Am J Hum Genet* **64**, 776–87.

19. Xu, J., Zheng, S. L., Hawkins, G. A., Faith, D. A., Kelly, B., Isaacs, S. D., Wiley, K. E., Chang, B., Ewing, C. M., Bujnovszky, P., Carpten, J. D., Bleecker, E. R., Walsh, P. C., Trent, J. M., Meyers, D. A. and Isaacs, W. B. (2001) Linkage and association studies of prostate cancer susceptibility: evidence for linkage at 8p22–23. *Am J Hum Genet* **69**, 341–50.

20. Lange, E. M., Gillanders, E. M., Davis, C. C., Brown, W. M., Campbell, J. K., Jones, M., Gildea, D., Riedesel, E., Albertus, J., Freas-Lutz, D., Markey, C., Giri, V., Dimmer, J. B., Montie, J. E., Trent, J. M. and Cooney, K. A. (2003) Genome-wide scan for prostate cancer susceptibility genes using families from the University of Michigan prostate cancer genetics project finds evidence for linkage on chromosome 17 near BRCA1. *Prostate* **57**, 326–34.

21. Amundadottir, L. T., Sulem, P., Gudmundsson, J., Helgason, A., Baker, A., Agnarsson, B. A., Sigurdsson, A., Benediktsdottir, K. R., Cazier, J. B., Sainz, J., Jakobsdottir, M., Kostic, J., Magnusdottir, D. N., Ghosh, S., Agnarsson, K., Birgisdottir, B., Le Roux, L., Olafsdottir, A., Blondal, T., Andresdottir, M., Gretarsdottir, O. S., Bergthorsson, J. T., Gudbjartsson, D., Gylfason, A., Thorleifsson, G., Manolescu, A., Kristjansson, K., Geirsson, G., Isaksson, H., Douglas, J., Johansson, J. E., Balter, K., Wiklund, F., Montie, J. E., Yu, X., Suarez, B. K., Ober, C., Cooney, K. A., Gronberg, H., Catalona, W. J., Einarsson, G. V., Barkardottir, R. B., Gulcher, J. R., Kong, A., Thorsteinsdottir, U. and Stefansson, K. (2006) A common variant associated with prostate cancer in European and African populations. *Nat Genet* **38**, 652–8.

22. Slager, S. L., Schaid, D. J., Cunningham, J. M., McDonnell, S. K., Marks, A. F., Peterson, B. J., Hebbring, S. J., Anderson, S., French, A. J. and Thibodeau, S. N. (2003) Confirmation of linkage of prostate cancer aggressiveness with chromosome 19q. *Am J Hum Genet* **72**, 759–62.

23. Schaid, D. J., Stanford, J. L., McDonnell, S. K., Suuriniemi, M., McIntosh, L., Karyadi, D. M., Carlson, E. E., Deutsch, K., Janer, M., Hood, L. and Ostrander, E. A. (2007) Genome-wide linkage scan of prostate cancer Gleason score and confirmation of chromosome 19q. *Hum Genet* **121**, 729–35.

24. Witte, J. S., Goddard, K. A., Conti, D. V., Elston, R. C., Lin, J., Suarez, B. K., Broman, K. W., Burmester, J. K., Weber, J. L. and Catalona, W. J. (2000) Genomewide scan for prostate cancer-aggressiveness loci. *Am J Hum Genet* **67**, 92–9.

25. Witte, J. S., Suarez, B. K., Thiel, B., Lin, J., Yu, A., Banerjee, T. K., Burmester, J. K., Casey, G. and Catalona, W. J. (2003) Genome-wide scan of brothers: replication and fine mapping of prostate cancer susceptibility and aggressiveness loci. *Prostate* **57**, 298–308.

26. Makridakis, N. M. and Reichardt, J. K. (2001) Molecular epidemiology of hormone-metabolic loci in prostate cancer. *Epidemiol Rev* **23**, 24–9.

27. Huggins, C. and Hodges, C. V. (2002) Studies on prostatic cancer: I. The effect of castration, of estrogen and of androgen injection on serum phosphatases in metastatic carcinoma of the prostate. 1941. *J Urol* **168**, 9–12.

28. Gnanapragasam, V. J., Robson, C. N., Leung, H. Y. and Neal, D. E. (2000) Androgen receptor signalling in the prostate. *BJU Int* **86**, 1001–13.

29. Hakimi, J. M., Schoenberg, M. P., Rondinelli, R. H., Piantadosi, S. and Barrack, E. R. (1997) Androgen receptor variants with short glutamine or glycine repeats may identify unique subpopulations of men with prostate cancer. *Clin Cancer Res* **3**, 1599–608.

30. Irvine, R. A., Yu, M. C., Ross, R. K. and Coetzee, G. A. (1995) The CAG and GGC microsatellites of the androgen receptor gene are in linkage disequilibrium in men with prostate cancer. *Cancer Res* **55**, 1937–40.

31. Lindstrom, S., Zheng, S. L., Wiklund, F., Jonsson, B. A., Adami, H. O., Balter, K. A., Brookes, A. J., Sun, J., Chang, B. L., Liu, W., Li, G., Isaacs, W. B., Adolfsson, J., Gronberg, H. and Xu, J. (2006) Systematic replication study of reported genetic associations in prostate cancer: strong support for genetic variation in the androgen pathway. *Prostate* **66**, 1729–43.

32. Ross, R. K., Pike, M. C., Coetzee, G. A., Reichardt, J. K., Yu, M. C., Feigelson, H., Stanczyk, F. Z., Kolonel, L. N. and Henderson, B. E. (1998) Androgen metabolism and prostate cancer: establishing a model of genetic susceptibility. *Cancer Res* **58**, 4497–504.

33. Mononen, N., Syrjakoski, K., Matikainen, M., Tammela, T. L., Schleutker, J., Kallioniemi, O. P., Trapman, J. and Koivisto, P. A. (2000) Two percent of Finnish prostate cancer patients have a germ-line mutation in the hormone-binding domain of the androgen receptor gene. *Cancer Res* **60**, 6479–81.

34. Simard, J., Durocher, F., Mebarki, F., Turgeon, C., Sanchez, R., Labrie, Y., Couet, J., Trudel, C., Rheaume, E., Morel, Y., Luu-The, V. and Labrie, F. (1996) Molecular biology and genetics of the 3 beta-hydroxysteroid dehydrogenase/delta5-delta4 isomerase gene family. *J Endocrinol* **150 Suppl**, S189–207.

35. Devgan, S. A., Henderson, B. E., Yu, M. C., Shi, C. Y., Pike, M. C., Ross, R. K. and Reichardt, J. K. (1997) Genetic variation of 3 beta-hydroxysteroid dehydrogenase type II in three racial/ethnic groups: implications for prostate cancer risk. *Prostate* **33**, 9–12.

36. Thigpen, A. E., Silver, R. I., Guileyardo, J. M., Casey, M. L., McConnell, J. D. and Russell, D. W. (1993) Tissue distribution and ontogeny of steroid 5 alpha-reductase isozyme expression. *J Clin Invest* **92**, 903–10.

37. Hochberg, Z., Chayen, R., Reiss, N., Falik, Z., Makler, A., Munichor, M., Farkas, A., Goldfarb, H., Ohana, N. and Hiort, O. (1996) Clinical, biochemical, and genetic findings in a large pedigree of male and female patients with 5 alpha-reductase 2 deficiency. *J Clin Endocrinol Metab* **81**, 2821–7.

38. Makridakis, N. M., di Salle, E. and Reichardt, J. K. (2000) Biochemical and pharmacogenetic dissection of human steroid 5 alpha-reductase type II. *Pharmacogenetics* **10**, 407–13.

39. Makridakis, N., Ross, R. K., Pike, M. C., Chang, L., Stanczyk, F. Z., Kolonel, L. N., Shi, C. Y., Yu, M. C., Henderson, B. E. and Reichardt, J. K. (1997) A prevalent missense substitution that modulates activity of prostatic steroid 5alpha-reductase. *Cancer Res* **57**, 1020–2.

40. Nam, R. K., Toi, A., Vesprini, D., Ho, M., Chu, W., Harvie, S., Sweet, J., Trachtenberg, J., Jewett, M. A. and Narod, S. A. (2001) V89L polymorphism of type-2, 5-alpha reductase enzyme gene predicts prostate cancer presence and progression. *Urology* **57**, 199–204.

41. Makridakis, N. M., Ross, R. K., Pike, M. C., Crocitto, L. E., Kolonel, L. N., Pearce, C. L., Henderson, B. E. and Reichardt, J. K. (1999) Association of mis-sense substitution in SRD5A2 gene with prostate cancer in African-American and Hispanic men in Los Angeles, USA. *Lancet* **354**, 975–8.

42. Van Den Akker, E. L., Koper, J. W., Boehmer, A. L., Themmen, A. P., Verhoef-Post, M., Timmerman, M. A., Otten, B. J., Drop, S. L. and De Jong, F. H. (2002) Differential inhibition of 17alpha-hydroxylase and 17,20-lyase activities by three novel missense CYP17 mutations identified in patients with P450c17 deficiency. *J Clin Endocrinol Metab* **87**, 5714–21.

43. Chung, B. C., Picado-Leonard, J., Haniu, M., Bienkowski, M., Hall, P. F., Shively, J. E. and Miller, W. L. (1987) Cytochrome P450c17 (steroid 17 alpha-hydroxylase/17,20 lyase): cloning of human adrenal and testis cDNAs indicates the same gene is expressed in both tissues. *Proc Natl Acad Sci USA* **84**, 407–11.

44. Haiman, C. A., Stampfer, M. J., Giovannucci, E., Ma, J., Decalo, N. E., Kantoff, P. W. and Hunter, D. J. (2001) The relationship between a polymorphism in CYP17 with plasma hormone levels and prostate cancer. *Cancer Epidemiol Biomarkers Prev* **10**, 743–8.

45. Yamada, Y., Watanabe, M., Murata, M., Yamanaka, M., Kubota, Y., Ito, H., Katoh, T., Kawamura, J., Yatani, R. and Shiraishi, T. (2001) Impact of genetic polymorphisms of 17-hydroxylase cytochrome P-450 (CYP17) and steroid 5alpha-reductase type II (SRD5A2) genes on prostate-cancer risk among the Japanese population. *Int J Cancer* **92**, 683–6.

46. Gsur, A., Bernhofer, G., Hinteregger, S., Haidinger, G., Schatzl, G., Madersbacher, S., Marberger, M., Vutuc, C. and Micksche, M. (2000) A polymorphism in the CYP17 gene is associated with prostate cancer risk. *Int J Cancer* **87**, 434–7.

47. Lunn, R. M., Bell, D. A., Mohler, J. L. and Taylor, J. A. (1999) Prostate cancer risk and polymorphism in 17 hydroxylase (CYP17) and steroid reductase (SRD5A2). *Carcinogenesis* **20**, 1727–31.

48. Habuchi, T., Liqing, Z., Suzuki, T., Sasaki, R., Tsuchiya, N., Tachiki, H., Shimoda, N., Satoh, S., Sato, K., Kakehi, Y., Kamoto, T., Ogawa, O. and Kato, T. (2000) Increased risk of prostate cancer and benign prostatic hyperplasia associated with a CYP17 gene polymorphism with a gene dosage effect. *Cancer Res* **60**, 5710–3.

49. Latil, A. G., Azzouzi, R., Cancel, G. S., Guillaume, E. C., Cochan-Priollet, B., Berthon, P. L. and Cussenot, O. (2001) Prostate carcinoma risk and allelic variants of genes involved in androgen biosynthesis and metabolism pathways. *Cancer* **92**, 1130–7.

50. Riegman, P. H., Vlietstra, R. J., van der Korput, J. A., Brinkmann, A. O. and Trapman, J. (1991) The promoter of the prostate-specific antigen gene contains a functional androgen responsive element. *Mol Endocrinol* **5**, 1921–30.

51. Cleutjens, K. B., van Eekelen, C. C., van der Korput, H. A., Brinkmann, A. O. and Trapman, J. (1996) Two androgen response regions cooperate in steroid hormone regulated activity of the prostate-specific antigen promoter. *J Biol Chem* **271**, 6379–88.

52. Xue, W., Irvine, R. A., Yu, M. C., Ross, R. K., Coetzee, G. A. and Ingles, S. A. (2000) Susceptibility to prostate cancer: interaction between genotypes at the androgen receptor and prostate-specific antigen loci. *Cancer Res* **60**, 839–41.

53. Lai, J., Kedda, M. A., Hinze, K., Smith, R. L., Yaxley, J., Spurdle, A. B., Morris, C. P., Harris, J. and Clements, J. A. (2007) PSA/KLK3 AREI promoter polymorphism alters androgen receptor binding and is associated with prostate cancer susceptibility. *Carcinogenesis* **28**, 1032–9.

54. Cheung, Y. L., Kerr, A. C., McFadyen, M. C., Melvin, W. T. and Murray, G. I. (1999) Differential expression of CYP1A1, CYP1A2, CYP1B1 in human kidney tumours. *Cancer Lett* **139**, 199–205.

55. Agundez, J. A. (2004) Cytochrome P450 gene polymorphism and cancer. *Curr Drug Metab* **5**, 211–24.
56. Hayes, C. L., Spink, D. C., Spink, B. C., Cao, J. Q., Walker, N. J. and Sutter, T. R. (1996) 17 beta-estradiol hydroxylation catalyzed by human cytochrome P450 1B1. *Proc Natl Acad Sci USA* **93**, 9776–81.
57. Spink, D. C., Eugster, H. P., Lincoln, D. W., 2nd, Schuetz, J. D., Schuetz, E. G., Johnson, J. A., Kaminsky, L. S. and Gierthy, J. F. (1992) 17 beta-estradiol hydroxylation catalyzed by human cytochrome P450 1A1: a comparison of the activities induced by 2,3,7,8-tetrachlorodibenzo-p-dioxin in MCF-7 cells with those from heterologous expression of the cDNA. *Arch Biochem Biophys* **293**, 342–8.
58. Crespi, C. L., Penman, B. W., Steimel, D. T., Smith, T., Yang, C. S. and Sutter, T. R. (1997) Development of a human lymphoblastoid cell line constitutively expressing human CYP1B1 cDNA: substrate specificity with model substrates and promutagens. *Mutagenesis* **12**, 83–9.
59. Cavalieri, E. L., Devanesan, P., Bosland, M. C., Badawi, A. F. and Rogan, E. G. (2002) Catechol estrogen metabolites and conjugates in different regions of the prostate of Noble rats treated with 4-hydroxyestradiol: implications for estrogen-induced initiation of prostate cancer. *Carcinogenesis* **23**, 329–33.
60. Williams, J. A., Martin, F. L., Muir, G. H., Hewer, A., Grover, P. L. and Phillips, D. H. (2000) Metabolic activation of carcinogens and expression of various cytochromes P450 in human prostate tissue. *Carcinogenesis* **21**, 1683–9.
61. Sissung, T. M., Price, D. K., Sparreboom, A. and Figg, W. D. (2006) Pharmacogenetics and regulation of human cytochrome P450 1B1: implications in hormone-mediated tumor metabolism and a novel target for therapeutic intervention. *Mol Cancer Res* **4**, 135–50.
62. Fukatsu, T., Hirokawa, Y., Araki, T., Hioki, T., Murata, T., Suzuki, H., Ichikawa, T., Tsukino, H., Qiu, D., Katoh, T., Sugimura, Y., Yatani, R., Shiraishi, T. and Watanabe, M. (2004) Genetic polymorphisms of hormone-related genes and prostate cancer risk in the Japanese population. *Anticancer Res* **24**, 2431–7.
63. Tang, Y. M., Green, B. L., Chen, G. F., Thompson, P. A., Lang, N. P., Shinde, A., Lin, D. X., Tan, W., Lyn-Cook, B. D., Hammons, G. J. and Kadlubar, F. F. (2000) Human CYP1B1 Leu432Val gene polymorphism: ethnic distribution in African-Americans, Caucasians and Chinese; oestradiol hydroxylase activity; and distribution in prostate cancer cases and controls. *Pharmacogenetics* **10**, 761–6.
64. Tanaka, Y., Sasaki, M., Kaneuchi, M., Shiina, H., Igawa, M. and Dahiya, R. (2002) Polymorphisms of the CYP1B1 gene have higher risk for prostate cancer. *Biochem Biophys Res Commun* **296**, 820–6.
65. Cicek, M. S., Liu, X., Casey, G. and Witte, J. S. (2005) Role of androgen metabolism genes CYP1B1, PSA/KLK3, and CYP11alpha in prostate cancer risk and aggressiveness. *Cancer Epidemiol Biomarkers Prev* **14**, 2173–7.
66. Chang, B. L., Zheng, S. L., Isaacs, S. D., Turner, A., Hawkins, G. A., Wiley, K. E., Bleecker, E. R., Walsh, P. C., Meyers, D. A., Isaacs, W. B. and Xu, J. (2003) Polymorphisms in the CYP1B1 gene are associated with increased risk of prostate cancer. *Br J Cancer* **89**, 1524–9.
67. Watkins, P. B., Wrighton, S. A., Maurel, P., Schuetz, E. G., Mendez-Picon, G., Parker, G. A. and Guzelian, P. S. (1985) Identification of an inducible form of cytochrome P-450 in human liver. *Proc Natl Acad Sci USA* **82**, 6310–4.
68. Rebbeck, T. R., Jaffe, J. M., Walker, A. H., Wein, A. J. and Malkowicz, S. B. (1998) Modification of clinical presentation of prostate tumors by a novel genetic variant in CYP3A4. *J Natl Cancer Inst* **90**, 1225–9.
69. Walker, A. H., Jaffe, J. M., Gunasegaram, S., Cummings, S. A., Huang, C. S., Chern, H. D., Olopade, O. I., Weber, B. L. and Rebbeck, T. R. (1998) Characterization of an allelic variant in the nifedipine-specific element of CYP3A4: ethnic distribution and implications for prostate cancer risk. Mutations in brief no. 191. Online. *Hum Mutat* **12**, 289.
70. Boiteux, S. and Radicella, J. P. (2000) The human OGG1 gene: structure, functions, and its implication in the process of carcinogenesis. *Arch Biochem Biophys* **377**, 1–8.
71. De Marzo, A. M., Marchi, V. L., Epstein, J. I. and Nelson, W. G. (1999) Proliferative inflammatory atrophy of the prostate: implications for prostatic carcinogenesis. *Am J Pathol* **155**, 1985–92.
72. Hussain, S. P. and Harris, C. C. (1998) Molecular epidemiology of human cancer: contribution of mutation spectra studies of tumor suppressor genes. *Cancer Res* **58**, 4023–37.
73. Xu, J., Zheng, S. L., Turner, A., Isaacs, S. D., Wiley, K. E., Hawkins, G. A., Chang, B. L., Bleecker, E. R., Walsh, P. C., Meyers, D. A. and Isaacs, W. B. (2002) Associations between hOGG1 sequence variants and prostate cancer susceptibility. *Cancer Res* **62**, 2253–7.
74. Weiss, J. M., Goode, E. L., Ladiges, W. C. and Ulrich, C. M. (2005) Polymorphic variation in hOGG1 and risk of cancer: a review of the functional and epidemiologic literature. *Mol Carcinog* **42**, 127–41.

75. Chen, L., Elahi, A., Pow-Sang, J., Lazarus, P. and Park, J. (2003) Association between polymorphism of human oxoguanine glycosylase 1 and risk of prostate cancer. *J Urol* **170**, 2471–4.

76. Frebourg, T. and Friend, S. H. (1993) The importance of p53 gene alterations in human cancer: is there more than circumstantial evidence? *J Natl Cancer Inst* **85**, 1554–7.

77. Ruijter, E., van de Kaa, C., Miller, G., Ruiter, D., Debruyne, F. and Schalken, J. (1999) Molecular genetics and epidemiology of prostate carcinoma. *Endocr Rev* **20**, 22–45.

78. Gumerlock, P. H., Chi, S. G., Shi, X. B., Voeller, H. J., Jacobson, J. W., Gelmann, E. P. and deVere White, R. W. (1997) p53 abnormalities in primary prostate cancer: single-strand conformation polymorphism analysis of complementary DNA in comparison with genomic DNA. The Cooperative Prostate Network. *J Natl Cancer Inst* **89**, 66–71.

79. Dumont, P., Leu, J. I., Della Pietra, A. C., 3rd, George, D. L. and Murphy, M. (2003) The codon 72 polymorphic variants of p53 have markedly different apoptotic potential. *Nat Genet* **33**, 357–65.

80. van Heemst, D., Mooijaart, S. P., Beekman, M., Schreuder, J., de Craen, A. J., Brandt, B. W., Slagboom, P. E. and Westendorp, R. G. (2005) Variation in the human TP53 gene affects old age survival and cancer mortality. *Exp Gerontol* **40**, 11–5.

81. Zhou, A., Hassel, B. A. and Silverman, R. H. (1993) Expression cloning of 2-5A-dependent RNAase: a uniquely regulated mediator of interferon action. *Cell* **72**, 753–65.

82. Zhou, A., Paranjape, J., Brown, T. L., Nie, H., Naik, S., Dong, B., Chang, A., Trapp, B., Fairchild, R., Colmenares, C. and Silverman, R. H. (1997) Interferon action and apoptosis are defective in mice devoid of 2',5'-oligoadenylate-dependent RNase L. *Embo J* **16**, 6355–63.

83. Castelli, J., Wood, K. A. and Youle, R. J. (1998) The 2-5A system in viral infection and apoptosis. *Biomed Pharmacother* **52**, 386–90.

84. Hassel, B. A., Zhou, A., Sotomayor, C., Maran, A. and Silverman, R. H. (1993) A dominant negative mutant of 2-5A-dependent RNase suppresses antiproliferative and antiviral effects of interferon. *Embo J* **12**, 3297–304.

85. Carpten, J., Nupponen, N., Isaacs, S., Sood, R., Robbins, C., Xu, J., Faruque, M., Moses, T., Ewing, C., Gillanders, E., Hu, P., Bujnovszky, P., Makalowska, I., Baffoe-Bonnie, A., Faith, D., Smith, J., Stephan, D., Wiley, K., Brownstein, M., Gildea, D., Kelly, B., Jenkins, R., Hostetter, G., Matikainen, M., Schleutker, J., Klinger, K., Connors, T., Xiang, Y., Wang, Z., De Marzo, A., Papadopoulos, N., Kallioniemi, O. P., Burk, R., Meyers, D., Gronberg, H., Meltzer, P., Silverman, R., Bailey-Wilson, J., Walsh, P., Isaacs, W. and Trent, J. (2002) Germline mutations in the ribonuclease L gene in families showing linkage with HPC1. *Nat Genet* **30**, 181–4.

86. Rokman, A., Ikonen, T., Seppala, E. H., Nupponen, N., Autio, V., Mononen, N., Bailey-Wilson, J., Trent, J., Carpten, J., Matikainen, M. P., Koivisto, P. A., Tammela, T. L., Kallioniemi, O. P. and Schleutker, J. (2002) Germline alterations of the RNASEL gene, a candidate HPC1 gene at 1q25, in patients and families with prostate cancer. *Am J Hum Genet* **70**, 1299–304.

87. Casey, G., Neville, P. J., Plummer, S. J., Xiang, Y., Krumroy, L. M., Klein, E. A., Catalona, W. J., Nupponen, N., Carpten, J. D., Trent, J. M., Silverman, R. H. and Witte, J. S. (2002) RNASEL Arg462Gln variant is implicated in up to 13% of prostate cancer cases. *Nat Genet* **32**, 581–3.

88. Xiang, Y., Wang, Z., Murakami, J., Plummer, S., Klein, E. A., Carpten, J. D., Trent, J. M., Isaacs, W. B., Casey, G. and Silverman, R. H. (2003) Effects of RNase L mutations associated with prostate cancer on apoptosis induced by 2',5'-oligoadenylates. *Cancer Res* **63**, 6795–801.

89. Wang, L., McDonnell, S. K., Elkins, D. A., Slager, S. L., Christensen, E., Marks, A. F., Cunningham, J. M., Peterson, B. J., Jacobsen, S. J., Cerhan, J. R., Blute, M. L., Schaid, D. J. and Thibodeau, S. N. (2002) Analysis of the RNASEL gene in familial and sporadic prostate cancer. *Am J Hum Genet* **71**, 116–23.

90. Nakazato, H., Suzuki, K., Matsui, H., Ohtake, N., Nakata, S. and Yamanaka, H. (2003) Role of genetic polymorphisms of the RNASEL gene on familial prostate cancer risk in a Japanese population. *Br J Cancer* **89**, 691–6.

91. Smith, G., Stanley, L. A., Sim, E., Strange, R. C. and Wolf, C. R. (1995) Metabolic polymorphisms and cancer susceptibility. *Cancer Surv* **25**, 27–65.

92. Hein, D. W., Doll, M. A., Fretland, A. J., Leff, M. A., Webb, S. J., Xiao, G. H., Devanaboyina, U. S., Nangju, N. A. and Feng, Y. (2000) Molecular genetics and epidemiology of the NAT1 and NAT2 acetylation polymorphisms. *Cancer Epidemiol Biomarkers Prev* **9**, 29–42.

93. Fukutome, K., Watanabe, M., Shiraishi, T., Murata, M., Uemura, H., Kubota, Y., Kawamura, J., Ito, H. and Yatani, R. (1999) N-acetyltransferase 1 genetic polymorphism influences the risk of prostate cancer development. *Cancer Lett* **136**, 83–7.

94. Lou, Y. R., Qiao, S., Talonpoika, R., Syvala, H. and Tuohimaa, P. (2004) The role of Vitamin D3 metabolism in prostate cancer. *J Steroid Biochem Mol Biol* **92**, 317–25.

95. Ma, J., Stampfer, M. J., Gann, P. H., Hough, H. L., Giovannucci, E., Kelsey, K. T., Hennekens, C. H. and Hunter, D. J. (1998) Vitamin D receptor polymorphisms, circulating vitamin D metabolites, and risk of prostate cancer in United States physicians. *Cancer Epidemiol Biomarkers Prev* **7**, 385–90.

96. Gann, P. H., Ma, J., Hennekens, C. H., Hollis, B. W., Haddad, J. G. and Stampfer, M. J. (1996) Circulating vitamin D metabolites in relation to subsequent development of prostate cancer. *Cancer Epidemiol Biomarkers Prev* **5**, 121–6.

97. Corder, E. H., Guess, H. A., Hulka, B. S., Friedman, G. D., Sadler, M., Vollmer, R. T., Lobaugh, B., Drezner, M. K., Vogelman, J. H. and Orentreich, N. (1993) Vitamin D and prostate cancer: a prediagnostic study with stored sera. *Cancer Epidemiol Biomarkers Prev* **2**, 467–72.

98. Braun, M. M., Helzlsouer, K. J., Hollis, B. W. and Comstock, G. W. (1995) Prostate cancer and prediagnostic levels of serum vitamin D metabolites (Maryland, United States). *Cancer Causes Control* **6**, 235–9.

99. Coughlin, S. S. and Hall, I. J. (2002) A review of genetic polymorphisms and prostate cancer risk. *Ann Epidemiol* **12**, 182–96.

100. Li, H., Stampfer, M. J., Hollis, J. B., Mucci, L. A., Gaziano, J. M., Hunter, D., Giovannucci, E. L. and Ma, J. (2007) A prospective study of plasma vitamin D metabolites, vitamin D receptor polymorphisms, and prostate cancer. *PLoS Med* **4**, e103.

101. Gudmundsson, J., Sulem, P., Manolescu, A., Amundadottir, L. T., Gudbjartsson, D., Helgason, A., Rafnar, T., Bergthorsson, J. T., Agnarsson, B. A., Baker, A., Sigurdsson, A., Benediktsdottir, K. R., Jakobsdottir, M., Xu, J., Blondal, T., Kostic, J., Sun, J., Ghosh, S., Stacey, S. N., Mouy, M., Saemunds-dottir, J., Backman, V. M., Kristjansson, K., Tres, A., Partin, A. W., Albers-Akkers, M. T., Godino-Ivan Marcos, J., Walsh, P. C., Swinkels, D. W., Navarrete, S., Isaacs, S. D., Aben, K. K., Graif, T., Cashy, J., Ruiz-Echarri, M., Wiley, K. E., Suarez, B. K., Witjes, J. A., Frigge, M., Ober, C., Jonsson, E., Einarsson, G. V., Mayordomo, J. I., Kiemeney, L. A., Isaacs, W. B., Catalona, W. J., Barkardottir, R. B., Gulcher, J. R., Thorsteinsdottir, U., Kong, A. and Stefansson, K. (2007) Genome-wide association study identifies a second prostate cancer susceptibility variant at 8q24. *Nat Genet* **39**, 631–7.

102. Gudmundsson, J., Sulem, P., Steinthorsdottir, V., Bergthorsson, J. T., Thorleifsson, G., Manolescu, A., Rafnar, T., Gudbjartsson, D., Agnarsson, B. A., Baker, A., Sigurdsson, A., Benediktsdottir, K. R., Jakobsdottir, M., Blondal, T., Stacey, S. N., Helgason, A., Gunnarsdottir, S., Olafsdottir, A., Kristinsson, K. T., Birgisdottir, B., Ghosh, S., Thorlacius, S., Magnusdottir, D., Stefansdottir, G., Kristjansson, K., Bagger, Y., Wilensky, R. L., Reilly, M. P., Morris, A. D., Kimber, C. H., Adeyemo, A., Chen, Y., Zhou, J., So, W. Y., Tong, P. C., Ng, M. C., Hansen, T., Andersen, G., Borch-Johnsen, K., Jorgensen, T., Tres, A., Fuertes, F., Ruiz-Echarri, M., Asin, L., Saez, B., van Boven, E., Klaver, S., Swinkels, D. W., Aben, K. K., Graif, T., Cashy, J., Suarez, B. K., van Vierssen Trip, O., Frigge, M. L., Ober, C., Hofker, M. H., Wijmenga, C., Christiansen, C., Rader, D. J., Palmer, C. N., Rotimi, C., Chan, J. C., Pedersen, O., Sigurdsson, G., Benediktsson, R., Jonsson, E., Einarsson, G. V., Mayordomo, J. I., Catalona, W. J., Kiemeney, L. A., Barkardottir, R. B., Gulcher, J. R., Thorsteinsdottir, U., Kong, A. and Stefansson, K. (2007) Two variants on chromosome 17 confer prostate cancer risk, and the one in TCF2 protects against type 2 diabetes. *Nat Genet* **39**, 977–83.

103. Yeager, M., Orr, N., Hayes, R. B., Jacobs, K. B., Kraft, P., Wacholder, S., Minichiello, M. J., Fearnhead, P., Yu, K., Chatterjee, N., Wang, Z., Welch, R., Staats, B. J., Calle, E. E., Feigelson, H. S., Thun, M. J., Rodriguez, C., Albanes, D., Virtamo, J., Weinstein, S., Schumacher, F. R., Giovannucci, E., Willett, W. C., Cancel-Tassin, G., Cussenot, O., Valeri, A., Andriole, G. L., Gelmann, E. P., Tucker, M., Gerhard, D. S., Fraumeni, J. F., Jr., Hoover, R., Hunter, D. J., Chanock, S. J. and Thomas, G. (2007) Genome-wide association study of prostate cancer identifies a second risk locus at 8q24. *Nat Genet* **39**, 645–9.

104. Zheng, S. L., Sun, J., Wiklund, F., Smith, S., Stattin, P., Li, G., Adami, H. O., Hsu, F. C., Zhu, Y., Balter, K., Kader, A. K., Turner, A. R., Liu, W., Bleecker, E. R., Meyers, D. A., Duggan, D., Carpten, J. D., Chang, B. L., Isaacs, W. B., Xu, J. and Gronberg, H. (2008) Cumulative association of five genetic variants with prostate cancer. *N Engl J Med* **358**, 910–9.

105. Eeles, R. A., Kote-Jarai, Z., Giles, G. G., Olama, A. A., Guy, M., Jugurnauth, S. K., Mulholland, S., Leongamornlert, D. A., Edwards, S. M., Morrison, J., Field, H. I., Southey, M. C., Severi, G., Donovan, J. L., Hamdy, F. C., Dearnaley, D. P., Muir, K. R., Smith, C., Bagnato, M., Ardern-Jones, A. T., Hall, A. L., O'Brien, L. T., Gehr-Swain, B. N., Wilkinson, R. A., Cox, A., Lewis, S., Brown, P. M., Jhavar, S. G., Tymrakiewicz, M., Lophatananon, A., Bryant, S. L., Horwich, A., Huddart, R. A., Khoo, V. S., Parker, C. C., Woodhouse, C. J., Thompson, A., Christmas, T., Ogden, C., Fisher, C., Jamieson, C., Cooper, C. S., English, D. R., Hopper, J. L., Neal, D. E. and Easton, D. F. (2008) Multiple newly identified loci associated with prostate cancer susceptibility. *Nat Genet* **40**, 316–21.

106. Thomas, G., Jacobs, K. B., Yeager, M., Kraft, P., Wacholder, S., Orr, N., Yu, K., Chatterjee, N., Welch, R., Hutchinson, A., Crenshaw, A., Cancel-Tassin, G., Staats, B. J., Wang, Z., Gonzalez-Bosquet, J., Fang, J., Deng, X., Berndt, S. I., Calle, E. E., Feigelson, H. S., Thun, M. J., Rodriguez, C., Albanes, D., Virtamo, J., Weinstein, S., Schumacher, F. R., Giovannucci, E., Willett, W. C., Cussenot, O., Valeri, A., Andriole, G. L., Crawford, E. D., Tucker, M., Gerhard, D. S., Fraumeni, J. F., Jr., Hoover, R., Hayes, R. B., Hunter, D. J. and Chanock, S. J. (2008) Multiple loci identified in a genome-wide association study of prostate cancer. *Nat Genet* **40**,310–5.
107. Gudmundsson, J., Sulem, P., Rafnar, T., Bergthorsson, J. T., Manolescu, A., Gudbjartsson, D., Agnarsson, B. A., Sigurdsson, A., Benediktsdottir, K. R., Blondal, T., Jakobsdottir, M., Stacey, S. N., Kostic, J., Kristinsson, K. T., Birgisdottir, B., Ghosh, S., Magnusdottir, D. N., Thorlacius, S., Thorleifsson, G., Zheng, S. L., Sun, J., Chang, B. L., Elmore, J. B., Breyer, J. P., McReynolds, K. M., Bradley, K. M., Yaspan, B. L., Wiklund, F., Stattin, P., Lindstrom, S., Adami, H. O., McDonnell, S. K., Schaid, D. J., Cunningham, J. M., Wang, L., Cerhan, J. R., St Sauver, J. L., Isaacs, S. D., Wiley, K. E., Partin, A. W., Walsh, P. C., Polo, S., Ruiz-Echarri, M., Navarrete, S., Fuertes, F., Saez, B., Godino, J., Weijerman, P. C., Swinkels, D. W., Aben, K. K., Witjes, J. A., Suarez, B. K., Helfand, B. T., Frigge, M. L., Kristjansson, K., Ober, C., Jonsson, E., Einarsson, G. V., Xu, J., Gronberg, H., Smith, J. R., Thibodeau, S. N., Isaacs, W. B., Catalona, W. J., Mayordomo, J. I., Kiemeney, L. A., Barkardottir, R. B., Gulcher, J. R., Thorsteinsdottir, U., Kong, A. and Stefansson, K. (2008) Common sequence variants on 2p15 and Xp11.22 confer susceptibility to prostate cancer. *Nat Genet* **40**,281–3.
108. Duggan, D., Zheng, S. L., Knowlton, M., Benitez, D., Dimitrov, L., Wiklund, F., Robbins, C., Isaacs, S. D., Cheng, Y., Li, G., Sun, J., Chang, B. L., Marovich, L., Wiley, K. E., Balter, K., Stattin, P., Adami, H. O., Gielzak, M., Yan, G., Sauvageot, J., Liu, W., Kim, J. W., Bleecker, E. R., Meyers, D. A., Trock, B. J., Partin, A. W., Walsh, P. C., Isaacs, W. B., Gronberg, H., Xu, J. and Carpten, J. D. (2007) Two genome-wide association studies of aggressive prostate cancer implicate putative prostate tumor suppressor gene DAB2IP. *J Natl Cancer Inst* **99**, 1836–44.

# 19 *GSTP1* Hypermethylation for Prostate Cancer Detection

*Rui Henrique and Carmen Jerónimo*

CONTENTS

## SUMMARY

The search for new prostate cancer markers, which might increase the accuracy of early detection, diagnosis, and prognosis prediction, constitutes an attractive and fast-growing research field. In recent years a new class of cancer molecular markers based on epigenetic alterations has emerged, among which aberrant DNA methylation of cancer-related genes has showed promise in the detection of several common malignant tumors. Since its first report in 1994, *GSTP1* hypermethylation has consistently proved its usefulness as a prostate cancer biomarker. Several independent studies provided convincing evidence that this epigenetic alteration constitutes a specific feature of most cancerous and pre-neoplastic prostate lesions. Moreover, the use of quantitative high-throughput techniques enables relatively easy and reproducible detection of *GSTP1* hypermethylation in routine clinical samples such as urine, blood, and prostate biopsy samples. Although limitations in sensitivity are recognized, the development of improved sampling and analytical techniques, as well as the addition of more target genes is likely to provide a valuable test for prostate cancer screening and management.

**Key Words:** Prostate cancer, Epigenetics, Hypermethylation, *GSTP1*, Biomarkers, Early detection.

From: *Current Clinical Urology: Prostate Cancer Screening*, Edited by: D. P. Ankerst et al.
DOI 10.1007/978-1-60327-281-0_19 © Humana Press, a part of Springer Science+Business Media, LLC 2009

# INTRODUCTION

Epigenetics refers to stable and heritable changes in gene expression patterns that do not involve modifications of the DNA sequence. In recent years, increased attention has been given to the role of epigenetic alterations in carcinogenesis as they seem to occur early in the process and provide an effective alternative mechanism to genetic alterations (e.g., mutations, deletions, LOH) in the development of cancer cells *(1–3)*. Among epigenetic alterations, aberrant methylation (often referred to as *hypermethylation*) of CpG-rich DNA sections (CpG islands), usually located at the regulatory regions of several cancer-related genes, has become an attractive target for research and development of new biomarkers for the most common types of human cancer *(4)*. Owing to the biological, pathological, and clinical peculiarities of prostate cancer, the hypermethylation model has been widely explored for the development of new strategies which might improve early detection, thus decreasing the morbidity and mortality rates associated with this highly prevalent malignancy. This chapter is devoted to *GSTP1* hypermethylation as a molecular tool for prostate cancer detection because it constitutes a paradigm of these research efforts and, in all probability, the most promising marker of its kind.

# BRIEF FUNCTIONAL AND STRUCTURAL CHARACTERIZATION OF THE *GSTP1* GENE

The *GSTP1* gene encodes for GST-π, an enzyme that belongs to the family of gluthathione-*S*-transferases, a class of enzymes involved in the conjugation of chemically reactive electrophiles with glutathione, thus abrogating their DNA damage ability and likely preventing the development of cancer *(5)*. Indeed, GST-π may be involved in the detoxification of heterocyclic amines which have been proposed as potential dietary prostate carcinogens *(6)*. It has been speculated that one of these compounds – 2-amino-1-methyl-6-phenylimidazo[4,5-*b*]pyridine (PhIP) – might be associated with the development of prostate cancer in humans owing to its genotoxic properties which induce prostate cancer in rats *(7)*. Thus, GST-π is likely to play an important role in preventing the development of prostate malignancy by means of genome protection. Eventually, this role would ascribe to *GSTP1* the status of tumor suppressor gene. Furthermore, because the induction of GST-π expression does not suppress cell growth in prostate cancer cell lines, a role of "caretaker gene" has been proposed *(8,9)*.

Although GST-π expression is frequently absent in prostate cancer, the region to which the *GSTP1* gene is mapped (11q13) is seldom lost or mutated in this neoplasm, a feature that raised the possibility that epigenetic mechanisms might be involved in gene silencing *(10)*. Indeed, this gene contains a typical CpG island spanning from −414 to +625, relative to the transcription start site *(11)*. In most normal tissues, including prostate, no methylation is found at CpG sites in the vicinity of the transcription start site (CpGs −43 to +30), although dense methylation is detected at CpG sites in the 5′-upstream region *(11)*. Remarkably, the boundary between these two regions is marked by a distinct (ATAAA)$_{19–24}$ repeat sequence, whereas the 3′-end of the CpG island shows heterogeneous CpG methylation, thus lacking a sharp transition *(11)*. However, in some prostate cancer cell lines and in most primary prostate carcinomas, there is dense methylation across the CpG island, including CpGs −43 to +30, and this feature is associated with loss of gene expression *(11,12)*. Hence, this region is critical for epigenetic regulation of *GSTP1* transcription and the term "*GSTP1* hypermethylation" refers specifically to methylation at those CpG dinucleotides.

There is ongoing debate about the process that initiates methylation and how it relates to gene silencing. Concerning the first question, some studies suggest that methylation progresses from the densely methylated regions flanking the promoter region *(13)* whereas others propose that methylation starts at "hypermethylation centers" located within the CpG island itself and progressively spreads across its extension *(14)*. Concerning gene silencing, there seems to be a close interaction between CpG methylation and chromatin remodeling *(15)*. In this model, the progressive methylation of CpG sites promotes methyl-binding domain 2 protein (MBD2) binding and recruits histone deacetylases and DNA methyltransferases, which result in histone deacetylation and additional DNA methylation *(15)*. After extensive methylation of the *GSTP1* CpG island, MeCP2 binding occurs and subsequent histone methyltransferase recruitment consolidates histone methylation in an inactive chromatin state *(15)*. Consequently, DNA methylation seems to constitute the "first layer" of epigenetic inactivation of the *GSTP1* gene, whereas histone modifications strengthen this mechanism through conformational changes in chromatin.

## METHODOLOGIES FOR DETECTION OF *GSTP1* PROMOTER METHYLATION

DNA methylation can be assessed using a variety of techniques (for detailed description see reference *(16)*, although most of them are expensive, cumbersome, insufficiently sensitive and/or specific to be used in the clinical setting. Most studies published to date about the role of *GSTP1* hypermethylation as a prostate cancer biomarker used assays based on the analysis of sodium bisulfite converted DNA *(17)*, mainly methylation-specific PCR (MSP) *(18)*. Because sodium bisulfite converts unmethylated cytosines to uracils, whereas methylated cytosines remain unchanged, it provides the conditions to discriminate methylated from unmethylated CpGs using appropriate sets of primers *(18)*. MSP is amenable to high-throughput analyses and seems ideal for the assessment of clinical samples because it is sensitive, relatively simple, and safe to perform and requires only minute amounts of DNA. However, there are two major limitations that might impair the use of MSP: the lack of quantitation of methylated sequences and DNA damage. The use of quantitative methodologies is a key feature for the analysis of clinical samples from prostate cancer suspects because non-cancerous cells might harbor low levels of methylation at several gene promoters, including *GSTP1 (19–22)*. The development of quantitative MSP-based assays, allowing the quantitation of methylated alleles amongst the total number of DNA copies in a given sample [e.g., MethyLight *(23)*] circumvents this problem. These methods, which might be collectively designated as quantitative MSP (QMSP), increase the specificity of the assay, are very sensitive and reliably detect one methylated allele in the presence of 10,000-fold excess of unmethylated alleles *(23)*. However, the use of a control to normalize the assay is required, i.e., an internal reference gene [e.g., *MYOD1* or *ACTB* (19,20)] or Alu sequences *(24)*. DNA damage induced by bisulfite conversion might impair the detection of methylated sequences if their quantity is very low in a given sample, thus reducing the sensitivity of the test. Moreover, as incompletely methylated target sequences will not be amplified, the actual methylation levels might be different than those determined by

QMSP. Recently, a new quantitative technique that does not require bisulfite conversion of template DNA has been developed (COMPARE-MS), which combines the use of methylation-sensitive restriction enzymes and methylated CpG binding domain proteins to assist capture and enrichment of methylated DNA *(25)*. Although it is claimed that this novel methodology does improve sensitivity and is less time-consuming than QMSP, it has been tested in only a limited number of samples and has not yet been validated by other research teams.

## PERFORMANCE OF *GSTP1* HYPERMETHYLATION IN PROSTATE CANCER SCREENING

*GSTP1* hypermethylation meets important requirements to be considered as a promising prostate cancer screening marker: (1) it is highly prevalent in primary prostate cancer, (2) it is detectable in most high-grade prostatic intraepithelial neoplasia, a putative prostate cancer precursor lesion, (3) it is seldom detected in benign lesions and morphologically normal prostate tissue, and (4) it is an uncommon alteration in other malignant tumors, with the exception of liver and breast cancers (although significantly less prevalent). Many studies have focused on the analysis of tissue samples in which *GSTP1* hypermethylation was successfully tested for the detection of prostate cancer, eventually providing a valuable ancillary tool for routine histopathological diagnosis *(19,20,26)*. However, if *GSTP1* hypermethylation testing is intended as a screening method, biopsy samples are not ideal candidates for this purpose. Because such a screening test must be non- or minimally invasive, efficient testing for *GSTP1* hypermethylation using body fluids, mainly urine and/or blood, is warranted. Ideally, the development of this test would be able to decrease the number of unnecessary prostate biopsies performed due to the limited specificity of the serum prostate-specific antigen (PSA) test, and might increase the detection of prostate cancer in individuals with below-threshold serum PSA, some of which carry aggressive forms of prostate adenocarcinoma *(27)*.

Several studies addressed the performance of *GSTP1* hypermethylation for detection of prostate cancer in body fluids *(28–34)* and their results are summarized in Table 1. It is immediately perceptible that the sensitivity of *GSTP1* hypermethylation is generally low, both in voided urine (18.8–38.9%) and serum/plasma (13.0–72.5%), although specificity is high (86.8–100%). It is noteworthy that the highest sensitivity values were obtained in studies that included a high proportion of patients with advanced disease, which is more likely to have circulating tumor cells *(28,29)*. These results are somewhat disappointing when compared with the power of *GSTP1* hypermethylation to detect even minute foci of prostate carcinoma in tissue samples *(26)*. However, it should be realized that all these studies limited their analyses to a single urine or blood sample. Because the amounts of DNA from neoplastic prostate cells shed in urine or circulating in the bloodstream are very low when the tumor is organ-confined, the increase in sampling volume would have a strong impact in the sensitivity of the test. This hypothesis is supported by the augmented rate of cancer detection when urine collection is performed after prostatic massage *(29,34)* or prostate biopsy *(32)* because these procedures increase the shedding of prostate cells in urine. It also remarkable that combined analysis of urine and plasma/serum increases the rate of prostate cancer detection, without compromising specificity, thus partially circumventing the limitations in the sensitivity of the test *(31)*. Moreover, further technical improvement of QMSP assays (e.g.,

Table 1
Performance of *GSTP1* Hypermethylation for Detection of Prostate Cancer
in Urine and Plasma/Serum

| Sample type, study (ref.) | Method | Sensitivity (%) | Specificity (%) | PPV (%) | NPV (%) |
|---|---|---|---|---|---|
| **Urine** | | | | | |
| Goessl et al. (2000) *(28)* | CMSP | 34.4 | 100 | 100 | 58.8 |
| Goessl et al. (2001) *(29)* | CMSP | 72.5 | 97.6 | 96.7 | 78.8 |
| Cairns et al. (2001) *(30)* | CMSP | 21.4 | ND | ND | ND |
| Jerónimo et al. (2002) *(31)* | CMSP | 30.4 | 96.8 | 95.5 | 34.1 |
| | QMSP | 18.8 | 96.8 | 92.9 | 34.9 |
| Gonzalgo et al. (2003) *(32)* | CMSP | 38.9 | ND | ND | ND |
| Hoque et al. (2005) *(33)* | QMSP | 48.1 | 100 | 100 | 77.1 |
| Rouprêt et al. (2007) *(34)* | QMSP | 83.2 | 86.8 | 94.0 | 67.3 |
| **Plasma/serum** | | | | | |
| Goessl et al. (2000) *(28)* | CMSP | 71.9 | 100 | 100 | 71.0 |
| Jerónimo et al. (2002) *(31)* | CMSP | 36.2 | 100 | 100 | 41.3 |
| | QMSP | 13.0 | 100 | 100 | 34.1 |

PPV, positive predictive value; NPV, negative predictive value; CMSP, conventional methylation-specific PCR; QMSP, quantitative methylation-specific PCR; ND, not determined.

reduction of DNA degradation and incremented efficiency of bisulfite conversion) might also contribute to increase the sensitivity of the *GSTP1* hypermethylation test, thus enabling its use as an efficient screening tool in body fluids. Finally, because there are reported differences in*GSTP1* promoter methylation prevalence among prostate cancer samples from African American, Caucasian, and Asian men *(35)* it should be realized that *GSTP1* hypermethylation testing might perform differently in distinct ethnic groups.

## FUTURE DIRECTIONS

### Beyond GSTP1 Hypermethylation: Multigene Methylation Analysis

The limited sensitivity of *GSTP1* hypermethylation as a prostate cancer marker is not only due to insufficient quantity of DNA from neoplastic cells available for analysis, but is also a consequence of the variable proportion of prostate cancer cases with low or null levels of methylation at the *GSTP1* promoter, which ranges from 5 to 20% in most studies *(36)*. To overcome this constraint methylation analysis of additional genes is warranted. Thus, several gene panels have been tested on independent prostate cancer series (summarized in Table 2) and were shown to increase prostate cancer detection rates both in tissue samples and body fluids *(33,34,37–41)*. Remarkably, multigene methylation analysis not only sustains high specificity and positive predictive value, but it also improves the negative predictive value of the test. These are very important findings because both sensitivity and negative predictive value are critical for assessing the accuracy of a screening test. However, the number of genes should be restricted and carefully selected because the simultaneous use of more than three or four markers is likely to compromise the specificity of the test, with only a marginal gain in sensitivity *(37)*.

## DNA Hypermethylation and the Identification of Clinically Relevant Prostate Cancer

An important question that arises from the potential use of molecular markers for prostate cancer detection is the identification of clinically relevant tumors. The main concern is that the development of more effective screening tests might increase the number of prostate carcinomas that would not influence survival, as reported for prostate carcinomas diagnosed due to PSA screening *(42)*. Although appropriately designed studies are needed to address this relevant issue, there are some indications that prostate cancers with high-methylation levels are more likely to be clinically aggressive and to influence the patient's lifespan because statistically significant associations between promoter methylation levels of several genes (including *GSTP1*) and clinicopathological parameters predictive of prognosis (e.g., Gleason score and pathological stage) have been reported *(39,43)*. Furthermore, a methylation score derived from the assessment of promoter methylation of a gene panel comprising *GSTP1*, *APC*, and *MDR1* was shown to discriminate organ-confined from locally advanced disease with 72.1% sensitivity and 67.8% specificity *(41)*. Interestingly, methylation analysis also seems to carry relevant prognostic information, as serum *GSTP1* hypermethylation was reported as the most relevant predictor of PSA recurrence in multivariate analysis in a series of patients with clinically localized prostate cancer treated with radical prostatectomy *(44)*. Taken together, these data strongly suggest that methylation-based markers might be able to stratify patients in different prognostic groups, adding relevant information to clinical and pathological parameters that influence the definition of current therapeutic strategies.

## Taking Hypermethylation from the Lab to the Clinics: Challenges and Caveats

Most, if not all, published reports on the role of *GSTP1* hypermethylation as a prostate cancer biomarker might be considered "discovery studies", corresponding to the definition of Phase 1 and Phase 2 biomarker studies *(45)*. Thus, before methylation tests are recommend for clinical use several steps need to be taken, constituting important challenges for researchers in the field. A critical matter is the definition of selection criteria to enroll prostate cancer suspects in large prospective, randomized, and controlled multi-institutional trials, which will also require the harmonization of sampling collection and storage. An additional key issue is the standardization of methodologies used to analyze methylation. It is this authors' opinion that quantitative assays will remain

## Table 2
### Diagnostic Information Provided by Hypermethylation Analysis of the Combination of *GSTP1* with Other *Loci*, in Tissue Samples and Urine

| Sample type, study (ref.) | Method | Sensitivity (%) | Specificity (%) | PPV (%) | NPV (%) |
|---|---|---|---|---|---|
| **Prostate tissue** | | | | | |
| Yegnasubramanian et al. (2004) (37) | QMSP | | | | |
| *GSTP1/MDR1* | | 97.3 | 100 | 100 | 92.6 |
| *GSTP1/MDR1/APC* | | 98.6 | 96.0 | 98.6 | 96.0 |
| *GSTP1/MDR1/APC/PTGS2* | | 100 | 92.0 | 97.3 | 100 |
| *GSTP1/MDR1/APC/PTGS2/RASSF1A* | | 100 | 92.0 | 97.3 | 100 |
| Tokumaru et al. (2004) (38) | QMSP | | | | |
| *GSTP1/TIG1* | | 88.5 | 100 | 100 | 61.1 |
| *GSTP1/APC* | | 85.2 | 100 | 100 | 55.0 |
| *GSTP1/RARB2* | | 90.2 | 100 | 100 | 64.7 |
| *GSTP1/TIG1/APC/RARB2* | | 96.7 | 100 | 100 | 93.8 |
| Jerónimo et al. (2004) (39) | QMSP | | | | |
| *GSTP1/APC* | | 98.3 | 100 | 100 | 93.8 |
| Bastian et al. (2005) (40) | QMSP | | | | |
| *GSTP1/PTGS2* | | 96.2 | 100 | 100 | 87.5 |
| *GSTP1/APC* | | 96.2 | 92.9 | 98.1 | 86.7 |
| *GSTP1/RASSF1A* | | 98.1 | 71.4 | 92.9 | 90.9 |
| *GSTP1/APC/PTGS2* | | 98.1 | 92.9 | 98.1 | 92.9 |
| Enokida et al. (2005) (41) | CMSP | | | | |
| *GSTP1/APC/MDR1* | | 75.9 | 84.1 | 92.1 | 58.6 |
| **Urine** | | | | | |
| Hoque et al. (2005) (33) | QMSP | | | | |
| *GSTP1/ARF/CDNK2A/MGMT* | | 86.5 | 100 | 100 | 92.9 |
| Rouprêt et al. (2007) (34) | QMSP | | | | |
| *GSTP1/APC/RASSF1A/RARB2* | | 86.3 | 89.5 | 95.3 | 72.3 |

PPV, positive predictive value; NPV, negative predictive value; CMSP, conventional methylation-specific PCR; QMSP, quantitative methylation-specific PCR.

the cornerstone of methylation analysis in this setting because there is no simple and straightforward match between "methylated" and "malignant" or between "unmethylated" and "benign".Indeed, as previously pointed out in Section "Brief Functional and Structural Characterization of the *GSTP1* Gene" of this chapter, promoter methylation is a dynamic process that occurs initially in a morphologically normal cell and progresses as the neoplastic phenotype develops. Hence, the definition of appropriate cutoff values is warranted to triage prostate cancer suspects for clinical surveillance or for further diagnostic procedures. It is expected that this definition of cutoff values will lead to accurate estimation of the proportion of prostate cancer patients with a negative hypermethylation test. Only then might hypermethylation testing be accurately compared with existing "screening" tests (e.g., serum PSA) or diagnostic procedures (e.g., histopathological assessment of prostate biopsies), thus proving the validity of *GSTP1* hypermethylation as a clinically useful prostate cancer biomarker.

## CONCLUSIONS

Existing data about *GSTP1* hypermethylation in prostate cancer demonstrate its potential as a specific cancer biomarker, supporting the development of quantitative methylation assays to increase the accuracy of prostate cancer detection and to stratify patients into different risk categories, allowing for improved patient management. In order to be useful for prostate cancer screening and/or diagnosis, these assays must be effective in blood and urine samples. However, appropriately designed studies, using standardized methods and enrolling significant numbers of prostate cancer suspects, are clearly needed to assess the clinical value of this novel molecular tool. Thus, a relatively long and fascinating journey remains ahead to demonstrate that *GSTP1* hypermethylation, eventually in combination with other genes, constitutes a valuable marker for prostate cancer screening and management.

**Acknowledgement** R.H. and C.J. are the recipients of a research grant from Liga Portuguesa Contra o Cancro – Núcleo Regional do Norte.

## REFERENCES

1. Jones P, Laird PW. Cancer epigenetics comes of age. Nat Genet 1999;21:163–167.
2. Esteller M, Herman JG. Cancer as an epigenetic disease: DNA methylation and chromatin alterations in human tumours. J Pathol 2002;196:1–7.
3. Herman JG, Baylin SB. Gene silencing in cancer in association with promoter hypermethylation. N Engl J Med 2003;349:2042–2054.
4. Jerónimo C, Henrique R, Sidransky D. Uses of DNA methylation in cancer diagnosis and risk assessment. In: Esteller M, ed. DNA methylation. Approaches, Methods and Applications. Boca Raton: CRC Press, 2004:11–26.
5. Coles B, Ketterer B. The role of glutathione and glutathione transferases in chemical carcinogenesis. Crit Rev Biochem Mol Biol 1990;25:47–70.
6. Nelson CP, Kidd LC, Sauvegeot J, Isaacs WB, De Marzo AM, Groopman JD, Nelson WG, Kensler TW. Protection against 2-hydroxyamino-1-methyl-6-phenylimidazo[4,5-b]pyridine cytotoxicity and DNA adduct formation in human prostate by glutathione S-transferase P1. Cancer Res 2001;61:103–109.
7. Stuart GR, Holcroft J, de Boer JG, Glickman BW. Prostate mutations in rats induced by the suspected human carcinogen 2-amino-1-methyl-6-phenylimidazo[4,5-b]pyridine. Cancer Res 2000;60:266–268.
8. Lin X, Asgari K, Putzi MJ, Gage WR, Yu X, Cornblatt BS, Kumar A, Piantadosi S, DeWeese TL, De Marzo AM, Nelson WG. Reversal of GSTP1 CpG island hypermethylation and reactivation of pi-class glutathione S-transferase (GSTP1) expression in human prostate cancer cells by treatment with procainamide. Cancer Res 2001;61:8611–8616.

9. Nelson WG, De Marzo AM, Deweese TL, Lin X, Brooks JD, Putzi MJ, Nelson CP, Groopman JD, Kensler TW. Preneoplastic prostate lesions: an opportunity for prostate cancer prevention. Ann N Y Acad Sci 2001;952:135–144.

10. Lee WH, Morton RA, Epstein JI, Brooks JD, Campbell PA, Bova GS, Hsieh WS, Isaacs WB, Nelson WG. Cytidine methylation of regulatory sequences near the pi-class glutathione S-transferase gene accompanies human prostatic carcinogenesis. Proc Natl Acad Sci USA 1994;91:11733–11737.

11. Millar DS, Paul CL, Molloy PL, Clark SJ. A distinct sequence (ATAAA)n separates methylated and unmethylated domains at the 5'-end of the GSTP1 CpG island. J Biol Chem 2000;275:24893–24899.

12. Lin X, Tascilar M, Lee WH, Vles WJ, Lee BH, Veeraswamy R, Asgari K, Freije D, van Rees B, Gage WR, Bova GS, Isaacs WB, Brooks JD, DeWeese TL, De Marzo AM, Nelson WG. GSTP1 CpG island hypermethylation is responsible for the absence of GSTP1 expression in human prostate cancer cells. Am J Pathol 2001;159:1815–1826.

13. Graff JR, Herman JG, Myohanen S, Baylin SB, Vertino PM. Mapping patterns of CpG island methylation in normal and neoplastic cells implicates both upstream and downstream regions in de novo methylation. J Biol Chem 1997;272:22322–22329.

14. Toth M, Lichtenberg U, Doerfler W. Genomic sequencing reveals a 5-methylcytosine-free domain in active promoters and the spreading of preimposed methylation patterns. Proc Natl Acad Sci USA 1989;86:3728–3732.

15. Stirzaker C, Song JZ, Davidson B, Clark SJ. Transcriptional gene silencing promotes DNA hypermethylation through a sequential change in chromatin modifications in cancer cells. Cancer Res 2004;64:3871–3877.

16. Fraga MF, Esteller M. DNA methylation: a profile of methods and applications. Biotechniques 2002;33:632–649.

17. Olek A, Oswald J, Walter J. A modified and improved method for bisulphite based cytosine methylation analysis. Nucleic Acids Res 1996;24:5064–5066.

18. Herman JG, Graff JR, Myohanen S, Nelkin BD, Baylin SB. Methylation-specific PCR: a novel PCR assay for methylation status of CpG islands. Proc Natl Acad Sci USA 1996;93: 9821–9826.

19. Jerónimo C, Usadel H, Henrique R, Oliveira J, Lopes C, Nelson WG, Sidransky D. Quantitation of GSTP1 methylation in non-neoplastic prostatic tissue and organ-confined prostate adenocarcinoma. J Natl Cancer Inst 2001;93:1747–1752.

20. Harden SV, Sanderson H, Goodman SN, Partin AA, Walsh PC, Epstein JI, Sidransky D. Quantitative GSTP1 methylation and the detection of prostate adenocarcinoma in sextant biopsies. J Natl Cancer Inst 2003;95:1634–1637.

21. Henrique R, Jerónimo C, Teixeira MR, Hoque MO, Carvalho AL, Pais I, Ribeiro FR, Oliveira J, Lopes C, Sidransky D. Epigenetic heterogeneity of high-grade prostatic intraepithelial neoplasia: clues for clonal progression in prostate carcinogenesis. Mol Cancer Res 2006;4:1–8.

22. Hanson JA, Gillespie JW, Grover A, Tangrea MA, Chuaqui RF, Emmert-Buck MR, Tangrea JA, Libutti SK, Linehan WM, Woodson KG. Gene promoter methylation in prostate tumor-associated stromal cells. J Natl Cancer Inst 2006;98:255–261.

23. Eads CA, Danenberg KD, Kawakami K, Saltz LB, Blake C, Shibata D, Danenberg PV, Laird PW. MethyLight: a high-throughput assay to measure DNA methylation. Nucleic Acids Res 2000;28:E32.

24. Weisenberger DJ, Campan M, Long TI, Kim M, Woods C, Fiala E, Ehrlich M, Laird PW. Analysis of repetitive element DNA methylation by MethyLight. Nucleic Acids Res 2005;33: 6823–6836.

25. Yegnasubramanian S, Lin X, Haffner MC, DeMarzo AM, Nelson WG. Combination of methylated-DNA precipitation and methylation-sensitive restriction enzymes (COMPARE-MS) for the rapid, sensitive and quantitative detection of DNA methylation. Nucleic Acids Res 2006;34:E19.

26. Harden SV, Guo Z, Epstein JI, Sidransky D. Quantitative GSTP1 methylation clearly distinguishes benign prostatic tissue and limited prostate adenocarcinoma. J Urol 2003;169:1138–1142.

27. Thompson IM, Goodman PJ, Tangen CM, Lucia MS, Miller GJ, Ford LG, Lieber MM, Cespedes RD, Atkins JN, Lippman SM, Carlin SM, Ryan A, Szczepanek CM, Crowley JJ, Coltman CA Jr. The influence of finasteride on the development of prostate cancer. N Engl J Med 2003;349: 215–224.

28. Goessl C, Krause H, Muller M, Heicappell R, Schrader M, Sachsinger J, Miller K. Fluorescent methylation-specific polymerase chain reaction for DNA-based detection of prostate cancer in bodily fluids. Cancer Res 2000;60:5941–5945.

29. Goessl C, Muller M, Heicappell R, Krause H, Straub B, Schrader M, Miller K. DNA-based detection of prostate cancer in urine after prostatic massage. Urology 2001;58:335–338.

30. Cairns P, Esteller M, Herman JG, Schoenberg M, Jerónimo C, Sanchez-Cespedes M, Chow NH, Grasso M, Wu L, Westra WB, Sidransky D. Molecular detection of prostate cancer in urine by GSTP1 hypermethylation. Clin Cancer Res 2001;7:2727–2730.

31. Jerónimo C, Usadel H, Henrique R, Silva C, Oliveira J, Lopes C, Sidransky D. Quantitative GSTP1 hypermethylation in bodily fluids of patients with prostate cancer. Urology 2002;60:1131–1135.

32. Gonzalgo ML, Pavlovich CP, Lee SM, Nelson WG. Prostate cancer detection by GSTP1 methylation analysis of postbiopsy urine specimens. Clin Cancer Res 2003;9:2673–2677.

33. Hoque MO, Topaloglu O, Begum S, Henrique R, Rosenbaum E, Van Criekinge W, Westra WH, Sidransky D. Quantitative methylation-specific polymerase chain reaction gene patterns in urine sediment distinguish prostate cancer patients from control subjects. J Clin Oncol 2005;23:6569–6575.

34. Rouprêt M, Hupertan V, Yates DR, Catto JW, Rehman I, Meuth M, Ricci S, Lacave R, Cancel-Tassin G, de la Taille A, Rozet F, Cathelineau X, Vallancien G, Hamdy FC, Cussenot O. Molecular detection of localized prostate cancer using quantitative methylation-specific PCR on urinary cells obtained following prostate massage. Clin Cancer Res 2007;13:1720–1725.

35. Enokida H, Shiina H, Urakami S, Igawa M, Ogishima T, Pookot D, Li LC, Tabatabai ZL, Kawahara M, Nakagawa M, Kane CJ, Carroll PR, Dahiya R. Ethnic group-related differences in CpG hypermethylation of the *GSTP1* gene promoter among African-American, Caucasian and Asian patients with prostate cancer. Int J Cancer 2005;116:174–181.

36. Henrique R, Jerónimo C. Molecular detection of prostate cancer: a role for GSTP1 hypermethylation. Eur Urol 2004;46:660–669.

37. Yegnasubramanian S, Kowalski J, Gonzalgo ML, Zahurak M, Piantadosi S, Walsh PC, Bova GS, DeMarzo AM, Isaacs WB, Nelson WG. Hypermethylation of CpG islands in primary and metastatic human prostate cancer. Cancer Res 2004;64:1975–1986.

38. Tokumaru Y, Harden SV, Sun DI, Yamashita K, Epstein JI, Sidransky D. Optimal use of a panel of methylation markers with *GSTP1* hypermethylation in the diagnosis of prostate adenocarcinoma. Clin Cancer Res 2004;10:5518–5522.

39. Jerónimo C, Henrique R, Hoque MO, Mambo E, Ribeiro FR, Varzim G, Oliveira J, Teixeira MR, Lopes C, Sidransky D. A quantitative methylation profile of prostate cancer. Clin Cancer Res 2004;10:8472–8478.

40. Bastian PJ, Ellinger J, Wellmann A, Wernert N, Heukamp LC, Muller SC, von Ruecker A. Diagnostic and prognostic information in prostate cancer with the help of a small set of hypermethylated gene loci. Clin Cancer Res 2005;11:4097–4106.

41. Enokida H, Shiina H, Urakami S, Igawa M, Ogishima T, Li LC, Kawahara M, Nakagawa M, Kane CJ, Carroll PR, Dahiya R. Multigene methylation analysis for detection and staging of prostate cancer. Clin Cancer Res 2005;11:6582–6588.

42. Etzioni R, Penson DF, Legler JM, di Tommaso D, Boer R, Gann PH, Feuer EJ. Overdiagnosis due to prostate-specific antigen screening: lessons from U.S. prostate cancer incidence trends. J Natl Cancer Inst 2002;94:981–990.

43. Jerónimo C, Henrique R, Hoque MO, Ribeiro FR, Oliveira J, Fonseca D, Teixeira MR, Lopes C, Sidransky D. Quantitative *RARβ2* hypermethylation: a promising prostate cancer marker. Clin Cancer Res 2004;10:4010–4014.

44. Bastian PJ, Palapattu GS, Lin X, Yegnasubramanian S, Mangold LA, Trock B, Eisenberger MA, Partin AW, Nelson WG. Preoperative serum DNA *GSTP1* CpG island hypermethylation and the risk of early prostate-specific antigen recurrence following radical prostatectomy. Clin Cancer Res 2005;11:4037–4043.

45. Pepe MS, Etzioni R, Feng Z, Potter JD, Thompson ML, Thornquist M, Winget M, Yasui Y. Phases of biomarker development for early detection of cancer. J Natl Cancer Inst 2002;93:1054–1061.

# 20 EPCA and EPCA-2 as Potential Biomarkers for Prostate Cancer Detection

*Eddy S. Leman and Robert H. Getzenberg*

CONTENTS

INTRODUCTION
THE NUCLEAR STRUCTURAL ELEMENTS (NUCLEAR MATRIX)
CONCLUDING REMARKS
REFERENCES

## SUMMARY

The detection of prostate cancer using a blood test has by many standards been extremely successful. Despite this remarkable success, there have been limitations attributed to the use of prostate-specific antigen (PSA) as a means for prostate cancer screening and detection. PSA is not specific for prostate cancer and as such is often found elevated in other conditions associated with the aging male such as benign prostatic hyperplasia (BPH) and prostatitis. The magnitude of this problem is large in that there are more than 25 million men who have had at least one negative biopsy due to an elevated PSA level. In many of these individuals it is uncertain whether cancer was missed upon the biopsy or actually not present. A more specific tool that could identify which individuals actually have prostate cancer and differentiate them from those without the disease would be of tremendous value.

Utilizing a focused proteomic approach, our laboratory has identified novel prostate cancer-associated biomarkers. One of the hallmarks of the cancer cell is alterations in the shape, size, and morphometry of the nucleus. Since nuclear changes are one of the key features the pathologist uses to identify cancer cells, our goal was to find something at the molecular level that would equal what the pathologist was seeing under the microscope. We therefore focused our effort on the nuclear structural elements termed the nuclear matrix. In doing so, we identified two prostate cancer biomarkers that are associated with the nuclear structure: Early Prostate Cancer Antigen (EPCA) and Early Prostate Cancer Antigen 2 (EPCA-2). These are distinct proteins with the only similarity being the technique that was used to identify them. While EPCA has been shown to be a potentially useful tissue-based marker for prostate cancer, EPCA-2 is a serum marker of the disease. In this chapter, we discuss the role of nuclear structural proteins as potential biomarkers of prostate cancer.

From: *Current Clinical Urology: Prostate Cancer Screening*, Edited by: D. P. Ankerst et al.
DOI 10.1007/978-1-60327-281-0_20 © Humana Press, a part of Springer Science+Business Media, LLC 2009

**Key Words:** Nuclear structural elements, Nuclear matrix, Prostate cancer, Biomarkers, EPCA, EPCA-2.

## INTRODUCTION

Current diagnostic tools for prostate cancer include the serum detection of prostate-specific antigen (PSA) and a digital rectal examination (DRE). Despite the widespread use of PSA, as well as increased awareness of prostate cancer, the mortality rate from prostate cancer remains high (second only to lung cancer), although it appears to be improving *(1)*. Nevertheless, the PSA assay alone has many shortcomings, and thus is not considered to be an ideal tumor marker. PSA is a normal prostatic protein that is not typically expressed at higher levels in cancer, but it is inappropriately released into the blood serum with the disease. PSA levels in the serum are also increased in men with benign conditions of the prostate, including benign prostatic hyperplasia (BPH) and prostatitis. In addition, abnormal serum PSA levels are detected in a number of individuals who may not have "clinically significant" prostate cancer, and therefore, may not require aggressive therapy. Finally, there are a number of men with prostate cancer who do not have elevated PSA levels. The limitations of the PSA assay, along with the clinical questions that remain in prostate cancer support the discovery of new tumor markers that will have clinical impact as well as provide opportunities for exploration of more efficacious treatment options.

Typically, diagnosis of cancer by a pathologist is indicated by architectural alterations to cells and/or tissues *(2)*. One of the cellular hallmarks of the transformed phenotype is an abnormal nuclear shape and the presence of abnormal nuclei. Neoplastic transformation of a cell results in comprehensive changes in the nuclear structure of the cells and their resulting morphology. These changes include increased nuclear size, deformed nuclear shape, presence of more prominent nucleoli, and larger clumps of heterochromatin, as well as alterations in the composition of nuclear matrix proteins (NMPs). Within the past decade, advances in proteomics have stimulated a search for new biomarkers with increased specificity. We used focused proteomics to profile the nuclear structural elements of prostate cancer cells and in so doing, have identified new biomarkers for the disease. Differences in the protein components of the nuclear structure (NMPs) have been demonstrated between cancer and normal rat prostates *(3)*, in a transgenic mouse model for prostate cancer *(4)*, as well as between BPH and prostate cancer *(5–7)*. Early Prostate Cancer Antigen (EPCA) and Early Prostate Cancer Antigen 2 (EPCA-2) are two unrelated prostate cancer biomarkers that were identified using this proteomics approach. In this section, the characteristics of nuclear structural elements (nuclear matrix), as well as the utilization of both EPCA and EPCA-2 as prostate cancer biomarkers will be highlighted.

## THE NUCLEAR STRUCTURAL ELEMENTS (NUCLEAR MATRIX)

The cell/tissue matrix system or the skeletal network in a tissue and/or cell is defined as an integrated three-dimensional skeletal network that organizes cellular structure and its functions from the peripheral network to the DNA *(8)*. These matrix systems are interactive and dynamic and consist of linkages and interactions of the nuclear matrix, the cytoskeleton, and the cell periphery, including the extracellular matrix. These interactive matrix systems organize and process spatial and temporal information to coordinate cell functions and gene expression *(8)*.

One of the characteristics of a transformed phenotype is the alteration in nuclear structure and architecture. As the dynamic scaffold of the nucleus, composition of the nuclear structure/architecture is different between normal and cancer cells. The differences in these nuclear structural elements between normal and cancer cells may play a role in the differences in gene expression during transformation. Since the nuclear structure/architecture plays a critical role in DNA organization, alterations in nuclear structure/architecture may result in altered DNA topology. Subsequently, this could lead to changes in interaction of various genes with the nuclear structure/architecture, which could play a role in modulating processes such as DNA replication, transcription, and RNA splicing. For example, the retinoblastoma (Rb) gene has been reported to associate with p84, a nuclear matrix protein *(9)*. The large T-antigen of the SV40 virus has been demonstrated to target the nuclear structure/architecture of cells that are infected or transformed by SV40 *(10)*.

There are several proposed rationales for utilizing the nuclear structural proteins as markers for prostate cancer. The first is utilization of the concept to focus on proteins believed to be crucial in the cancer process – the nuclear matrix proteins, which represent some of the fundamental changes that occur within a cancer cell. Secondly, because these are low abundance proteins in the nuclear matrix, representing less than 1% of the total protein composition of the cell and approximately 10% of the nuclear proteins, they would have minimal potential to be identified through some of the more general approaches and hence often be missed. Furthermore, the relatively insoluble nature of many of these proteins makes them difficult to separate through common approaches. By focusing on the nuclear matrix, we were able to eliminate some of the highly abundant and interfering proteins which often exist in resolving complex protein mixtures; for example, those of the blood and/or tissue. Although the exact mechanisms of how these nuclear structural proteins can be detected in blood are not yet known, we speculate that they are released into the blood by cellular breakdown or apoptosis and are quite stable once they get there *(11)*.

Differences in the proteins within the nuclear structural elements have been found between cancer and normal rat prostates *(3,7)*, as well as between human BPH and prostate cancer *(5,7,12)*. Using tumor cells derived from the Dunning rat prostatic adenocarcinoma, our laboratory identified a set of proteins in the Dunning sublines: G, H, AT2, AT6, and MLL *(3)*. Utilizing a proteomics approach for resolving these nuclear structural proteins, which involves high-resolution two-dimensional gel electrophoresis, two unique proteins (G-1 and G-2) were identified to be specific for the androgen-sensitive and non-metastatic G and H tumor sublines *(3)*. Two other nuclear structural proteins, AM-1 and AM-2, were found in the highly metastatic androgen insensitive lines AT2, AT6, and MLL *(3)*. In addition, three other proteins (D1–D3) were specific to all the Dunning tumors and were not found in the normal dorsal prostate *(3)*.

## *Early Prostate Cancer Antigen (EPCA)*

EPCA is a nuclear matrix protein that has been demonstrated to be expressed in prostate cancer tissues. Immunohistochemical analyses reveal that EPCA is expressed throughout the prostate and represents a "field effect" associated with prostate cancer

*(13,14)*. Using tissues from negative biopsies, subsequent biopsies, and prostatectomy specimens, Dhir et al. estimated sensitivity of the EPCA immunohistochemical analysis at 84% with a specificity of 85% *(13)*. The expression of EPCA in the "negative biopsies" of men can help reveal if prostate cancer is located within the prostate. Furthermore, EPCA could serve as an adjunct to the current diagnostic approach for patients undergoing prostate needle biopsies, with the potential of identifying men with prostate cancer as much as 5 or more years earlier than the current diagnostic approach. The EPCA immunohistochemical analysis was further validated by Uetsuki et al. *(14)*. In this study, EPCA staining was positive in 94% of prostate cancer tissues and negative in the prostates of men with bladder cancer. There was no correlation of EPCA staining intensity with Gleason score or stage *(14)*. EPCA staining was positive in 86% of noncancerous tissues adjacent to major cancer foci *(14)*. These studies suggest that EPCA may reflect alterations in the nuclear structure that occur in earlier stages of prostate cancer.

EPCA was also measured in the plasma of 46 individuals, including prostate cancer, normal-healthy, prostatitis, spinal cord injury victims, as well as those with other types of cancer *(15)*. With a predetermined cut-off of 1.7 absorbance level at 450 nm, only the prostate cancer patients showed plasma EPCA levels above the 1.7 cut-off *(15)*. Overall, EPCA was demonstrated as a plasma-based marker for prostate cancer with sensitivity and specificity of 92 and 94%, respectively *(15)*. Although larger trials are still required to validate this study, the plasma-based ELISA assays for EPCA show great potential of this marker as a highly specific blood-based marker for detection of prostate cancer. This marker, though, has not been shown to be as robust of a blood-based marker as described below for EPCA-2.

### *Early Prostate Cancer Antigen-2 (EPCA-2)*

Although unrelated to EPCA with the exception of its name and the technique used to identify it, EPCA-2 is a more recently studied marker associated with prostate cancer. Unlike EPCA, EPCA-2 is not associated with a "field effect" and appears only in the prostate cancer tissue. We are currently studying EPCA-2 for its potential to serve as a highly specific and sensitive serum-based marker for prostate cancer. Utilizing antibodies raised against EPCA-2, our laboratory developed ELISA assays which detect the biomarker in the blood and demonstrate its ability to specifically identify prostate cancer patients versus men who are considered normal under several different categories *(16)*. In a study of more than 300 men, antibodies against EPCA-2 were used to evaluate the sera of a number of groups, including normal men, men with BPH, or prostate cancer, as well as other benign diseases and cancer. Included were groups of men who had normal PSA levels and no reason for further follow up. Another group of men had elevated PSA levels, but repeated negative biopsies indicating that they did not have prostate cancer. We also looked at a set of men with BPH who had not undergone prostate biopsies and men with prostatitis. Finally, we wanted to examine a large number of other types of conditions to determine whether EPCA-2 was indeed found principally in prostate cancer versus other cancer types or disease states. EPCA-2 at a pre-determined cut-off of 30 ng/ml is highly specific for prostate cancer. In our study, the specificity was 97% *(16)*. With this high specificity, EPCA-2 detected 94% of the prostate cancers *(16)*.

In order to address one of the important clinical questions described above, we determined that serum EPCA-2 levels differentiated between the prostate cancers that at the time of surgery were contained within the prostate from the cancers that had escaped the prostate at surgery. Based on an ROC (Receiver Operator Characteristic) analysis, the area under the curve of 0.89 indicated that EPCA-2 is highly accurate at differentiating between organ-confined and non-organ-confined prostate cancer *(16)*. Taken together, our current findings demonstrate that EPCA-2, a prostate cancer-associated nuclear protein, can be utilized as a potential serum-based biomarker for prostate cancer. We have recently demonstrated that EPCA-2 can detect prostate cancer even in men with "normal" PSA levels *(17)*. In addition, men with prostatitis do not give false positive findings *(17)*. We have also been successful at lowering the background of the assay which has tightened the values of those without prostate cancer close to zero *(17)*. Further validations using larger sample sizes in multi-center studies are clearly warranted, but it appears that EPCA-2 may indeed serve as a desperately needed highly specific marker of prostate cancer.

## CONCLUDING REMARKS

Since its introduction in the 1980s, PSA has been used for prostate cancer detection. In 1990, a cut-off point of 4.0 ng/ml was established for PSA *(18)*. However, the use of this cut-point has been questioned. Serum PSA measurement along with digital rectal examination (DRE) continue to be the most recommended and performed tests by physicians for prostate cancer detection. The cut-off value for PSA has been lowered from 4.0 to 2.5 ng/ml in many major health care practices. PSA has also changed the countenance of prostate cancer. Today, at the time of presentation few men have metastatic disease. This "stage migration" has been a major advance. The principal limitation of PSA is its lack of specificity for prostate cancer. This has led to a large number of unnecessary biopsies and confusion as to who should be treated.

The use of proteomics to develop more specific biomarkers to detect prostate cancer has permitted us to focus on the molecular correlates of what the pathologist sees. Through this search, we were able to identify both EPCA and EPCA-2. EPCA has been demonstrated in tissue studies to be highly specific in separating men with prostate cancer from those without and EPCA-2 has been shown to have high sensitivity and specificity as a blood-based marker in detecting men with prostate cancer. It is important to note that at this point, studies of EPCA-2 are proof of principle that these markers appear to be highly specific for prostate cancer and may differentiate between organ-confined and non-organ-confined disease. Studies have examined the performance of EPCA-2 in relevant patient populations but the sensitivity and specificity values obtained are not necessarily reflective of a screening population. Therefore, larger studies from multi-center institutions are clearly required. If the results from these further validation studies support our initial findings, both EPCA and EPCA-2 will have a major impact on men as they age in helping to identify specifically who has prostate cancer, and perhaps, which have a more aggressive form of the disease.

**Acknowledgements**  This work is generously supported by the Patana Fund through a grant from the Prostate Cancer Research Foundation.

# REFERENCES

1. Jemal A, Siegel R, Ward E, Murray T, Xu J, Thun MJ. Cancer statistics, 2007. CA Cancer J Clin 2007;57(1):43–66.
2. Nickerson JA. Nuclear dreams: the malignant alteration of nuclear architecture. J Cell Biochem 1998;70(2):172–80.
3. Getzenberg RH, Pienta KJ, Huang EY, Coffey DS. Identification of nuclear matrix proteins in the cancer and normal rat prostate. Cancer Res 1991;51(24):6514–20.
4. Leman ES, Arlotti JA, Dhir R, Greenberg N, Getzenberg RH. Characterization of the nuclear matrix proteins in a transgenic mouse model for prostate cancer. J Cell Biochem 2002;86(2):203–12.
5. Lakshmanan Y, Subong EN, Partin AW. Differential nuclear matrix protein expression in prostate cancers: correlation with pathologic stage. J Urol 1998;159(4):1354–8.
6. Partin AW, Getzenberg RH, CarMichael MJ, et al. Nuclear matrix protein patterns in human benign prostatic hyperplasia and prostate cancer. Cancer Res 1993;53(4):744–6.
7. Pienta KJ, Lehr JE. A common set of nuclear matrix proteins in prostate cancer cells. Prostate 1993;23(1):61–7.
8. Getzenberg RH. Nuclear matrix and the regulation of gene expression: tissue specificity. J Cell Biochem 1994;55(1):22–31.
9. Durfee T, Mancini MA, Jones D, Elledge SJ, Lee WH. The amino-terminal region of the retinoblastoma gene product binds a novel nuclear matrix protein that co-localizes to centers for RNA processing. J Cell Biol 1994;127(3):609–22.
10. Staufenbiel M, Deppert W. Different structural systems of the nucleus are targets for SV40 large T antigen. Cell 1983;33(1):173–81.
11. Miller TE, Beausang LA, Winchell LF, Lidgard GP. Detection of nuclear matrix proteins in serum from cancer patients. Cancer Res 1992;52(2):422–7.
12. Partin AW, Yoo J, Carter HB, et al. The use of prostate specific antigen, clinical stage and Gleason score to predict pathological stage in men with localized prostate cancer. J Urol 1993;150(1):110–4.
13. Dhir R, Vietmeier B, Arlotti J, et al. Early identification of individuals with prostate cancer in negative biopsies. J Urol 2004;171(4):1419–23.
14. Uetsuki H, Tsunemori H, Taoka R, Haba R, Ishikawa M, Kakehi Y. Expression of a novel biomarker, EPCA, in adenocarcinomas and precancerous lesions in the prostate. J Urol 2005;174(2):514–8.
15. Paul B, Dhir R, Landsittel D, Hitchens MR, Getzenberg RH. Detection of prostate cancer with a blood-based assay for early prostate cancer antigen. Cancer Res 2005;65(10):4097–100.
16. Leman ES, Cannon GW, Trock BJ, et al. EPCA-2: a highly specific serum marker for prostate cancer. Urology 2007;69(4):714–20.
17. Leman ES, Cannon GW, Trock BJ, et al. Further analysis of serum based EPCA-2 as a specific prostate cancer associated biomarker. In: The American Urological Association May 19–24, 2007, Anaheim, CA.
18. Cooner WH, Mosley BR, Rutherford CL, Jr., et al. Prostate cancer detection in a clinical urological practice by ultrasonography, digital rectal examination and prostate specific antigen. J Urol 1990;143(6):1146–52; discussion 52–4.

# V DESIGN AND METHODOLOGIC CONSIDERATIONS IN BIOMARKER STUDIES

# 21 Toward a Robust System for Biomarker Triage and Validation – EDRN Experience

*Ziding Feng, Jacob Kagan and Sudhir Srivastava*

## Contents

## Summary

The Early Detection Research Network (EDRN) has the mission to identify and validate biomarkers for clinical use. The Genitourinary Collaborative Group within EDRN has developed a robust triage and validation system that serves both "facilitator" and "brake" roles. The system consists of the establishment of a reference set of specimens collected under Prospective-specimen-collection-Retrospective-Blinded-Evaluation (PRoBE) design criteria, use of this reference set to pre-validate candidate biomarkers before committing a full-scale validation study, and expansion of this reference set for a full-scale validation study for future biomarkers. This reference set could also be expanded for biomarker discovery purposes.

**Key Words:** Reference set, Biomarkers, Validation, Pre-validation, Early diagnosis, Prognosis.

The Early Detection Research Network (EDRN) is a research consortium established in 1999 with the mission to translate biomarkers to clinics for cancer risk prediction, diagnosis, early detection, and prognosis. The main motivation for establishing such a consortium is based on the fact that although thousands of cancer biomarkers have been published in the literature, few have been used in clinics. With the tremendous advances

From: *Current Clinical Urology: Prostate Cancer Screening*, Edited by: D. P. Ankerst et al.
DOI 10.1007/978-1-60327-281-0_21 © Humana Press, a part of Springer Science+Business Media, LLC 2009

in genomics and proteomics, one hopes that many of these will lead to improvement in the early diagnosis of cancer and reduce cancer burden in the US population.

Over the 9-year period since its inception, EDRN investigators have learnt a great deal about the process of validating biomarkers for clinical utility. Translational research requires a broad spectrum of research interests and activities to be coordinated, including molecular biology research, epidemiologic and population research, and clinical care of patients. The research methodology differs between disciplines but our goal should be focusing on establishing a robust system for biomarker triage and validation so that good biomarkers will be chosen and be validated. Describing the process of establishing such a system will serve as an example of how to validate biomarkers for clinical application.

## SELDI VALIDATION STUDY EXPERIENCE

During 2000–2002, there were many reports on protein profiling using surface-enhanced laser desorption/ionization (SELDI) for cancer diagnosis, many of which strongly indicated potential clinical utility (1–3). Therefore, the EDRN decided to validate SELDI protein profiling for prostate cancer diagnosis. Because the technology is unconventional in that it does not identify informative proteins but relies on protein mass spectrum pattern to distinguish cancer patients from controls, investigators designed a three-stage validation process (4). The first stage required demonstration that SELDI protein profiles are reproducible across different labs, when applied to the same serum pool. After many standardization efforts, this stage was successfully completed (5), demonstrating that the profiles are indeed reproducible. The second stage required validation of the profile on high-quality specimens from a well-designed multi-center study. Results were negative (6), the study could not reproduce informative peaks or even identify new informative peaks that distinguish prostate cancer patients from patients with negative biopsies for prostate cancer. The third stage, which would have been based on Prostate Cancer Prevention Trial (PCPT) sera, was then not pursued.

The first two stages of the SELDI validation taught investigators several important lessons. The first was identification of an important source of bias that could have explained the early "promising" results, a difference in serum storage lengths and conditions between prostate cancer cases and non-prostate cancer controls (7). Figure 1 and Color Plate 8, generated from discovery data from which outstanding performance was observed (3), indicates that protein peak intensities were negatively associated with storage length (7). It is unfortunate that sera for cancer patients tend to be collected over many years and used multiple times while sera for controls tend to be collected recently and have smaller number of freeze thaws. In the stage-2 validation study cases and controls were well-balanced in storage length and number of freeze thaws (no more than one freeze thaw), as well as other clinical and epidemiologic factors (age and race). Although the source of bias was identified before the launching of the stage-2 validation study, high-quality specimens were not readily available to do an intermediate step validation before committing to stage 2. For the stage-2 validation study (6), it took long time to obtain the required number of specimens satisfying the tight inclusion and exclusion criteria from the existing repositories. These observations pointed to the crucial importance of the availability of high-quality specimens.

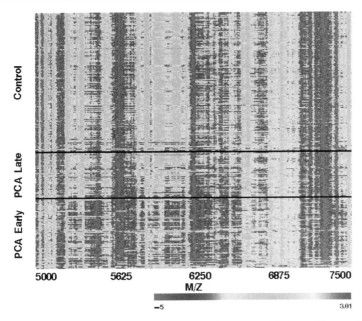

**Fig. 1.** Heat map ordered by blood draw date. "PCA Late" group and "Control" group had blood draw 1995–2001. "PCA Early" group had blood draw date prior to 1995. (*see* Color Plate 8)

## ESTABLISHING A PROSTATE CANCER REFERENCE SET

At 2004 EDRN meeting in Houston, after lengthy discussion, the GU Collaborative Group decided to establish a prostate cancer reference set that could address all issues identified in the SELDI validation study. The first decision was that the reference set should be designed with a clear clinical application in mind and that specimens be collected from the clinical target population without potential bias. Three clinical application settings were identified. The first was to develop a test to help men make the initial biopsy decision, addressing the question whether under current clinical guidelines, the number of unnecessary biopsies would be reduced for the population of men undergoing their first biopsy. The second setting was to help men to make a biopsy decision if the initial biopsy is negative. The third was to aid men in making treatment decisions after a positive biopsy for prostate cancer. While the third need is probably the most important in the clinical care of prostate cancer, it requires long-term follow up to collect mortality data. The GU Group decided to initially focus on the first biopsy population. PSA would not be a good marker in this population as these men most likely decided to have a biopsy due to elevated PSA. This comprehensive clinical application presents a realistic and practical problem with population and individual impact.

One major advantage of the study design is that serum samples could be collected prior to biopsy with outcomes available shortly thereafter. This feature eliminates common sources of biases in case–control designs where specimens are collected after the disease status is known.

The second decision was that the reference set be used for triaging biomarkers. Investigators would be invited, within or outside of the EDRN, to submit their biomarkers to be evaluated in blinded fashion on the reference set, a pre-validation step. Note that if such a reference set had been available, the full-scale SELDI validation study could have been avoided. If no large discrepancy is observed between the performance on the initial discovery at the local lab and the performance in the reference set, a full-scale validation study would be committed to validate this marker.

The third decision was that although the pre-validation reference set sample size is 120 (60 men with positive biopsy, 60 men with negative biopsy), recruitment would continue to allow a validation study to be completed timely if some markers merit such validation. The unbiased selection of cases and controls, the sera collection, and the fact that the same type of specimens are used for pre-validation and validation studies ensure the high probability that performance on the marker observed on the pre-validation set will hold up in the full-scale validation study and the biomarker, if validated, will have clinical utility.

## USE OF THE REFERENCE SET TO TRIAGE BIOMARKERS FOR VALIDATION

The pre-validation set was quickly established by specimens contributed from three EDRN Clinical, Epidemiologic, and Validation Centers (CEVC). Biomarker discovery labs were invited to give a presentation of their markers, the group ranked them and voted for access to the pre-validation set. Markers from four labs were approved and aliquots were sent to each of them in a blinded fashion. The markers approved for

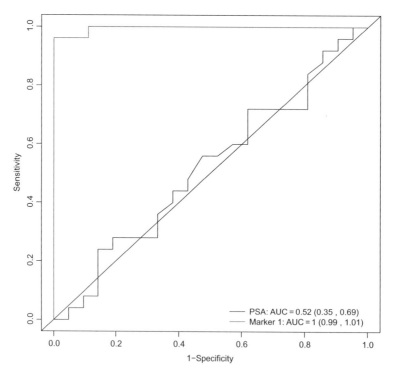

**Fig. 2.** ROC curves and 95% confidence intervals for Marker 1 and PSA on discovery data (highly promising). The low AUC value for PSA is due to the fact that biopsy is often triggered by elevated PSA. (*see* Color Plate 9)

pre-validation included hk2, hk4, hk11, TSP-1, %[−2]proPSA, and EPCA2. Assay results were sent back to the EDRN Data Management and Coordinating Center (DMCC) for summary and comparisons.

Two "highly promising and novel biomarkers" at discovery phase had drastically lower performance on this pre-validation reference set as indicated in Figs. 2, 3, 4 and Color Plates 9, 10, 11 . A further investigation with the biomarker discovery investigator and specimen provider revealed that for one of them, the specimen storage length was again a possible reason for the discrepancy. In the reference set, the storage length was well-balanced. In the specimens used for discovery, it was confounded that with prostate cancer status, sera from cancer patients had much longer storage time than serum from negative biopsy controls. Note that in a case–control study design, there could be many sources of biases and it is impossible to identify all of them. Therefore, the pre-validation reference set served an important "brake" role, sparing investigators false leads.

Widespread PSA screening complicates biomarker evaluation for prostate cancer risk prediction or diagnosis because biopsy work up is usually triggered by elevated PSA. The above three clinical applications were proposed for practical reasons given the reality of PSA screening. If PSA screening patterns or criteria for post-PSA work up changed, the target population for intended application might also change. The validation results then might not generalize. On the other hand, constructing a reference set for general population screening would require negative biopsy confirmation

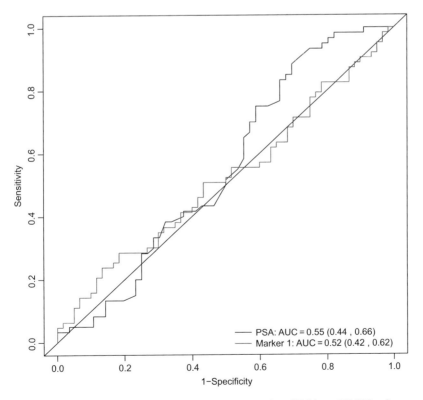

**Fig. 3.** ROC curves and 95% confidence intervals for Marker 1 and PSA on EDRN reference set data (not promising). (*see* Color Plate 10)

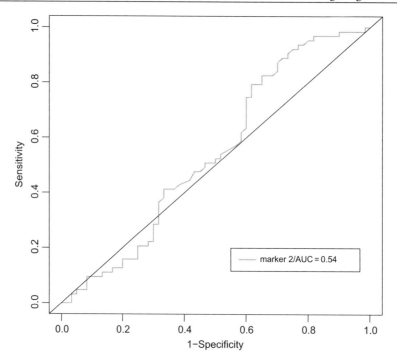

**Fig. 4.** ROC curve of Marker 2 on EDRN reference set (not promising), performance drastically decreased on EDRN reference set. On discovery data both sensitivity and specificity were above 90%. (*see* Color Plate 11)

for men who by current practice would not undergo biopsy. This is only feasible in some large prostate cancer prevention trials that require biopsy for all participants regardless of their PSA values, such as Prostate Cancer Prevention Trial (PCPT). Teaming up with such large cohorts will allow EDRN to address that question. Another difficulty in designing a reference set for general population screening of prostate cancer is the high prevalence of indolent prostate cancers. It seems more efficient to first address the third clinical application proposed above and learn more about aggressive prostate cancer before designing a general population screening biomarker study. Focusing on the clinical applications that are more feasible and more likely to get fruitful results is an important lesson learned in EDRN – "go for lower-hanging fruits".

## DESIGN OF A FULL-SCALE VALIDATION STUDY – PROBE DESIGN

One biomarker, %[−2]proPSA, indicated consistent performance (Fig. 5 and Color Plate 12) on the reference set with that at the initial discovery phase *(8)*. A protocol was therefore developed, reviewed, and approved for a validation study. Sera were collected from about 680 men who underwent biopsy for prostate cancer diagnosis after the activation of the reference set protocol and met the inclusion criteria from four recruitment centers. Study sera were sent to Johns Hopkins University EDRN Biomarker Reference Lab (BRL) to perform the %[−2]proPSA assay. Disease status of the specimens was blinded to the assay lab and the sequence of subject aliquots was randomized so no bias

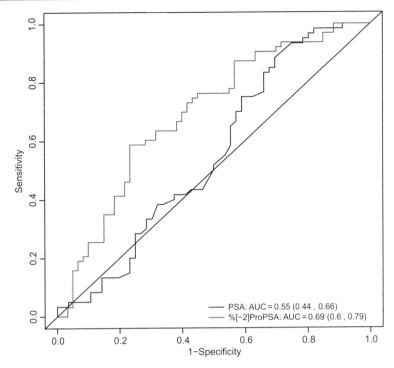

**Fig. 5.** ROC curves and 95% confidence intervals for %[−2]proPSA and PSA: Confirmed moderate performance for %[−2]proPSA consistent to that observed in initial discovery studies. (*see* Color Plate 12)

could be introduced during the assay process. The ROC curve of the test was moderate with an AUC = 0.69. However, the test might have clinical utility in better stratifying the risk for men who are biopsy candidates under current clinical practice, particular for men with PSA 2–10 ng/mL as a further stratified analyses for men with PSA 2–10 ng/mL indicated even better performance (AUC = 0.73), consistent to the discovery study report *(9)*.

One important aspect of this study design is that the protocol development of this validation study was after the recruitment of most of the study participants. This differs from the designs we often see in randomized clinical trials in which the recruitment always starts after the protocol activation. However, this Prospective-specimen-collection-Retrospective-Blinded-Evaluation (PRoBE) study *(10)* design makes no compromise to study rigor and is very efficient. This is because of the prospective specimen collection, i.e., specimens collected from a clinically well-defined cohort in the absence of knowledge about patient outcome. The lengthy specimen collection starts earlier and could be used for validation studies for future biomarkers with the same clinical application potential. The industrial partner who owns the license of %[−2]proPSA had Food and Drug Administration (FDA) approval on including a subset of the data from this study (mainly due to the restriction on the range of PSA) in their pivotal FDA register trial. We believe that this PRoBE design is very attractive for diagnostic test validation trial due to its efficiency, rigor, and ethic consideration (test results at the time of recruitment will have implication on the clinical management of the patients while analyzing retrospective repository does not have such implication). Pepe et al. *(10)* provide extensive discussion on the PRoBE design.

## FUTURE DIRECTIONS

In recent years promising urine-based biomarkers for prostate diagnosis have emerged *(11,12)*. The EDRN GU group is developing a protocol to validate PCA3. Although PCA3 is assayed using urine, serum will also be collected from the patients participating in the study so that both urine- and serum-based markers can be compared on the same set of patients and their complementary properties assessed. The idea is again that in addition to the task of validating a promising marker, the design considers the possibility of validating other markers for the same clinical application. The study design includes both the initial and repeat biopsy population. The latter will address the second clinical application proposed at the 2004 Houston meeting.

To partly address the third clinical application, EDRN is teaming up with Canary Foundation to conduct a Prostate Cancer Active Surveillance Study (PASS). PASS is a multi-center prospective cohort study that recruits prostate cancer patients who fit radical prostatectomy (RP) criteria but elect to adopt active surveillance instead of RP at the baseline. Patients will be followed, with blood and biopsy tissues collected longitudinally. The outcome is prostate cancer progression. The main objective of the study is to validate promising existing or future markers for prostate cancer progression. This cohort does not fully address the third question because men who elected active surveillance comprise a small portion of the men who had a positive biopsy and need guidance on treatment options. An obvious and useful expansion is to include all men who meet RP criteria, regardless of their treatment at baseline. That will form a well-defined target population for which a test could be applied in order to help patients and their doctors make treatment decisions. Note the difference in the target populations. The PASS design focuses on men who already elected to do active surveillance; therefore markers validated do not necessarily provide a test for all men who meet RP criteria and need to make a treatment decision. Though resource does not permit such an expansion, a retrospective Tissue Microarray (TMA) study using archived tissue blocks from RP was initiated to examine tissue-based biomarkers predicting prostate recurrence for this group of patients.

Discussion is underway on expanding the reference set for biomarker discovery. One striking observation in our reference set experience is the drastic decrease in performance of several biomarkers that showed the most promising results at the discovery phase. As we have observed, bias from specimens used in discovery studies is difficult to disentangle if the specimen collection does not meet PRoBE design criteria. Although it is important that the EDRN has reference sets to pre-validate these markers and eliminate false leads, it is more efficient if biomarkers that were moved out of the discovery phase have a higher chance to retain their performance. Using high-quality specimens at the discovery phase from the target population for intended clinical application will increase the chance of more biomarkers moving into the validation pipeline, increasing the chance of a successful validation.

Reference sets have their own limitations and using them for both discovery and validation will limit the general applicability of the findings. For the EDRN prostate cancer reference set, the prevalence of positive biopsy is above 40%, probably higher than that in the general population of men who currently undergo biopsy for prostate cancer diagnosis at their local clinics. For rare cancers such as ovarian cancer, or cancers such as pancreatic cancer for which the knowledge of risk factors is inadequate to identify a high-risk group to enrich the prevalence of cancer, prospective collection would not be feasible at the discovery stage or even at a non-pivotal validation trial stage. However, with that limitation acknowledged, the specimens from a carefully designed reference set, collected multi-center per protocol, will most likely have better quality than specimens used in most discovery labs. The blinding and randomization can be reliably implemented centrally whereas in many published biomarker discovery papers, one cannot tell how it had been done.

There should be a policy for access to these high-quality specimens for biomarker discovery. The policy could be similar to that for access to pre-validation sets except that for the discovery purpose, one does not need the preliminary data to have performance indicating a potential clinical application. However, the policy should have elements including a strong rationale for the approach, strong study design, evidence of a robust assay, and agreement that samples are blinded when performing assay, unblinded only after sending assay results to the central data repository, and archived by the EDRN for building a maker panel, and for dissemination after a certain period of time.

# REFERENCES

1. Petricoin, E. F., Ardekani, A. M., , Hitt, B. A., Levine, P. J., Fusaro, V. A., Steinberg, S. M., Mills, G. B., Simone, C., Fishman, D. A., Kohn, E. C., and Liotta, L. A.. (2002) Use of proteomic patterns in serum to identify ovarian cancer. *Lancet* **359**, 572–7.
2. Petricoin, E. F. 3rd, Ornstein, D. K., Paweletz, C. P., Ardekani, A., Hackett, P. S., Hitt, B. A., Velassco, A., Trucco, C., Wiegand, L., Wood, K., Simone, C. B., Levine, P. J., Linehan, W. M., Emmert-Buck, M. R., Steinberg, S. M., Kohn, E. C., and Liotta, L. A.(2002) Serum proteomic patterns for detection of prostate cancer. *J Natl Cancer Inst* **94**, 1576–8.
3. Adam, B. L., Qu, Y., Davis, J. W., Ward, M. D., Clements, M. A., Cazares, L. H., Semmes, O. J., Schellhammer, P. F., Yasui, Y., Feng, Z., and Wright, G. L. Jr. (2002) Serum protein fingerprinting coupled with a pattern-matching algorithm distinguishes prostate cancer from benign prostate hyperplasia and healthy men. *Cancer Res* **62**, 3609–14.
4. Grizzle, W. E., Adam, B. L., Bigbee, W. L., Conrads, T. P., Carroll, C., Feng, Z., Izbicka, E., Jendoubi, M., Johnsey, D., Kagan, J., Leach, R. J., McCarthy, D. B., Semmes, O. J., Srivastava, S., Srivastava, S., Thompson, I. M., Thornquist, M. D., Verma, M., Zhang, Z., and Zou, Z. (2003) Serum protein expression profiling for cancer detection: validation of a SELDI-based approach for prostate cancer. *Dis Markers* **19**, 185–95.
5. Semmes, O. J., Feng, Z., Adam, B.-L., Banez, L. L., Bigbee, W. L., Campos, D., Cazares, L. H., Chan, D. W., Grizzle, W. E., Izbicka, E., Kagan, J., Malik, G., McLerran, D., Moul, J. W., Partin, A., Prasanna, P., Rosenzweig, J., Sokoll, L. J., Srivastava, S., Srivastava, S., Thompson, I., Welsh, M. J., White, N., Winget, M., Yasui, Y., Zhang, A., and Zhu, L. (2005) Evaluation of serum protein profiling by surface-enhanced laser desorption/ionization time-of-flight mass spectrometry for the detection of prostate cancer: I. Assessment of platform reproducibility. *Clin Chem* **51**, 102–12.
6. McLerran, D., Grizzle, W. E., Feng, Z., Thompson, I. M., Bigbee, W. L., Cazares, L. H., Chan, D. W., Dahlgren, J., Diaz, J., Kagan, J., Lin, D. W., Malik, G., Oelschlager, D., Partin, A., Randolph, T. W., Sokoll, L. Srivastava, S., Srivastava, S., Thornquist, M., Troyer, D., Wright, G. L., Zhang, Z., Zhu, L., and Semmes, O. J. (2008) SELDI-TOF MS whole serum proteomic profiling with IMAC surface does not reliably detect prostate cancer. *Clin Chem* **54**, 53–60.
7. McLerran, D., Grizzle, W. E., Feng, Z., Bigbee, W. L., Banez, L. L., Cazares, L. H., Chan, D. W., Diaz, J., Izbicka, E., Kagan, J., Malehorn, D. E., Malik, G., Oelschlager, D., Partin, A., Randolph, T., Rosenzweig, N., Srivastava, S., Srivastava, S., Thompson, I. M., Thornquist, M., Troyer, D., Yasui, Y., Zhang, Z., Zhu, L., and Semmes, O. J. (2008). Analytical validation of serum proteomic profiling for diagnosis of prostate cancer: sources of sample bias. *Clin Chem* **54**, 44–52.
8. Sokoll, L. J., Wang, Y., Feng, Z., Kagan, J., Partin, A. W., Sanda, M. G., Thompson, I. M., and Chan, D. W. (2008) [-2]Proenzyme Prostate Specific Antigen for Prostate Cancer Detection: A National Cancer Institute Early Detection Research Network Validation Study. *J Urology* **180**, 539–43.

9. Catalona, W. J., Bartsch, G., Rittenhouse, H. G., Evans, C. L., Linton, H. J., Amirkhan, A., Horninger, W., Klocker, H., and Mikolajczyk, S. D. (2003) Serum pro prostate specific antigen improves cancer detection compared to free and complexed prostate specific antigen in men with prostate specific antigen 2 to 4 ng/ml. J Urology, **170,** 2181–5.

10. Pepe, M., Feng, Z., Janes, H., Bossuyt, P., Potter, J. (2008) Pivotal Evaluation of the Accuracy of a Biomarker used for Classification or Prediction: Standards for Study Design. *J Natl Cancer Inst* **100**, 1432–38.

11. Tomlins, S. A., Rhodes, D. R., Perner, S., Dhanasekaran, S. M., Mehra, R., Sun, W.-W., Varambally, S., Cao, X., Tchinda, J., Kuefer, R., Lee, C., Montie, J. E., Shah, R. B., Pienta, K. J., Rubin, M. A., and Chinnaiyan, A. M. (2005) Recurrent fusion of TMPRSS2 and ETS transcription factor genes in prostate cancer. *Science* **310**, 644–8.

12. van Gils, M. P., Cornel, E. B., Hessels, D., Peelen, W. P., Witjes, J. A., Mulders, P. F., Rittenhouse, H. G., and Schalken, J. A. (2007) Molecular PCA3 diagnostics on prostatic fluid. *Prostate* **67**, 881–7.

# 22

# Statistical Evaluation of Markers and Risk Tools for Prostate Cancer Classification and Prediction

*Yingye Zheng and Donna P. Ankerst*

## Contents

## Summary

Adopting novel biomarkers for use in prostate cancer screening requires rigorous scientific evaluation. The predictive accuracy of the markers must be quantified and compared with other potential markers. In this chapter we focus on the statistical approaches commonly used for evaluating biomarkers in the context of early detection for prostate cancer. We cover statistical methods for estimating accuracy summaries for both disease classification and risk prediction, including the true positive fraction (TPF), false positive fraction (FPF), positive predictive value (PPV), negative predictive value (NPV), receiver-operating characteristic (ROC) curve, and predictiveness curve. We also provide methods for combining multiple biomarker tests and comparing biomarkers. An example from the San Antonio Center of Biomarkers Of Risk for Prostate Cancer (SABOR) cohort is used to illustrate these methods.

**Key Words:** True positive fraction (TPF), False positive fraction (FPF), Positive predictive value (PPV), Negative predictive value (NPV), Receiver-operating characteristic (ROC) curve, Predictiveness curve, Combining multiple tests, Comparing markers.

From: *Current Clinical Urology: Prostate Cancer Screening*, Edited by: D. P. Ankerst et al.
DOI 10.1007/978-1-60327-281-0_22 © Humana Press, a part of Springer Science+Business Media, LLC 2009

# INTRODUCTION

New technological advances, including microarrays and proteomics, promise to identify new molecular signatures for early detection of prostate cancer and risk stratification. Most biomarker tests for most diseases are not perfect. Serum prostate-specific antigen (PSA), a widely used biomarker for screening and early detection of prostate cancer, still has important limitations in predicting the outcome of individual patients due to disease heterogeneity *(1,2)*, and its true impact in terms of reducing the disease burden is still largely unknown. Therefore rigorous evaluation of biomarkers for prostate cancer screening is a high priority. Prior to adoption of a biomarker for use in prostate cancer screening its predictive accuracy must be quantified and compared with other potential markers, including existing diagnostic systems, such as the digital rectal examination (DRE), and with established risk factors, such as family history of prostate cancer in a first-degree relative.

In this chapter we focus on the statistical approaches commonly used for evaluating biomarkers in the context of early detection of prostate cancer. Note here we use the term biomarker, or marker, in a generic sense, to mean any measure that could signal the onset of the disease or could be used for risk prediction. Examples of markers include the DRE, molecular genomic signatures, serum measures such as PSA, risk scores developed from epidemiological research such as the Prostate Cancer Prevention Trial (PCPT) risk score *(3)*, or sometimes even a combination of these. Biomarkers are used for multiple purposes. For screening, biomarkers are sought that have the capacity to discriminate diseased populations from healthy ones, i.e., that classify people as "healthy" or "having prostate cancer." For risk prediction, biomarkers are sought that can identify patients at high or low risk of developing prostate cancer or progression of the disease, in the latter case so that individual-tailored monitoring plans or treatment strategies can be employed. As such, different statistical approaches should be considered for biomarkers serving different clinical goals. The focus of biomarker research for screening is on the operating characteristics or predictive performance of the biomarker in the targeted population. Therefore it requires different statistical tools than those developed for therapeutic or epidemiological studies.

To illustrate the statistical methods, we use an example from the San Antonio Center of Biomarkers Of Risk for Prostate Cancer (SABOR) in this chapter. SABOR is a clinical and epidemiologic validation center of the Early Detection Research Network (EDRN) of the National Cancer Institute (NCI) and is charged with the discovery, development, and validation of biomarkers for the detection of genitourinary cancers *(4)*. Since 2000, SABOR has recruited 3,379 men without a diagnosis of prostate cancer into a longitudinal follow-up study. Extensive demographic, family history, dietary, and other data are obtained as well as biologic samples including serum. The cohort of men is unique in its ethnic/racial constitution, including 1,712 (49.1%) non-Hispanic Caucasians, 1,296 (37.2%) Hispanics, 472 (13.5%) African Americans, and 8 (0.2%) of other minorities enrolled from several areas in south Texas. Participants are followed annually with DRE and PSA measurements, with prostate biopsies offered for PSA greater than or equal to 2.5 ng/mL, abnormal DRE, or a positive family history of disease. This cohort was established to provide specimens for prospective evaluation of the performance of prostate cancer biomarkers in the general population and represents a screened cohort of men, similar to the PCPT. A group of 446 SABOR participants were identified who had a prostate biopsy performed as part of the study and a PSA and DRE measured within 2.5 years prior to the biopsy.

## EVALUATING BIOMARKERS FOR DISEASE CLASSIFICATION

There are various methods for defining the accuracy of a diagnostic test for predicting a disease outcome, such as prostate cancer versus no prostate cancer, with the different methods addressing different clinical questions; Pepe*(5)* provides a more detailed reference to that here. To define the measures let $D$ denote prostate cancer status ($D = 1$ in the presence of prostate cancer, and $D = 0$ in the absence of prostate cancer), and $Y$ the result of a diagnostic test. If $Y$ is dichotomous, then $Y = 1$ (test positive) is indicative of disease, and $Y = 0$ (test negative) is indicative of no disease. A marker $Y$ measured on a continuous scale can first be dichotomized as positive if it exceeds some threshold value and negative otherwise, assuming high values of the marker are more indicative of the disease. For example, positive tests for prostate cancer based on the continuous marker PSA are defined when PSA exceeds 2.5 or 4.0 ng/mL.

### *Measures of Discrimination: True/False Positive Fraction and Receiver-Operating Characteristic Curve*

A key question in diagnostic medicine is how well a test can distinguish people with a dichotomized state of health, e.g., those with prostate cancer versus those free of cancer. There are two key aspects that characterize the discriminatory ability of a marker. First, an accurate marker should be able to "rule in" those who truly have cancer. Failing to treat a diseased subject timely due to misdiagnosis can have grave consequences. Second, an accurate marker should be able to "rule out" subjects that are in fact healthy. An incorrect positive result can generate severe burden for the subject both emotionally and financially. Ideally a positive marker result should be able to identify all the subjects who are in true diseased states without including any one that is truly healthy. However, such a perfect test is quite rare in practice.

For a dichotomous marker, the discriminatory accuracy is commonly described by a pair of quantities: the true and false positive fractions (TPF and FPF) defined as follows:

$$\text{TPF} = P[Y = 1 | D = 1],$$
$$\text{FPF} = P[Y = 1 | D = 0],$$

where here and throughout the text "$P$" denotes probability and "|" denotes "in the subset of" the quantity that follows. So, TPF is the probability of a positive test in the subset of subjects who truly have the disease and FPF is the probability of a positive test in the subset of subjects who do not have disease. The TPF is also referred to as the sensitivity, the fraction of the population with cancer who test positive, while the FPF is often referred to as 1 – specificity, where specificity is the fraction of the healthy population that test negative ($P[Y=0|D=0]$). A perfect test has TPF equal to 1 and FPF equal to 0. A non-informative test has both TPF and FPF equal to $P[Y = 1]$, the probability of a positive test across the whole population. Both summaries TPF and FPF are important, as they reflect two different types of errors in medical decision-making, which may have different consequences in terms of benefit and cost.

**Example:** Of the 446 SABOR participants, 129 (28.9%) had a positive DRE and 148 (33.2%) had prostate cancer on biopsy. The TPF of DRE for prostate cancer was 26.4%, indicating only approximately a quarter of prostate cancer cases tested positive by DRE. The FPF was 30.2%, indicating approximately one third of non-cancer cases underwent an unnecessary biopsy. The TPF is too low and the FPF too high for DRE to be useful for screening on the general public scale.

When the outcome of a test is continuous with higher values corresponding to disease, a binary test is defined by choosing a cutpoint $c$ such that a test is called positive if the test result $Y$ is greater than $c$ and negative otherwise. Sensitivity and specificity associated with such a binary test can be used to characterize the accuracy of a continuous test at a particular $c$. Clearly, the accuracy of a test can change depending on the choice of $c$. A receiver-operating characteristic (ROC) curve provides a summary measure of accuracy for a continuous test as a plot of sensitivity on the $y$-axis versus 1 minus specificity on the $x$-axis evaluated at all possible choices of $c$.

The ROC curve has been widely applied in diagnostic medicine as a standard summary of diagnostic accuracy since its origination from signal detection theory in psychophysics (6–9). There are many appealing features of an ROC curve. First, it provides a way to visualize the notion of diagnostic accuracy in a straightforward way. An ROC curve very close to the 45 degree line indicates a test with virtually little discriminatory ability. The higher the ROC curve, the better its capacity for distinguishing diseased from non-diseased subjects. Second, ROC curves are invariant with respect to measurement scales, for example, PSA and the logarithm of PSA will yield the same ROC curve. This makes ROC curves also particularly useful when comparing tests on completely different measurement scales. Finally, ROC curves are by definition independent of disease prevalence and hence can be applied to the case–control study situation in addition to prospective studies.

A few summaries from the ROC curve are of interest. The area under the ROC curve (AUC):

$$\mathrm{AUC} = \int_0^1 \mathrm{ROC}(u)du,$$

is the most popular summary, where in the notation above, $\mathrm{ROC}(u)$ is the value of the ROC curve (TPF) at FPF $= u$, and the AUC is the integral of the ROC curve over all possible FPF values from 0 to 1. The AUC ranges from 0.5 for a non-informative test to 1 for a perfect test. Using probability theory it can be shown that it equals the probability that a test result from a randomly selected diseased subject exceeds that from a randomly selected non-diseased subject. Hence the AUC has an intuitive interpretation beyond being a mathematical integral of the ROC curve.

Other useful measures include $\mathrm{ROC}(u_0)$, the TPF value at a specific FPF value $= u_0$, or the partial area under the ROC curve, $p\mathrm{AUC}(u_0)$, defined by the integral form of AUC above, but replacing the upper limit of integration of 1 with $u_0$. For a marker to be useful for prostate cancer screening, only low FPF values are clinically relevant, e.g. $u_0=0.20$, and therefore it could be argued that attention should be restricted to $p\mathrm{AUC}(0.20)$, the region of the ROC curve with false positive fractions less than or equal to 20%.

To estimate the ROC curve suppose we have $n_D$ test results from the diseased population represented as $\{Y_{Di} : i = 1, \ldots, n_D\}$ and $n_H$ test results from the disease-free population represented as $\{Y_{Hj} : j = 1,\ldots, n_H\}$. We can estimate the ROC curve non-parametrically with the empirical ROC curve by plotting the following quantities for all possible cut points $c$:

$$\widehat{\text{TPF}}(c) = \sum\nolimits_{i=1}^{n_D} I(Y_{Di} \geq c)/n_D$$

$$\widehat{\text{FPF}}(c) = \sum\nolimits_{j=1}^{n_H} I(Y_{Hj} \geq c)/n_H,$$

where $I(Y_{Di} \geq c)$ equals 1 if $Y_{Di} \geq c$ and 0 otherwise and similarly for $I(Y_{Hj} \geq c)$. The AUC is calculated from the empirical ROC curve by averaging across $c$. Alternatively, the AUC by definition is $P(Y_D > Y_H)$ where $Y_D$, $Y_H$ are marker values from randomly selected cases and controls, respectively, and can therefore be calculated by the Mann–Whitney $U$-statistic:

$$A\widehat{U}C = \sum_{j=1}^{n_D} \sum_{i=1}^{n_H} I[Y_{Di} \geq Y_{Hj}]/n_D n_H.$$

Since the Mann–Whitney statistic is a simple function of the Wilcoxon rank sum statistic, it follows that the non-parametric Wilcoxon test can be used for testing the null hypothesis that the AUC equals 0.5 versus the alternative that it exceeds 0.5. The standard deviation of the AUC is more complicated to compute, requiring the $U$-statistic approach of DeLong et al. *(10)*, or the bootstrap resampling method*(11)*.

**Example:** In the SABOR example the ROC curve for PSA is shown in Fig. 1. It obtains an AUC of 0.640 (standard deviation 0.027) and $p$-value $< 0.0001$ for a test of the null hypothesis that it equals 0.500. Although highly significant, an AUC of 64% does not in general indicate a marker useful for screening.

The empirical ROC curve in Fig. 1 is not smooth but has steps at all biomarker values in the dataset. If a smooth ROC curve is desired a parametric model can be fit to it. The most popular form of a parametric ROC curve is the binormal ROC model:

$$\text{ROC}(u) = \Phi(a + b\Phi^{-1}(u)),$$

where $\Phi(.)$ is the cumulative distribution function of the standard normal distribution, $\Phi^{-1}$ is the inverse of the function, and $a$ and $b$ are parameters to be estimated. The

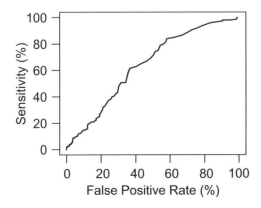

**Fig. 1.** Receiver-operating characteristic curve for PSA from the SABOR study.

binormal model assumes that for some strictly increasing transformation $h$, $h(Y_D)$, and $h(Y_H)$ have normal distributions, and provides a good approximation to a wide range of ROC curves that occur in practice *(12,13)*. For a binormal ROC curve the AUC has a simple analytic form

$$AUC = \Phi \left( \frac{a}{\sqrt{1 + b^2}} \right).$$

Several authors have proposed methods for estimating the binormal ROC curve *(14, 15)*. One approach is the ROC-GLM procedure based on binary regression *(16,17)*.

The level of a marker, and hence its accuracy, can be affected by other covariates, $Z$. For example PSA increases with age and its accuracy for prostate cancer diagnosis may vary by age. One can calculate separate ROC curves stratified by values of a covariate, such as for different age groups, but this results in a loss of power and efficiency when the number of covariate groups is large. Detailed algorithms for fitting *covariate-specific* ROC curves have been proposed *(18–20)*. If a matched design pairs cases with controls based on specific-covariate values, then a covariate-*adjusted* ROC analysis should be performed, by standardizing case observations with respect to the appropriate covariate-specific control distribution *(21,* software can be found in http://www.fhcrc.org.science/lab/pepe/dabs). Otherwise estimates from the ROC curve, including the AUC, will be attenuated.

### Positive and Negative Predictive Values

Positive and negative predictive values are another set of commonly used accuracy measures. They reflect how well the test result predicts true disease state. For a binary marker result, the positive predictive value (PPV) can be written as

$$PPV = P(D = 1|Y = 1),$$

and is the probability that a person with a positive marker test has the disease. The negative predictive value (NPV) can be written as

$$NPV = P(D = 0|Y = 0),$$

and is the probability that a person who tests negative for the marker does not have the disease. Compared to sensitivity and specificity, predictive values may be more relevant to the end users, clinicians, as well as to patients, as they often want to know the likelihood of having the disease when presented with the result of a marker test.

It is important to recognize that for any given study, both components, PPV *and* NPV, are needed to fully characterize the accuracy of a biomarker (similarly for TPF and FPF). There are trade-offs between each of the two components: an improvement in one component may imply a decline for the other. This is essentially different from the methods of evaluating disease association which usually focus on one-dimensional summaries such as the odds ratio.

The two types of accuracy summaries (TPF, FPF vs. PPV, NPV) are directly related. For example, if the population prevalence of disease $P(D = 1) = \rho$, is available, PPV is related to (TPF, FPF) by

$$PPV = \rho TPF/[\rho TPF + (1 - \rho)FPF].$$

Conversely, if the probability of a positive test $\phi = P[Y = 1]$ is available, TPF can be obtained by

$$\text{TPF} = \phi\text{PPV}/[\phi\text{PPV} + (1 - \phi)\text{PPV})].$$

However, in general the summaries (TPF, FPF) and (PPV, NPV) address different questions in practice. The set of classification probability measures, TPF and FPF, are important tools in retrospective studies where subjects are selected based on their disease status, as they quantify how well the marker reflects their disease status. These are often of interest in early phases of biomarker studies and can be calculated with a relatively small case–control study *(22)*. The predictive values PPV and NPV, however, depend on the population disease prevalence. For this reason, predictive values are often calculated when prior knowledge of the true prevalence in the population is available or from a prospective cohort study.

**Example:** In the SABOR example the PPV and NPV of DRE are 30.2 and 65.6%, respectively. The DRE does not have good positive predictive value: if the DRE test is positive there is only a 30% chance of prostate cancer on biopsy. If the DRE is negative, the chance that a prostate biopsy would also be negative is somewhat higher at 65%.

PPV and NPV are defined for dichotomous tests. No standard definition exists when the biomarker $Y$ is continuous. Moskowitz and Pepe*(23)* proposed to define for $0 \leq v \leq 1$, PPV$(v) = P(D=1 \mid F(y) \geq v)$ and NPV$(v) = P(D = 0 \mid F(y) < v)$, where $F(y)$ is the cumulative distribution function of $Y$ in the population. By this definition subjects with marker values at or above the $v$th population percentile ($F(y) \geq v$) are regarded as biomarker positive and those below are regarded as negative. By this formulation NPV$(v)$ is a simple function of $v$, PPV$(v)$, and the disease prevalence $\rho$: NPV$(v)$ $=1-\{\rho- [1-\text{PPV}(v)](1-v)\}/v$.

The PPV curve, a plot PPV$(v)$ versus $v$, is a natural analogue of the ROC curve for generalizing the notion of predictive value to continuous markers. Importantly, using $v$ as the $x$-axis rather than the raw marker value provides a common scale for different markers that may be incomparable with respect to their raw values. Moreover, since $v$ is the proportion of the population testing negative with the marker, it makes sense to compare the PPVs of markers when they are rescaled to have equal $v$'s.

**Example:** The empirical PPV and NPV plots of Moskowitz and Pepe *(23)* for PSA are shown in Fig. 2. The PPV remains nearly constant at 45% for all cut-off values of

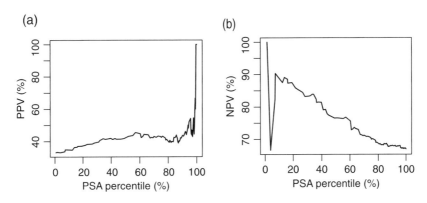

**Fig. 2.** Empirical (**a.**) PPV and (**b.**) NPV curves for PSA from the SABOR study.

PSA. The NPV of PSA is higher and drops from 90% at lower PSA thresholds to 70% at higher PSA thresholds. The sharp drops in the *right side* of Fig. 2a and *left side* of Fig. 2b are due to numeric difficulties from low sample sizes and are not meaningful.

## EVALUATING RISK PREDICTION MARKERS

Biomarkers can also be used for risk prediction. Rather than directly classifying patients in terms of their disease status, the goal is to identify patients at different levels of risk, such as high, intermediate, or low risk, for individual-tailored treatment strategies or monitoring plans. Different statistical approaches to evaluating a marker for screening might be appropriate in this setting *(24,25)*. While maintaining the false positive fraction at a low level is paramount in primary screening, a high true positive fraction is often more important for individual prediction. The corresponding risk threshold is a subjective aspect to consider in order to ensure that decisions are satisfying to individuals.

One simple way to evaluate biomarkers for risk prediction is to examine their effect on risk of cancer conditional on other predictors in a logistic regression. The relative risk calculated from such a model, however, is not sufficient for quantifying the predictive performance of the marker in the population. To fully describe the utilities of a risk prediction marker, one needs to consider (1) absolute risk, i.e., whether the risk as predicted by the marker can reach a level that is of clinical importance, and (2) the prevalence of the marker, i.e., what fraction of the population can be identified as "high risk."

### *Predictiveness Curve*

Pepe et al.*(26)* recently proposed a new graphical tool, the predictiveness curve, which attempts to combine both the notion of risk modeling and population performance in evaluating a biomarker for risk prediction. The curve is a plot of risk associated with the $v$th quantile of the marker, $P\{D = 1|Y = F^{-1}(v)\}$ versus $v$ for $v$ ranging from 0 to 1, with $F(\cdot)$ as the cumulative distribution of the marker. Similar to the PPV curve, there are two advantages of using the scale $v = F(y)$ on the $x$-axis. First, it facilitates the comparison of multiple biomarkers that may be originally measured on different scales. Second, it highlights the importance of the distribution of risk in the population when considering the predictive performance of a marker. Different from the PPV curve, whereas the PPV curve shows classification errors by fraction of subjects testing positive in the population, the predictiveness curve directly displays the distribution of risk in the population (predictiveness).

The predictiveness curve can be calculated by the steps in Table 1.

### Table 1
#### Steps for Calculating the Predictiveness Curve for a Marker $Y$

---

1. Estimate the absolute risk of $Y$ from the data using logistic regression: $\text{Risk}(Y) = \exp(\beta_0 + \beta_1 Y)/(1 + \exp(\beta_0 + \beta_1 Y))$.
2. Estimate the marker quantiles $y$ using the equation: $v = 1/N \Sigma_i I(Y_i \leq y)$, where $Y_i$ are the observed marker values across cases and controls.
3. Plot Risk $(F^{-1}(v))$ versus $v$ for $v$ in (0, 1).

---

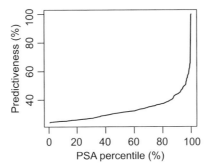

**Fig. 3.** The predictiveness plot.

**Example:** The predictiveness curve of PSA from the SABOR data is shown in Fig. 3. It shows the distribution of risks. To create the curve we ordered the risks from lowest to highest and plotted their values. We see that at 90% on the *x*-axis the risk value is approximately 0.40. This indicates that based on PSA, 90% of subjects in the cohort have calculated risks below 0.40 and 10% have risks above 0.40 (Fig. 3).

Other measures for evaluating risk predictions have been proposed. Cook *(27)* compares risk models by evaluating the number of subjects reclassified into different risk categories. Similar to the predictiveness curve, these calculations emphasize the marginal or conditional distributions of risk in the population and conclusions depend on the goodness-of-fit of the risk model. While it is important to consider risk thresholds to ensure that medical decisions are satisfying at individual levels, ultimately one needs to consider the public health impact of the marker, which lies in the marker's capacity to rule in diseased subjects (sensitivity) and rule out healthy subjects (specificity). This calls for a multifaceted approach for evaluating the population performance of biomarkers. Pepe et al. *(26)* advocate use of an integrated plot, which aligns the ROC curve with the predictiveness curve by the risk threshold criterion, to get a comprehensive summary of the population performance of the risk model. They maintain that "by simultaneously displaying predictiveness and classification performance with the integrated plot, we believe that biomarker researchers are better equipped to understand the potential utility of a risk model applied in the population."

## COMBINING MULTIPLE TEST RESULTS

Compared with a single clinical or genetic marker alone, a panel of multiple biomarkers may contain a higher level of discriminatory information, particularly across large heterogeneous patient populations and for complex diseases such as prostate cancer. For example, Wang et al. *(28)* constructed a 22-phage-peptide detector based on full autoantibody signatures and showed it had increased discriminatory accuracy for prostate cancer compared to PSA.

Construction of optimal prognostic indices has received increasing interest in recent years *(29–31)*. A simple yet elegant result for finding the optimal combination rule of multiple markers $Y = (Y_1, \ldots, Y_m)$ is based on the likelihood ratio function

$$LR(Y) = \frac{P[Y|D = 1]}{P[Y|D = 0]}.$$

The likelihood ratio is optimal in the sense that the decision rule based on $LR(Y) > c$ maximizes the TPF among all rules with $FPF = p$, for each $p$ in $(0,1)$, or equivalently, has the highest ROC curves (29,30). Furthermore, since the risk score $Risk(Y) = P[D = 1|Y]$ is a monotonic function of $LR(Y)$, it has the same ROC curve as $LR(Y)$ and is also optimal. This implies that in practice the optimal combinatory rule can be found by estimating the risk score, as done for the PCPT risk score using logistic regression (3).

Often in the early stage of biomarker development, an independent dataset to validate the performance of the newly derived combinatory rule is not yet available, in which case accuracy summaries or error rates are calculated based on outcome information from the same data. Since the same data were used to develop the prediction rule, such accuracy measures are over-optimistic, yielding better performance than if they were calculated on an external sample (32). When the number of markers combined to form the rule is large relative to the sample size, such as in genomic studies, the problem of overfitting can be magnified. One solution is to use cross-validation methods to estimate the prediction error. The commonly used $K$-fold cross-validation randomly splits the data into $K$ approximately equal-sized sets, $S_k$, $k = 1, \ldots, K$. For each $S_k$ classification error $E_{(k)}$ is estimated using the rules derived on all observations not in $S_k$ applied to all observations in $S_k$ as the "external validation sample." The cross-validated classification error is the sample average of the $K$ estimates of error rate:

$$\hat{E}_{cv} = \frac{1}{K} \sum_{k=1}^{K} E_{(k)}.$$

Standard errors for the cross-validated error rate can be approximated by the standard errors estimated from the original data (33). Note that this approach does not take into account uncertainty in the model selection procedure and to do so requires re-performing the model selection procedure at each of the $K$ model-fitting steps. In practice even when $K$-fold cross-validation is performed external validation of the prediction rule is still essential due to the over-optimism; Parekh et al. (4) performed the first external validation of the PCPT risk score.

## COMPARING TWO MARKERS

Comparison of the classification or predictive accuracy of two biomarkers $Y_1$ and $Y_2$ can be based on pairs of measures TPF/FPF or PPV/NPV via several quantities. Using PPV as an example, one may consider the absolute difference,

$$\Delta PPV = PPV_{Y1} - PPV_{Y2},$$

odds ratio

$$oPPV = \frac{PPV_{Y1}/(1 - PPV_{Y1})}{PPV_{Y2}/(1 - PPV_{Y2})},$$

or the relative measure

$$rPPV = \frac{PPV_{Y1}}{PPV_{Y2}}.$$

Pepe (2003) recommended the relative measure because of its simple interpretation. For example, if markers $Y_1$ and $Y_2$ have similar NPV but rPPV>1, given similar performance of NPV, $Y_1$ would be preferred as more predictive than $Y_2$. As for the usual relationship between relative risk and odds ratio, when the prevalence of the disease is low, rPPV is approximately equal to oPPV.

Typically marker data arise from study designs where competing markers are measured for each individual. This yields paired data and formal statistical inference needs to take into account the correlation between markers measured on the same individual, using for example the bootstrap resampling method at the individual level. A biomarker may also be used in combination with a panel of other known diagnostic factors, raising the question of whether the marker has added discriminatory accuracy over the existing system. The increased accuracy is quantified by comparing the ROC curve for the risk score combining the marker with other risk factors to the ROC curve for the other risk factors alone. The difference between the AUCs of the two corresponding ROC curves can be considered as one measure of incremental value of the marker.

# REFERENCES

1. Thompson, I.M., Pauler, D.K., Goodman, P.J., Tangen, C.M., Lucia, S.M., Parnes, H.L., Minasian, L.M., Ford, L.G., Lippman, S.M., Crawford, E.D., Crowley, J.J., and Coltman, C.A., Jr. (2004) Prevalence of prostate cancer among men with a prostate-specific antigen level $\leq 4.0$ ng per milliliter *New England Journal of Medicine* **350**, 2239–46.
2. Thompson I.M., Ankerst D.P., Chi C., Lucia M.S., Goodman P., Crowley J.J., Parnes H.L., and Coltman C.A., Jr. (2005) The operating characteristics of prostate-specific antigen in a population with initial PSA of 3.0 ng/ml or lower *Journal of the American Medical Association* **294**, 66–70.
3. Thompson, I.M., Ankerst, D.P., Chi, C., Goodman, P.J., Tangen, C.M., Lucia, M.S., Feng, Z., Parnes, H.L., and Coltman, C.A., Jr. (2006) Assessing prostate cancer risk: Results from the Prostate Cancer Prevention Trial *Journal of the National Cancer Institute* **98**, 529–34.
4. Parekh, D.J., Ankerst D.P., Higgins, B.A., Hernandez, J., Canby-Hagino, E., Brand, T., Troyer, D.A., Leach, R.J., and Thompson, I.M. (2006) External validation of the Prostate Cancer Prevention Trial Risk Calculator in a screened population *Urology* **68**, 1153–55.
5. Pepe, M.S. (2003) The statistical evaluation of medical tests for classification and prediction *Oxford University Press* (Oxford).
6. Swets, John A. and Pickett, Ronald M. (1982) Evaluation of diagnostic systems: Methods from signal detection theory *Academic Press* (New York; London).
7. Hanley, J.A. (1989) Receiver operating characteristic (ROC) methodology: The state of the art *Critical Reviews in Diagnostic Imaging*, **29**, 307–35.
8. Begg, Colin B. (1991) Advances in statistical methodology for diagnostic medicine in the 1980's *Statistics in Medicine* **10**, 1887–95.
9. Zweg, M.H. and Campbell, G. (1993) Receiver-operating characteristic (ROC) plots: A fundamental evaluation tool in clinical medicine *Clinical Chemistry* **39**, 561–77.
10. DeLong E.R., DeLong D.M., and Clarke-Pearson D.L. (1988) Comparing the areas under two or more correlated receiver operating characteristic curves: a nonparametric approach *Biometrics* **44**, 837–45.
11. Efron, B. and Tibshirani, R. (1993) An introduction to the bootstrap *Chapman & Hall Ltd* (London; New York).
12. Swets, J.A. (1986) Indices of discrimination or diagnostic accuracy: Their ROCs and implied models *Psychological Bulletin*, **99**, 100–117.
13. Hanley, J.A. (1996) The use of the `binormal' model for parametric ROC analysis of quantitative diagnostic tests *Statistics in Medicine*, **15**, 1575–85.
14. Metz, C.E., Herman, B.A., and Shen, J. (1998) Maximum likelihood estimation of receiver operating characteristic (ROC) curves from continuously-distributed data *Statistics in Medicine* **17**, 1033–53.
15. Cai, T. and Moskowitz, C. (2004) Semiparametric Estimation of the Binormal ROC Curve *Biostatistics* **5**, 573–86.

16. Pepe, M.S. (1997) A regression modelling framework for receiver operating characteristic curves in medical diagnostic testing *Biometrika* **84** , 595–608.

17. Pepe, M.S. (2000) An interpretation for the ROC curve and inference using GLM procedures *Biometrics* **56** , 352–59.

18. Zheng, Y. and Heagerty, P. (2004) Semi-parametric regression quantile methods for ROC analysis *Biostatistics* **5**, 615–32.

19. Alonzo, T.A. and Pepe, M.S. (2002) Distribution-free ROC analysis using binary regression techniques *Biostatistics* **3**, 421–32.

20. Pepe, M.S. and Cai, T. (2004) The analysis of placement values for evaluating discriminatory measures *Biometrics* **60**, 528–35.

21. Janes, H. and Pepe, M.S. (2008) Matching in studies of classification accuracy: Implications for bias, efficiency, and assessment of incremental value *Biometrics* **64**, 1–9.

22. Pepe, M.S., Etzioni, R, Feng, Z, Potter, J.D., Thompson, M.L., Thornquist, M., Winget, M., and Yasui, Y. (2001) Phases of biomarker development for early detection of cancer *Journal of the National Cancer Institute* **93**, 1054–61.

23. Moskowitz, C.S. and Pepe, M.S. (2004) Quantifying and comparing the predictive accuracy of continuous prognostic factors for binary outcomes *Biostatistics* **5**, 113–27.

24. Gail, M.H. and Pfeiffer, R.M. (2005) On criteria for evaluating models of absolute risk *Biostatistics* **6**, 227–239.

25. Cook, N. (2007) Use and misuse of the receiver operating characteristic curve in risk prediction *Circulation* **115**, 928–35.

26. Pepe, M.S., Feng, Z., Huang, Y, Longton, G., Prentice, R., Thompson, I.M., and Zheng, Y. (2007) Integrating the Predictiveness of a Marker with its Performance as a Classifier. Technical Report 283, *UW biostatistics Working Paper Series.* Available at: http://www.bepress.com/uwbiostat/paper289.

27. Cook, N.R., Buring, J.E., and Ridker, P.M. (2006) The effect of including C-reactive protein in cardiovascular risk prediction models for women. *Annals of Internal Medicine* **145**, 21–9.

28. Wang, X., Yu, J., and Sreekumar, A. et al. (2005) Autoantibody signatures in prostate cancer *N Engl J Med* **353**, 1224–35.

29. Baker, S.G. (2000) Identifying combinations of cancer markers for further study as triggers of early intervention, *Biometrics* **56**, 1082–7.

30. McIntosh, M.W. and Pepe, M.S. (2002) Combining several screening tests: Optimality of the risk score *Biometrics,* **58**, 657–64.

31. Pepe, M.S., Cai, T., and Longton, G. (2006) Combining predictors for classification using the area under the ROC curve, *Biometrics* **62**, 221–9.

32. Copas, J.B. and Corbett, P. (2002) Overestimation of the receiver operating characteristic curve for logistic regression *Biometrika* **89**, 315–31.

33. Tian, L., Cai, T., Goetghebeur E., and Wei, L.J. (2007) Model Evaluation Based on the Distribution of Estimated Absolute Prediction Error *Biometrika* **94**, 297–311.

# 23 Pitfalls in Prostate Cancer Biomarker Evaluation Studies

*Donna P. Ankerst*

## CONTENTS

## SUMMARY

Biomarker studies in prostate cancer research aim to discover new markers or novel uses of prostate-specific antigen (PSA) to complement or replace PSA as the existing standard for screening. These studies often report as primary endpoint the operating characteristics of the new marker and in some cases, make a direct comparison to PSA on the same subject population. Due to the widespread use of PSA for referral to more definitive prostate cancer diagnosis in the United States, it is easy to encounter pitfalls in the design and analysis of such studies, including failure to assess the incremental value of a new marker to PSA or failure to adjust for verification bias (use of PSA for disease ascertainment). This chapter covers four such commonly seen pitfalls in biomarker studies in prostate cancer screening and provides methods for avoiding or correcting the associated biases.

**Key Words:** Verification bias, Multiple imputation, Logistic regression, Prostate-specific antigen.

## INTRODUCTION

While serum prostate-specific antigen (PSA) is the most widely used biomarker for screening for early detection of prostate cancer, its limitations in terms of operating characteristics are recognized *(1,2)*. Therefore biomarker studies investigating novel

From: *Current Clinical Urology: Prostate Cancer Screening*, Edited by: D. P. Ankerst et al.
DOI 10.1007/978-1-60327-281-0_23 © Humana Press, a part of Springer Science+Business Media, LLC 2009

alternative uses of PSA and new markers from emerging technology remain an active area of research vital to the improvement of prostate cancer screening programs. These studies typically evaluate the operating characteristics of the new markers in isolation or in comparison to PSA on a selected population, using some metric, such as sensitivity or specificity, as the primary endpoint for evaluating performance. As the number of reports from such biomarker studies has grown, so too has the apparent discrepancies among study findings, such as a range of reported area underneath the receiver-operating characteristic (ROC) curves (AUC) or differences in sensitivities and specificities, even among studies evaluating the same marker ostensibly for the same endpoint (3–5).

Variability in reports of the operating characteristics of PSA and other markers across studies can partially be attributed to heterogeneous populations. As a post-hoc systematic review, such differences can be characterized by the inspection of the study results by specific participant characteristics in each study, such as by plots of study-reported AUCs, versus percent abnormal digital rectal exams (DRE) or median age in each study.

Of greater concern is the systematic biases in operating characteristics due to study design, such as whether the study was prospective or retrospective, the protocol by which a prospective population was verified for disease status, or how cases and controls were selected for a retrospective study. Due to widespread utility of PSA for diagnosis, study design can be dependent upon PSA, and when so, studies of operating characteristics of PSA, PSA derivatives, or new markers correlated with PSA can be systematically biased. The purpose of this chapter is to identify these potential pitfalls in biomarker studies and to outline analytic strategies for dealing with them.

## METHODS

To better clarify the analytic pitfalls encountered in biomarker studies the commonly used statistical methods in these studies are first outlined.

### *Logistic Regression*

The first is the familiar logistic regression, which is a forward look of the association between a marker or group of risk factors and prostate cancer status. The log odds of prostate cancer are modeled as a linear regression with exponentiated regression coefficients equal to the odds ratio of disease for a unit increase in the marker or covariate values:

$$\log \frac{P(\text{Cancer}|X)}{1 - P(\text{Cancer}|X)} = \beta'X,$$

where "$P(\cdot)$" denotes probability, "|" denotes conditioning on the factors following it, $X$ is a set of markers or risk factors, and $\beta$ is the associated set of log odds ratios.

### *Operating Characteristics*

Definitions of operating characteristics for a continuous marker, such as PSA, are dependent on the cut-off $c$ used to identify a participant as testing positive for prostate cancer. If the marker is overexpressed in cancer cases then a test based on the marker is defined as positive when the marker exceeds $c$ and negative otherwise, if the marker is underexpressed in cancer cases it is defined by the reverse. For presentation we will assume the case of PSA, where the marker is overexpressed in cancer cases. Since there are many choices for the cut-off $c$ for defining a positive test, operating characteristics are evaluated for a range of choices in order to find the optimal one. Given a set of cancer cases and controls, sensitivity is the proportion of participants with prostate cancer who have PSA values greater than $c$ and specificity is the proportion of non-cancer cases (controls) with PSA values less than or equal to $c$:

$$\text{Sensitivity} = \frac{\text{No. cases with marker} > c}{\text{No. cases}}$$

$$\text{Specificity} = \frac{\text{No. controls with marker} \leq c}{\text{No. controls}}$$

Sensitivity and specificity give the proportion of correctly tested participants for cases and controls separately, and the goal is to find a cut-off $c$ such that both are high. Because the denominators entail the disease status and the computed fractions refer back to who tested positive or negative, sensitivity and specificity are referred to as retrospective measures. Sensitivity and specificity refer to different sub-populations so do not sum to one, but they do change in reverse directions for changing cut-off $c$. For $c$ equal to the minimum marker value sensitivity is essentially the maximum value 1.0 (100%) and specificity the minimum, 0.0 (0%). Then as $c$ increases sensitivity decreases while specificity increases. So selecting the optimal cut-off $c$ that simultaneously maximizes both measures is not possible, but rather a $c$ is chosen for which both measures do not fall below some unacceptable value for each. For example, for PSA to be feasible in a screening program a specificity greater than 80% is typically required. Therefore $c$ is chosen that obtains the maximum sensitivity under this requirement. Since sensitivity decreases with increasing $c$, the minimum $c$ that obtains specificity of 80% is the optimal cut-off.

Often the false positive rate, the proportion of non-cases who test positive ($1-$specificity) is reported instead of the specificity. The false negative rate ($1-$sensitivity) is analogously defined:

$$\text{False negative rate} = \frac{\text{No. cases with marker} \leq c}{\text{No. cases}}$$

$$\text{False positive rate} = \frac{\text{No. controls with marker} > c}{\text{No. controls}}$$

The objective is to minimize these quantities.

The receiver-operating characteristic (ROC) curve summarizes sensitivity and specificity across all cut-off values of $c$, and hence gives a global report of the operating characteristics of a marker. It is constructed as a plot of the false positive rate on the $x$-axis versus sensitivity on the $y$-axis for all possible cut-offs $c$ and summarized by the area underneath the curve (AUC). The maximal AUC is 100% and tests are preferred which maximize the AUC. The minimal AUC is 50% and corresponds to a marker that does not distinguish cases from controls better than the flip of a coin. As a rank-based measure, the AUC provides a method to compare two or more different markers that is independent of the scales of the markers. A test of the null hypothesis that the AUCs from two different markers are equal can be performed using the $U$-statistic approach *(6)*.

In contrast to the retrospective measures of sensitivity and specificity, positive and negative predictive values (PPV, NPV) provide a prospective measure of marker performance by examining the proportion of persons with marker exceeding $c$ that are cancer cases and the proportion with marker less than or equal to $c$ that are controls:

$$\text{Positive predictive value} = \frac{\text{No. cases with marker} > c}{\text{No. with marker} > c}$$

$$\text{Negative predictive value} = \frac{\text{No. controls with marker} \leq c}{\text{No. with marker} \leq c}$$

The objective is to maximize these quantities.

## PITFALLS

The above statistical definitions are sensitive to the study design and to how cancer cases and controls are verified. Some easily encountered pitfalls are summarized in this section along with solutions for avoiding or post-hoc correcting them.

## PITFALL 1

Pitfall 1: Failure to evaluate the independent diagnostic information of a new biomarker or PSA derivative against the standard, PSA.

For evaluating new therapies for a disease the gold standard is the randomized clinical trial comparing the new therapy to the existing standard of care on subjects from the same population. It is noteworthy that many studies of new biomarkers do not additionally measure the existing standard, PSA, so that a within-study comparison can be made. In such cases the operating characteristics of a marker may look promising but an additional study will be required to ascertain whether it has actually improved upon PSA. This particularly applies to markers that are PSA derivatives, such as PSA velocity (change in PSA over time), PSA doubling time (time until the PSA doubles), and PSA density (ratio of PSA to prostate volume) *(7–12)*. These derivatives tend to be highly correlated with PSA and the few studies that have appropriately evaluated their independent diagnostic contribution to PSA, by simultaneously including both PSA and the proposed derivative in the same risk model, have found no to little incremental value above PSA; see, for example, Refs. *(3–5,13–16)*. Since most PSA derivatives are more difficult to measure than PSA (PSA density requiring a transurethral ultrasound, for example) it can be argued that they must not only outperform PSA, but do so substantially before they would be considered for replacing or complementing PSA.

New PSA assays have recently been developed, including percent-free (unbound) PSA, percent-complexed PSA, and PSA isoforms, such as precursor PSA (proPSA) and benign PSA (BPSA), but thus far have produced only minor improvement in operating characteristics along restricted ranges of PSA *(17–20)*. Etzioni and colleagues (21) appropriately evaluated complexed PSA and PSA on a single cohort of participants and found only modest improvements in accuracy attributable to complexed PSA over that provided by PSA.

The design of studies for new biomarkers should include whenever possible the measurement of PSA. The sample correlation between PSA and the new marker should be reported and its statistical significance assessed. If the predictive capability of the marker is the primary endpoint, such as by odds ratio in a logistic regression, then three analyses should be performed: univariate logistic regression for the new marker, logistic regression for PSA, and a combined multivariable logistic regression simultaneously including the new marker and PSA (Table 1).

As for PSA in Test 1, if the new marker is statistically significant in Test 2 it is predictive of prostate cancer status and if not, it is not worth further consideration as a marker. For calibration of the new marker it is of interest in its own right to assess the statistical significance and extent of effect of PSA in the same cohort. Depending on the sample size, Tests 1 and 2 can also be adjusted by other covariates or risk factors, such as family history or digital rectal exam, so that whether the new marker of interest remains statistically significant after adjusting for these risk factors can also be assessed.

Even if statistically significant in Test 2, the new marker may fail to be statistically significant in Test 3, and in this case it provides no independent diagnostic information to PSA. Transformations of the new marker or inclusion of interaction terms between the new marker and PSA, allowing the new marker to have different effects at different ranges of PSA, may lead to incremental value. The model in Test 3 or any new derived combination will need to be validated in a different external cohort to the one used in the current study.

### *Example: PSA velocity versus PSA in the PCPT*

When evaluated by a univariable logistic regression in the absence of the PCPT risk factors on 5,519 PCPT placebo participants used to develop the PCPT risk calculator, PSA velocity was statistically significantly associated with prostate cancer, with odds ratio indicating a nearly sixfold increase in the odds of prostate cancer per unit increase in velocity *(13)*. But in a multivariable logistic regression model containing both PSA and PSA velocity, PSA remained statistically significant for association with prostate cancer while PSA velocity did not, and the odds ratio for association of PSA velocity with prostate cancer dropped below 1.2.

As for odds ratio analyses, for operating characteristic analyses such as by the AUC, the AUC for both the new marker and PSA should be reported. *U*-statistic methods *(6)* can be used to assess whether the two AUCs statistically differ. Simple combined rules can be formulated, such as test positive if PSA exceeds a threshold and/or the new marker exceeds a threshold and then also evaluated via the AUC. Etzioni et al. *(21)* entertained a variety of such logic "and/or" rules for combining PSA and percent-free

Table 1
**Three Logistic Regressions to Assess the Independent Diagnostic
Value of a New Marker to PSA**

Logistic regression of outcome on covariate
Test 1: Cancer status on PSA
Test 2: Cancer status on Marker
Test 3: Cancer status on PSA + marker

PSA and used an AUC analysis to conclude that percent-free PSA did not improve upon PSA. An advantage of the AUC or other operating characteristics for comparing markers is that they can be done without a statistical model and do not depend on the scale or transformation selected for the marker.

## PITFALL 2

Pitfall 2: Failure to adjust for verification bias in the assessment of the operating characteristics of a marker.

Since the PSA era where PSA has become commonly used to refer men to biopsy or more definitive prostate cancer testing, verification bias has become an issue in studies of the operating characteristics of PSA (2,22). The problem arises since the definitions of sensitivity and specificity require a population where prostate cancer is definitively verified, by biopsy for instance, but this population is nearly always that referred by clinical indication, including a high PSA. And as can be seen in the definitions of sensitivity and specificity in the Section "Methods", the operating characteristics depend directly on the PSA distribution of the selected population. For example, suppose one prospective study used a population of men who had prostate biopsy to define cancer cases and controls where only men with PSA exceeding 2.5 ng/mL had been referred to biopsy. Another study was similar to the PCPT and had a required biopsy for all men regardless of PSA. Both studies report the sensitivity of the cut-off 2.5 ng/mL but the two studies will differ in their reports merely due to subject selection. In the first study the sensitivity of the cut-off 2.5 ng/mL is 100% because all cases have PSA > 2.5 ng/mL. In fact, all controls from the study also have PSA > 2.5 ng/mL. In the second study, the sensitivity of 2.5 ng/mL will be less (only 40.5% from the PCPT, (2)). One may argue that this is an extreme example and only cut-offs higher than 2.5 ng/mL should be compared between the two studies, but the above bias and difference between the two studies will persist for all cut-offs higher than 2.5 ng/mL and between any two studies that have different PSA distributions, even if both contain PSA values below 2.5 ng/mL. Specificity will also differ systematically between the two studies so that the overall AUCs reported by the two studies will also differ. That verified participants used in studies of the operating characteristics of PSA are biased with respect to their PSA distributions has led to a diverse range of reported AUCs for PSA (3). The PSA-referral bias can also arise when evaluating the operating characteristic of a new marker as long as the new marker is correlated with PSA.

The same statistical solutions to handle missing data in longitudinal studies can be used to correct for verification bias in studies of operating characteristics of a marker. These solutions entail including all men from the prospective or retrospective study who have the marker of interest measured into the operating characteristic evaluation regardless of whether or not the prostate cancer status was ascertained. Those with "missing" prostate cancer status essentially have their prostate cancer status multiply imputed based on a model fit to participants who did have the cancer status verified (23). The operating characteristic of interest is evaluated over all imputed datasets with the sample average or median taken as the point estimate; the sample variation of the operating characteristic across imputed datasets is used to correctly inflate the standard error of the point estimate. The method hinges on a requirement that enough risk factors have been measured on all participants, including those without cancer verification, so that the probability of cancer can be accurately predicted. When this is not the case more

Table 2
## Multiple Imputation Procedure for Performing a Verification Bias Adjustment

Imputation method for verification bias

Step 1: Fit a logistic regression of prostate cancer status on all available risk factors $X$, including the marker of interest, in the group of participants who have their prostate cancer status verified, obtaining odds ratios $\beta$.

Step 2: For each non-verified participant estimate their individual probability of prostate cancer based on their individual risk factors $X_i$ and the odds ratios $\beta$ from Step 1 using the inverse logistic function:

$$\text{Probability Cancer Individual}_i = \frac{\exp(\beta X_i)}{1 + \exp(\beta X_i)}$$

and draw a random binary variable (0/1) with this probability. This imputes the missing cancer status (1 = prostate cancer, 0 = control) for the non-verified participant.

Step 3: Calculate the operating characteristic of interest for the complete cohort using the imputed cancer statuses from Step 2.

Step 4: Repeat Steps 2–3 for $N = 10$–100 iterations. For each iteration store the calculated operating characteristic and its standard error.

Step 5: The verification-bias adjusted estimate of the operating characteristic is the average over the $N$ operating characteristics from Step 4 and the standard error is the sum of the average of the $N$ standard errors in Step 4 and the sample variance of the $N$ operating characteristics in Step 4.

complicated methods accounting for what is termed non-ignorable missing data must be used *(24)*. The multiple imputation method, which can be implemented using standard statistical software, is summarized in Table 2.

## Example: Verification bias in the receiver-operating characteristic curves for the PCPT

There was concern over verification bias in the ROC curve for PSA in the PCPT because interim biopsies were prompted for those men who had a PSA that exceeded 4 ng/mL *(2)*. However, the analysis also included a large number of unprompted end-of-study biopsies, which could minimize the impact of verification bias. Therefore ROC curves for PSA were computed both with and without a verification bias adjustment using an algorithm similar to Table 2.

As reported in *(2)*, out of 8,575 PCPT placebo arm participants who had a PSA and DRE available for an ROC analysis, 5,587 (65.2%) received a prostate biopsy, either during or at the end of the study. The 5,587 men who got a biopsy (verified) in the PCPT were statistically significantly older, more likely to have a family history, more likely to be white, and more likely to have elevated PSA (> 4 ng/mL) or an abnormal DRE than the remainder of the 8,575 placebo participants who did not get a biopsy. Figure 1 shows ROC curves on just the 5,587 verified placebo participants, after applying the verification bias adjustment to obtain the median ROC curve for all 8,575 placebo participants, and for individual imputations for the 2,988 missing

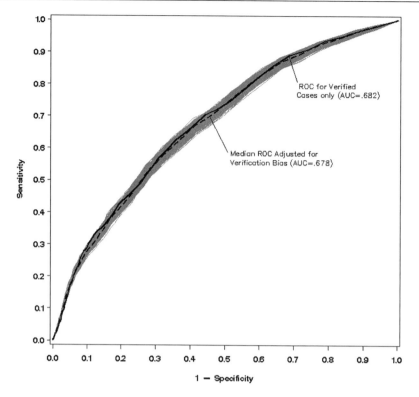

**Fig. 1.** Receiver-operating characteristic curves for $N = 5,587$ verified PCPT placebo participants (*solid line*), $N = 8,575$ verified and unverified PCPT placebo participants (*dashed line*), and corresponding to the individual imputations for the 2,988 PCPT placebo participants who were not verified (*gray lines*).

prostate cancer statuses. The verified-only curve is nearly identical to the one adjusting for verification bias (both AUCs near 68%), suggesting verification bias was not a problem in the PCPT. The individually imputed ROC curves give a sense of variation due to missing prostate cancer statuses. It was suggested that the required end-of-study biopsy of the PCPT could be credited for removing the verification bias. To investigate this more formally prostate cancer statuses for all men who had PSA $\leq 4$ ng/mL were switched to unknown to create a hypothetical cohort where only men with PSA $> 4$ ng/mL were verified. Instead of 5,587 out of 8,575 men verified (65.2%) the new cohort had only 637 out of 8,575 verified (7.4%). This may seem at first glance extreme, but a sample size of 637 is in accordance with many of the biomarker study sample sizes and recently Punglia and colleagues performed a verification bias adjustment on a cohort with only 11% verified (22). The analogous figure of verified-only to verified-adjusted ROC curves for the hypothetical cohort is shown in Fig. 2. For the verified-only cases the AUC is grossly underestimated at 50% compared to the correct 68% of Fig. 1. In this case the verification bias adjusted curve differs more dramatically from the verified-only curve, and even falls below the 50% line. There is much more uncertainty among the individual imputed curves due to the larger amounts of missing prostate cancer statuses. Figures 1 and 2 illustrate the impact of subject selection in an ROC analysis.

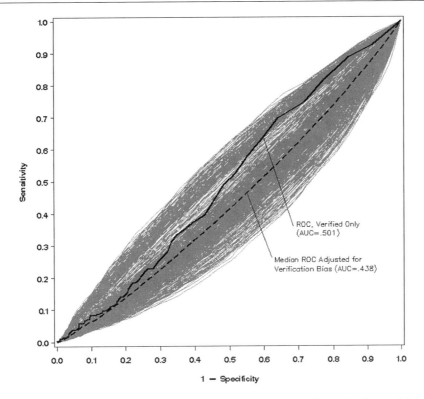

**Fig. 2.** Receiver-operating characteristic curves for $N = 637$ verified PCPT placebo participants with PSA $> 4$ ng/mL (*solid line*), $N = 8,575$ verified and unverified PCPT placebo participants with all verified participants with PSA $\leq 4$ ng/mL set to unverified (*dashed line*), and corresponding to the individual imputations for any participants set to unverified (*gray lines*).

## PITFALL 3

Pitfall 3: Comparing a new marker against PSA in a restricted range of PSA.

Many studies evaluate a new marker at limited ranges of PSA, such as the "uncertain" range between 4.0 and 10.0 ng/mL, with the idea of focusing attention on ranges where PSA has failed; see for example, *(15)*. Operating characteristics of the new marker and PSA are then compared. This sort of comparison suffers the same subject selection bias as for verification bias. For example, the sensitivity of PSA for cut-off 10.0 ng/mL will be 0% for such a sample merely because of selection. The sensitivity estimate for the new marker may also be biased by subject selection if the new marker is correlated with PSA. Therefore, it is not clear that the results of a test of operating characteristics between the new marker and PSA will be reproducible in other studies, and neither the estimates of the operating characteristics of the new marker nor of PSA will be comparable to estimates in other studies. In and of themselves, these studies do not provide direct evidence that the new biomarker will outperform PSA when used in practice for all PSA values and the complete test that incorporates both markers over their full ranges will still need to be developed and validated in a new study.

Given the resources it would be more informative to conduct a study that evaluates all ranges of PSA and defines a conditional test based on the new marker for PSA values in the uncertain range, such as the combined rules for PSA and complexed PSA evaluated in *(21)*. Such conditional tests can then be compared against PSA across the whole range of values, also using the ROC curve. Indeed an advantage of the ROC curve is that different tests of single or multiple biomarkers can be compared without regard to units. In studies where the new marker is evaluated on a restricted range of PSA, such as values between 4.0 and 10.0 ng/mL, the operating characteristics of PSA in the same restricted subset should not be reported or used for comparison since these are biased and do not correspond to usual definitions.

## PITFALL 4

Pitfall 4: Defining controls based on low values of PSA.

A final pitfall mentioned concerns the practice of defining controls for a marker evaluation study as those with a low value of PSA. This practice induces at least three forms of biases. First, as shown by *(1)*, it is now accepted that there is no lower bound of PSA below which prostate cancer is negligible so that a fraction of the controls in the study may have the incorrect cancer status. Second, there is subject selection bias by inserting more low PSAs into the study than expected, i.e., by oversampling low PSAs for controls, and this will affect the operating characteristics as described in Pitfall 2. Third, there is verification bias present in this study in that cancer cases are verified but controls are not.

To avoid this pitfall not select controls on the basis of PSA less than a threshold but rather include these participants as non-verified participants and run a verification bias adjustment algorithm as in Table 2 to calculate the operating characteristics.

## DISCUSSION

It is easy to fall into the pitfalls described above due to the predominant use of the leading marker PSA for prostate cancer verification. Some of the proposed methodologies for avoiding or correcting the pitfalls may not be feasible for a particular study at hand, for instance when risk factors have not been measured on all participants for use in a verification bias adjustment analysis. In this case, it is worth emphasizing in the discussion of study findings the nature of the potential biases. As pointed out in *(3)* knowledge of such biases helps to explain the often conflicting reports of operating characteristics of PSA, its relatives, and correlated biomarkers across different studies.

## REFERENCES

1. Thompson, I.M., Pauler, D.K., Goodman, P.J., Tangen, C.M., Lucia, S.M., Parnes, H.L., Minasian, L.M., Ford, L.G., Lippman, S.M., Crawford, E.D., Crowley, J.J., and Coltman, C.A., Jr. (2004) Prevalence of prostate cancer among men with a prostate-specific antigen level ≤ 4.0 ng per milliliter *New England Journal of Medicine* **350**, 2239–46.
2. Thompson, I.M., Ankerst, D.P., Chi, C., Lucia, M.S., Goodman, P., Crowley, J.J., Parnes, H.L., and Coltman, C.A., Jr. (2005) The operating characteristics of prostate-specific antigen in a population with initial PSA of 3.0 ng/ml or lower *Journal of the American Medical Association* **294**, 66–70.
3. Ankerst, D.P., Thompson, I.M. (2007) Understanding mixed messages about prostate specific antigen: biases in the evaluation of cancer biomarkers *Journal of Urology* **177**, 426–7.
4. Etzioni, R.D., Ankerst, D.P., Thompson, I.M. (2007) Re: Detection of life-threatening prostate cancer with prostate-specific antigen velocity during a window of curability *Journal of the National Cancer Institute* **99**, 489–90.

5. Etzioni, R.D., Ankerst, D.P., Thompson, I.M., et al. (2007b) Is PSA velocity useful in early detection of prostate cancer? A critical appraisal of the evidence *Journal of the National Cancer Institute*, **99**, 1510–5.

6. DeLong E.R., DeLong D.M., Clarke-Pearson D.L. (1988) Comparing the areas under two or more correlated receiver operating characteristic curves: a nonparametric approach *Biometrics* **44**, 837–45.

7. Benson, M.C., Whang, I.S., Olsson, C.A., et al. (1992) The use of prostate specific antigen density to enhance the predictive value of intermediate levels of serum prostate specific antigen *Journal of Urology* **147**, 817–21.

8. Carter, H.B., Pearson, J.D., Metter, E.J. et al. (1992) Longitudinal evaluation of prostate-specific antigen levels in men with and without prostate disease *Journal of the American Medical Association* **267**, 2215–20.

9. Schmid, H.P. (1995) Tumour markers in patients on deferred treatment: prostate specific antigen doubling times *Cancer Surveys* **23**, 157–67.

10. Carter, H.B., Ferrucci, L., Ketterman, A., Landis, P., Wright, E.J., Epstein, J.I., Trock, B.J., Metter, E.J. (2006) Detection of life-threatening prostate cancer with prostate-specific antigen velocity during a window of curability *Journal of the National Cancer Institute* **98**, 1521–7.

11. Kundu, S.D., Roehl, K.A., Yu, X, Antenor, J.A., Suarez, B.K., Catalona, W.J. (2007) Prostate specific antigen density correlates with features of prostate cancer aggressiveness *Journal of Urology* **177**, 505–9.

12. Moul, J.W., Sun, L., Hotaling, J.M., et al. (2007) Age adjusted prostate specific antigen and prostate specific antigen velocity cut points in prostate cancer screening *Journal of Urology* **177**, 499–503.

13. Thompson, I. M., Ankerst, D.P., Chi, C., Goodman, P.J., Tangen, C.M., Lucia, M.S., Feng, Z., Parnes, H.L., and Coltman, C.A., Jr. (2006) Assessing prostate cancer risk: Results from the Prostate Cancer Prevention Trial *Journal of the National Cancer Institute* **98**, 529–34.

14. Fall, K., Garmo, H., Andren, O., Bill-Axelson, A., Adolfsson, J., Adami, H.O., Johansson, J.E., Holmberg, L. (2007) Prostate specific antigen levels as a predictor of lethal prostate cancer *Journal of the National Cancer Institute* **99**, 526–32.

15. Roobol, M.J., Kranse, R., de Koning, H.J., Schroeder, F.H. (2004) Prostate-specific antigen velocity at low prostate-specific antigen levels as screening tool for prostate cancer: results of second screening round of ERSPC (Rotterdam) *Urology* **63**, 309–15.

16. Schroeder, F.H., Roobol, M.J., van der Kwast, T.H., Kranse, R., and Bangma, C.H. (2006) Does PSA velocity predict prostate cancer in pre-screened populations? *European Urology* **49**, 460–5.

17. Catalona, W.J., Smith, D.S., Wolfert, R.L. et al. (1995) Evaluation of percentage of free serum prostate-specific antigen to improve specificity of prostate cancer screening *Journal of the American Medical Association* **274**, 1214–20.

18. Partin, A.W., Brawer, M.K., Bartsch, G. et al. (2003) Complexed prostate specific antigen improves specificity for prostate cancer detection: results of a prospective multicenter clinical trial *Journal of Urology* **170**, 1787–91.

19. Mikolajczyk, S.D., Rittenhouse, H.G. (2004) Tumor-associated forms of prostate specific antigen improve the discrimination of prostate cancer from benign disease *Rinsho Byori* **52**, 223–30.

20. Khan, M.A., Sokoll, L.J., Chan, D.W. et al. (2004) Clinical utility of proPSA and "benign" PSA when percent free PSA is less than 15% *Urology* **64**, 1160–4.

21. Etzioni, R., Falcon, S., Gann, P.H., Kooperberg, C.L., Penson, D.F., Stampfer, M.J. (2004) Prostate-specific antigen and free prostate-specific antigen in the early detection of prostate cancer: do combination tests improve detection? *Cancer Epidemiology, Biomarkers and Prevention* **13**, 1640–5.

22. Punglia, R.S., D'Amico, A.V., Catalona, W.J., Roehl, K.A., Kuntz, K.M. (2003) Effect of verification bias on screening for prostate cancer by measurement of prostate-specific antigen *New England Journal of Medicine* **349**, 335–42.

23. Fitzmaurice GM, Laird NM, Ware JH (2004) *Applied Longitudinal Analysis*. New Jersey: John Wiley & Sons.

24. Rotnitzky A., Faraggi D., Schisterman E. (2006) Doubly robust estimation of the area under the receiver-operating characteristic curve in the presence of verification bias *Journal of the American Statistical Association* **101**, 1276–88.

25. Wang, X., Yu, J., Sreekumar, A. et al. (2005) *Autoantibody signatures in prostate cancer* *New England Journal of Medicine*, **353**, 1224–35.

# VI Building upon Recently Completed and Ongoing Prospective Trials

# 24 Prostate-Specific Antigen and Its Role on the Prostate Cancer Prevention Trial

*Catherine M. Tangen and Phyllis J. Goodman*

## CONTENTS

INTRODUCTION
PCPT RESULTS
MONITORING OF PSA ON STUDY
THE EFFECT OF FINASTERIDE ON PSA'S
    ABILITY TO DETECT PROSTATE CANCER
LONG-TERM EFFECTS OF FINASTERIDE ON PSA
REFERENCES

## SUMMARY

One of the primary challenges in the Prostate Cancer Prevention Trial was how to incorporate examinations and tests that men were regularly undergoing when these tests (such as PSA) were affected by the intervention (finasteride). The potential for finasteride to influence the *detection* of prostate cancer was a major hurdle to overcome This chapter will report on three different aspects of PSA in the PCPT. The first section describes the methods that were used in the trial to minimize the potential detection bias with finasteride. Summary data are reported that provide some assessment of the effectiveness of those methods. The second section provides a comparison of the properties of PSA to predict prostate cancer and high-grade disease in the finasteride and placebo treatment groups. The last section provides a summary of the longitudinal characteristics of PSA during the course of the trial, stratified by the subject's treatment group assignment and final disease status.

**Key Words:** PCPT, Prostate-specific antigen, Detection bias, Sensitivity, ROC.

From: *Current Clinical Urology: Prostate Cancer Screening*, Edited by: D. P. Ankerst et al.
DOI 10.1007/978-1-60327-281-0_24 © Humana Press, a part of Springer Science+Business Media, LLC 2009

## INTRODUCTION

In the Prostate Cancer Prevention Trial (PCPT) we randomly assigned 18,882 men aged 55 or older with a normal digital rectal examination, a prostate-specific antigen (PSA) level of 3.0 ng/mL or lower and with no significant chronic co-morbid diseases, especially severe BPH (AUA symptom score < 20) to treatment with finasteride (5 mg/day) or placebo for 7 years. Prostate biopsy was recommended if the annual PSA level, or the PSA level adjusted for the effect of finasteride, was greater than 4.0 ng/ml or if the digital rectal examination (DRE) was abnormal. It was anticipated that 60% of participants would have an endpoint determined; either prostate cancer diagnosed during the study or a biopsy at the end of the study. The primary endpoint was the prevalence of prostate cancer during the 7 years of the study. Secondary endpoints included the side effects of finasteride, quality of life measures, grade and stage distribution of prostate cancers detected, testing parameters of PSA and DRE, the incidence of BPH, and total and prostate-cancer specific mortality.

After randomization, men were contacted every 3 months. The 3-month and 9-month contacts were by telephone; the 6-month and annual contacts were visits to the Study Center. At the annual visit, a physical exam included a DRE and a blood draw for PSA. An abnormal DRE and/or an elevated PSA would prompt a recommendation for a prostate biopsy. After 7 years of treatment all participants who had not previously been determined to have prostate cancer, were scheduled for a prostate biopsy. A study schema is presented in Fig. 1.

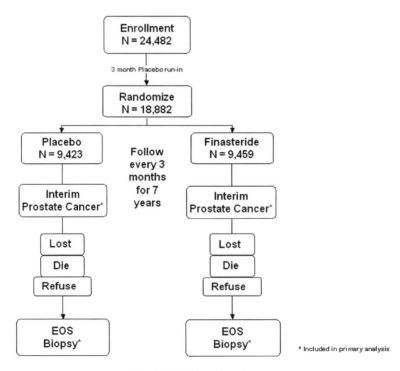

**Fig. 1.** PCPT study schema.

# PCPT RESULTS

Accrual to PCPT began in October 1993. Three years later, after having met the accrual goal, the trial was closed to further randomizations. A total of 18,882 men were randomized at 221 sites across the United States. Throughout the study, an independent Data and Safety Monitoring Committee (DSMC) held regular meetings to review the trial data. Based on sensitivity analyses, the DSMC determined that the study conclusions were extremely unlikely to change with the addition of further endpoints, and recommended the study be closed approximately 1 year earlier than planned. The paper was published in the online version of the *NEJM* on June 24, 2003 *(1)*. The analysis of the data showed a 24.8% reduction in the number of prostate cancers detected in the finasteride group versus placebo (18.4% of men evaluated on finasteride had prostate cancer vs. 24.4% of men evaluated on placebo). However, while men taking finasteride had fewer prostate cancers, they had an increased number of high-grade prostate cancers (Gleason 7–10). In the entire group of men assigned to finasteride who had their disease evaluated, 6.4% had high-grade disease while 5.1% of those evaluated in the placebo group had high-grade disease. The vast majority of the cancers detected were low stage. A total of 97.7% of cancers in men in the finasteride group were classified as T1 or T2 as were 98.4% of those tumors found in men in the placebo group. Reductions were seen in both prostate cancers detected as a result of a biopsy for cause (elevated PSA or abnormal DRE) (435 vs. 571) or end of study (368 vs. 576). The differences in high-grade disease were seen in the biopsies for cause (188 vs. 148) but not in end-of-study biopsies (92 vs. 89).

# MONITORING OF PSA ON STUDY

The design of the PCPT presented many challenges some of which are described in Feigl, et al. *(2)*. Although survival was considered the most clinically relevant endpoint, it was not feasible because of the required sample size and study duration needed. The endpoint chosen for the study was the period prevalence of prostate cancer. Period prevalence includes prostate cancers diagnosed during the course of the study as well as point prevalence as determined by a prostate biopsy at 7 years.

Much of the following information is based on two publications by Goodman et al. *(3,4)*. As those investigators point out, one particular study design challenge centered on the effect of finasteride on PSA and the use of PSA as a screening and diagnostic test for prostate cancer prior to the 7-year biopsy. Finasteride lowers the PSA value by approximately 50% on average *(5)*. Finasteride also had the known effect of shrinking the size of the prostate *(4)*. This shrinkage could affect prostate cancer detection in ways that were not known. It was unclear whether this prostate shrinkage would introduce a DRE-detection bias that would favor the finasteride or the placebo group. In a simple finasteride versus placebo study that relied only on cancer detection using community defined standard methods, it was possible that finasteride administration could affect how prostate cancers were detected by both PSA *and* DRE. For these reasons, it was not possible to rely on the difference in cancer detection in general practice using PSA and DRE over the 7-year course of the study. These "interim" or "for cause" cancers, as they were termed in the PCPT, could be affected by significant detection biases.

The increasing use of PSA in the community to monitor for prostate cancer led to a decision that men on the trial would have their PSA levels analyzed yearly. However, because of the lowering effect of finasteride and the need for the study to remain blinded, the analyses needed to be performed by a central laboratory with the result adjusted for treatment prior to reporting from the SWOG Statistical Center. The central laboratory performed the pre-enrollment and annual PSA values. Each participant had his serum drawn and PSA analyzed prior to enrollment and annually thereafter. The enrollment PSA value was used to determine eligibility ($\leq 3.0$ ng/ml) and the annual PSA was used as a monitoring tool for the detection of prostate cancers that might occur before the end-of-study biopsy. Finasteride lowers the PSA value by approximately 50%. During the planning stages of the trial, the standard was that PSA values of >4 ng/ml prompted a prostate biopsy. Due to the lowering effect of finasteride, a PSA value of approximately > 2 ng/ml would prompt a recommendation for a biopsy for those participants on finasteride. The Statistical Center reported the biopsy recommendation based on the (adjusted) PSA value of >4.0 ng/ml and if a biopsy was recommended, also reported the adjusted value to the Sites. If the participant had a biopsy and the result was negative, future biopsy recommendations were made if the PSA had risen 50% above the value that prompted the recommendation of the original biopsy or if the adjusted PSA value was > 10 ng/ml. Based on DSMC review of the indexing (adjustment) value and the rates of biopsy recommendations in the two study groups, and a trend of decreasing biopsy recommendations (due to both PSA and DRE), the initial indexing PSA value was changed from 2.0 to 2.3 at the participant's 4th year on study *(4)*.

Even with the monitoring and the change in the PSA adjustment factor, there was still the inability to completely control the number of biopsy recommendations during routine clinical follow-up over the course of the study. Therefore, the interim prostate cancer rate was not an acceptable endpoint for this trial. The results of such an analysis would be un-interpretable due to known and other potential biases. Ultimately, the only method to avoid these biases was determined to be an end-of-study (EOS) biopsy for all participants after 7 years of study treatment. EOS biopsy was recommended for all men who reached the 7-year mark without a prostate cancer diagnosis regardless of whether or not they had an elevated PSA or abnormal DRE (Fig. 2).

One critical assumption regarding PSA in the PCPT was that finasteride would produce a monotonic downward shift of PSA – that is, the indexing factor would work equally across all men on finasteride so that it "preserved the rank" of a man's PSA

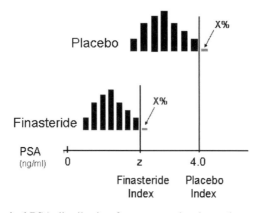

**Fig. 2.** Theoretical PSA distribution for men on placebo and men on finasteride.

value when compared to the rank of all the other men. The monotonic shift assumption must be qualified by the fact that an unknown fraction of the men will have a PSA change due to physiologic changes that are independent of finasteride and the variability in the PSA measurement itself. On average, a PSA level is reduced by 50% but for an individual man, there is a range of how much the PSA value is reduced. This was evaluated by examining normalized rank plots for the placebo and finasteride groups. These plots can be seen in Goodman et al. *(4)*. The conclusion based on examining these plots was that the assumption of monotonicity appeared to be reasonable in the PCPT.

It became apparent that prior to releasing PSA results to a study site, adherence to study drug and potential off-study use of finasteride needed to be determined. CRAs were instructed to assess adherence to study drug in the immediate 2-week period prior to the blood draw. If the participant was non-adherent (took less than one pill in the 2 weeks prior to the blood draw) or had any other condition that could have affected PSA, they were instructed to delay the blood draw. The pill count data for men who had an elevated PSA were also reviewed by a data coordinator at the Statistical Center prior to release of the PSA result to ensure that the adjustment factor had been correctly applied.

Figure 3 displays the trend of biopsy recommendations, either from PSA or DRE, over time for each arm. The figure demonstrates that in the 2nd and 3rd years, there were a decreasing number of biopsy recommendations for men receiving finasteride (an individual may be represented more than once). Had the PSA index not been changed at year 4, there would have been 222 fewer biopsy recommendations in the finasteride study group. The number of biopsy recommendations averaged 471 per arm per year with a low of 367 and a high of 553. The total number of biopsy recommendations, including men at year 7 (end-of-study) was 3,309 recommendations in 2,122 men on finasteride and 3,544 biopsy recommendations in 2,348 men on placebo ($p = 0.29$ for difference in total number of prompts; $p = 0.10$ in number of men) *(4)*.

In addition to trying to equalize the number of interim biopsies, and thus chances for prostate cancer detection in each group by adjusting the PSA values in the finasteride

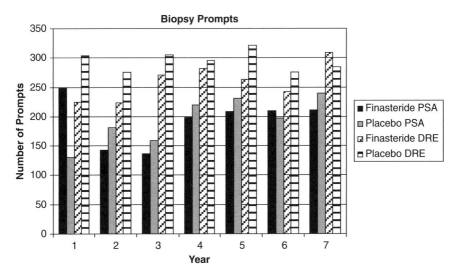

**Fig. 3.** Biopsy prompts over time by type of prompt and treatment arm on PCPT.

group, an important consideration was whether or not the men being prompted for a biopsy were comparable in the two study groups. The men prompted for a biopsy were also compared in terms of reason for biopsy prompt and baseline characteristics. See *(4)* for more details. While an attempt was made to equalize the total number of interim biopsy recommendations in the two study arms, another potential source of bias was a differential interim biopsy refusal rate and the reasons for biopsy refusal. It was necessary to assume that the factors affecting loss to biopsy would be the same in both groups of the study. This was important because we needed to lose participants in as comparable a manner as possible in the two arms. The reasons that interim biopsies were not done included participant (and primary care physician) refusal, death, and loss of participant to follow-up.

The reasons that interim biopsies were refused are equally distributed on the two arms *(4)*. There had been some concern that for participants on finasteride, an additional repeat PSA test done outside of the PCPT would be done. Such PSA values would not have been adjusted for the finasteride effect and could have appeared in the normal range. This does not appear to have happened as the number of refusals due to "Negative Repeat Test" is equal on the two treatment arms. Overall, the completion rates were 49.0% on finasteride and 52.3% on placebo.

Presented in Fig. 4 are the annual percent of for-cause biopsy prompts by either an elevated PSA or abnormal DREs that were performed. In the first year, approximately 62% of the biopsies were performed on both arms and this percent decreased over time to a low of approximately 40% at year 6. At year 7, over 80% of for-cause biopsies (in addition to being an end-of-study biopsy) were done, most likely because this was also the required end-of-study biopsy time point.

Even with the vigilant PSA indexing procedure that was in place, it was possible that PSA could be more or less sensitive in men on finasteride versus placebo. In that

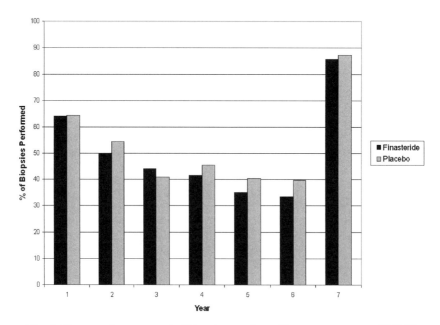

**Fig. 4.** Percent of recommended biopsies conducted by treatment arm of PCPT.

situation, the probability to detect prostate cancer or high-grade disease would have been different on the two treatment arms. The question of differential sensitivity of PSA is the topic of the next section.

## THE EFFECT OF FINASTERIDE ON PSA'S ABILITY TO DETECT PROSTATE CANCER

Several observations from PCPT data have suggested that the increase in high-grade disease (Gleason grade 7 or higher) may have been the effect of detection bias rather than a change in the biology of the disease. As noted in the introduction of this chapter, subjects in the finasteride group who underwent a for-cause biopsy had more high-grade tumors diagnosed ($n = 188$) than subjects in the placebo group ($n = 148$), whereas the numbers of biopsies revealing high-grade disease in the end-of-study biopsies were similar in the two groups ($n = 92$ for finasteride, $n = 89$ for placebo group) (1). The increased hazard ratio for high-grade tumor detection with finasteride appeared early in the study and did not increase with time (1). These observations raise the possibility that the increased detection of high-grade disease by PSA- and DRE-prompted biopsies in the finasteride group could have been due in part to the higher sensitivity of the PSA test for high-grade disease in the finasteride group. Thompson, Chi, Ankerst et al. (6) analyzed the results of prostate cancer detection in PCPT participants to determine whether finasteride treatment may have affected the performance characteristics of PSA as a diagnostic test.

Their analysis included all participants in the placebo and finasteride groups who underwent prostate biopsy at any of the seven annual visits, were on treatment at the time of the PSA measurement, and had a PSA measure and DRE within 1 year prior to the biopsy. For participants with multiple biopsies, the most recent biopsy was used. The receiver operating characteristics (ROC) of PSA for the placebo and finasteride groups were summarized in terms of the sensitivity and specificity for a number of cutoff values of PSA, and the ROC curve was calculated for prostate cancer versus no prostate cancer, for Gleason grade 7 or higher prostate cancer versus Gleason grade less than 7 or no prostate cancer, and for Gleason grade 8 or higher prostate cancer versus Gleason grade less than 8 or no prostate cancer. The sensitivity was defined as the proportion of men with prostate cancer whose PSA value exceeded each cutoff value, and the specificity as the proportion of men without prostate cancer whose PSA value was equal to or less than each cutoff value.

A total of 5,676 men in the finasteride group had at least one biopsy during study, either for-cause or as required at the end of study. Of these men, 357 were excluded from this analysis because no PSA or DRE result within a year of biopsy was available, and 740 were excluded because they were off-treatment when their PSA level was measured. A total of 5,947 men in the placebo group had at least one biopsy during the study; 360 of these men were excluded from this analysis because of a missing PSA or DRE result and 475 because they were off-treatment when their PSA was measured. Therefore, 4,579 men in the finasteride group (3,584 with a for-cause biopsy and 995 with an end-of-study biopsy) and 5,112 men in the placebo group (3,967 with a for-cause biopsy and 1,145 with an end-of-study biopsy) were included in the analysis.

Thompson, Chi, Ankerst et al. (6) provide a comparison of the participants included in their analysis and those that were excluded (Table 1). In both the finasteride and

Table 1
Characteristics of Participants in the Prostate Cancer Prevention Trial Who Were Included and Not Included in the PSA ROC Analysis*

| Characteristic | Placebo group | | Finasteride group | |
| --- | --- | --- | --- | --- |
| | Included (n = 5,112) | Not included (n = 4,347) | Included (n = 4,579) | Not included (n = 4,844) |
| Age at baseline (years) | | | | |
| Less than 60 | 1,654 (32.4) | 1,303 (30.0) | 1,433 (31.3) | 1,522 (31.4) |
| 60–64 | 1,589 (31.1) | 1,235 (28.4) | 1,472 (32.1) | 1,498 (30.9) |
| 65–69 | 1,189 (23.3) | 1,032 (23.7) | 1,043 (22.8) | 1,067 (22.0) |
| 70 or older | 680 (13.3) | 777 (17.9) | 631 (13.8) | 757 (15.6) |
| | $p < 0.001$ | | $p = 0.07$ | |
| Family history of prostate cancer | | | | |
| No | 4,256 (83.3) | 3,748 (86.2) | 3,843 (83.9) | 4,122 (85.1) |
| Yes | 856 (16.7) | 599 (13.8) | 736 (16.1) | 722 (14.9) |
| | $p < 0.001$ | | $p = 0.12$ | |
| Race | | | | |
| White | 4,893 (95.7) | 4,035 (92.8) | 4,355 (95.1) | 4,533 (93.6) |
| African American | 158 (3.1) | 202 (4.6) | 168 (3.7) | 204 (4.2) |
| Other | 61 (1.2) | 106 (2.4) | 56 (1.2) | 103 (2.1) |
| Missing | 0 (0.0) | 4 (0.1) | 0 (0.0) | 4 (0.1) |
| | $p < 0.001$ | | $p = 0.001$ | |
| No. of PSA measures[†] | | | | |
| 0 | 0 (0.0) | 500 (11.5) | 0 (0.0) | 614 (12.7) |
| 1–3 | 210 (4.1) | 1,111 (25.6) | 144 (3.1) | 1,327 (27.3) |
| 4–6 | 849 (16.6) | 1,697 (39.0) | 738 (16.1) | 1,704 (35.2) |
| ≥7 | 4,053 (79.3) | 1,039 (23.9) | 3,697 (80.7) | 1,199 (24.8) |
| | $p < 0.001$ | | $p < 0.001$ | |

**Table 1**
**(Continued)**

| Characteristic | Placebo group | | Finasteride group | |
|---|---|---|---|---|
| | Included (n = 5,112) | Not included (n = 4347) | Included (n = 4579) | Not included (n = 4844) |
| No. of DRE measures[‡] | | | | |
| 0 | 0 (0.0) | 486 (11.2) | 0 (0.0) | 599 (12.4) |
| 1–3 | 201 (3.9) | 1,118 (25.7) | 141 (3.1) | 1,320 (27.3) |
| 4–6 | 760 (14.9) | 1,693 (38.9) | 606 (13.2) | 1,753 (36.2) |
| ≥7 | 4,151 (81.2) | 1,050 (24.2) | 3,832 (83.7) | 1,172 (24.2) |
| | $p < 0.001$ | | $p < 0.001$ | |
| Reason for biopsy | | | | |
| End-of-study | 3,967 (77.6) | | 3,584 (78.3) | |
| For-cause | 1,145 (22.4) | | 995 (21.7) | |
| No. of previous biopsies | | | | |
| 0 | 4,393 (85.9) | | 3,962 (86.5) | |
| ≥1 | 719 (14.1) | | 617 (13.5) | |
| ≥2 | 127 (2.5) | | 107 (2.3) | |
| Age at biopsy (years) | | | | |
| Less than 60 | 35 (0.7) | | 36 (0.8) | |
| 60-64 | 1,061 (20.8) | | 902 (19.7) | |
| 65-69 | 1,595 (31.2) | | 1,416 (30.9) | |
| 70 or older | 2,421 (47.4) | | 2,225 (48.6) | |

*Comparisons between included and not included participants and are from chi-square test.
[†] $p = 0.03$ from chi-square for placebo included men versus finasteride included men.
[‡] $p = 0.003$ for placebo included men versus finasteride included men.

placebo groups, there were statistically significantly greater proportions of white participants in the included group than in the not-included group. In both treatment groups, there was more screening among the men included in the analysis, and there were slightly more screens (PSA and DRE) performed in the finasteride group than in the placebo group. There were no statistically significant differences between the included men in the finasteride and placebo groups with respect to age at study entry, family history, or race (*p*-values not shown). The two treatment groups also did not differ in terms of proportions of the biopsies that were performed for the two reasons (i.e., for cause or end of study), number of previous biopsies, and age at biopsy.

Of the 5,112 men in the placebo group included in their analysis, 1,111 (21.7%) were diagnosed with prostate cancer. Information on tumor grade was available for 1,100 of these men, of whom 240 had Gleason score 7 or higher (21.8% of evaluable cancers) and 55 had Gleason score 8 or greater (5% of evaluable cancers). Of the 4,579 men who received finasteride, 695 (15.2%) were diagnosed with prostate cancer. Information on tumor grade was available for 686 of these men, of whom 264 had Gleason score 7 or higher (38.5% of evaluable cancers) and 81 had Gleason score 8 or higher (11.8% of evaluable cancers).

Comparisons between the finasteride and placebo groups of the ROC curves of PSA for detection of prostate cancer versus no prostate cancer, of Gleason grade $\geq 7$ versus Gleason grade $\leq 6$ or no cancer, and of Gleason grade $\geq 8$ versus Gleason grade $\leq 7$ or no cancer (Fig. 5) showed that in every case the AUCs of PSA were greater for the finasteride group than the placebo group. For detection of prostate cancer overall, the AUCs were 0.757 in the finasteride group and 0.681 in the placebo group ($p < 0.001$); for detection of Gleason grade $\geq 7$ disease, the AUCs were 0.838 and 0.781, respectively ($p = 0.003$), and for detection of Gleason grade $\geq 8$ disease, the AUCs were 0.886 and 0.824, respectively ($p = 0.071$).

Thompson, Chi, Ankerst et al. *(6)* compared the specificities and sensitivities of a series of PSA cutoffs for detecting the three categories of disease – prostate cancer, Gleason $\geq 7$ prostate cancer, and Gleason $\geq 8$ prostate cancer – in the placebo and finasteride arms (Table 2). For the placebo group commonly used PSA cutoffs were used; for the finasteride group cutoffs were matched to obtain the same specificities as the placebo group. Finasteride reduces PSA by an unknown, possibly nonlinear factor exceeding 50% *(7)*. In order to make an accurate comparison between sensitivities, and to correspond to vertical differences between the ROC curves, the PSA cutoffs for the finasteride group were defined as those that yielded the same specificity as the corresponding PSA cutoffs for the placebo group (see Table 2). An adjustment for verification bias was not made by the investigators because in an earlier analysis of the placebo arm PSA properties, AUCs with and without verification bias adjustment were practically identical *(8)*, probably due in large part to the end-of-study biopsy for the PCPT.

The PSA cutoff of 4.0 ng/ml in the placebo group and the matched cutoff in the finasteride group achieved specificities exceeding 90% for each of the three categories of prostate cancer. However, the sensitivities of PSA were uniformly greater in the finasteride group: 37.8, 53.0, and 64.2% for prostate cancer, Gleason grade $\geq 7$ disease, and Gleason grade $\geq 8$ disease, respectively, compared with 24.0, 39.2, and 49.1%, respectively, in the placebo arm.

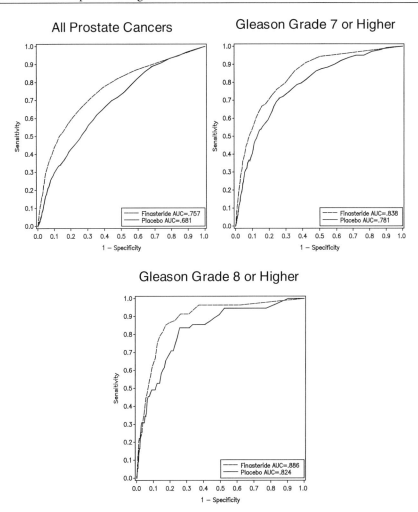

**Fig. 5.** Receiver operating characteristic (ROC) curves for PSA detection of all prostate cancer and high-grade cancer.

Thompson, Chi, Ankerst et al.'s analysis of PCPT data found that finasteride introduces detection bias for both prostate cancer and for high-grade prostate cancer by increasing the sensitivity of PSA for these endpoints. They suggest that the statistically significantly greater AUC for detection of prostate cancer overall as well as for detection of high-grade disease in men treated with finasteride is important for two reasons: (1) it is unusual for a single factor to statistically significantly improve the AUC of PSA and (2) the effect of finasteride on the sensitivity of PSA may have been at least in part responsible for the increased detection of high-grade disease that was observed in the PCPT.

It is well known in the medical community that higher PSA values in healthy men are more often associated with benign prostate conditions (e.g., prostatitis and benign prostatic hyperplasia) than with prostate cancer *(9)*. Because finasteride reduces the symptoms of BPH, and initiation of finasteride therapy causes a substantial fall in PSA,

Table 2

Sensitivity of PSA on Placebo and Finasteride for Detection of Prostate Cancer,
Gleason ≥ 7 Grade Disease, and Gleason ≥ 8 Grade Disease in the Placebo and
Finasteride Arms of the PCPT for Standard PSA Cutoffs and Finasteride Cutoffs
Chosen to Match PSA Specificities in the Placebo Group

| PSA placebo cutoff (mg/ml) | PSA finasteride (unadjusted) | Specificity of placebo and finasteride♣ | Sensitivity of placebo | 95% CI Sensitivity of placebo | Sensitivity of finasteride | 95% CI sensitivity of finasteride |
|---|---|---|---|---|---|---|
| \multicolumn{7}{c}{Prostate cancer versus no prostate cancer} |
| 1.0 | 0.4 | 40.8 | 81.8 | (79.5, 84.1) | 86.8 | (84.3, 89.3) |
| 1.5 | 0.6 | 59.0 | 67.0 | (64.2, 69.8) | 77.3 | (74.2, 80.4) |
| 2.0 | 0.9 | 71.2 | 53.5 | (50.6, 56.4) | 66.0 | (62.5, 69.5) |
| 2.5 | 1.1 | 80.0 | 42.8 | (39.9, 45.7) | 56.8 | (53.1, 60.5) |
| 3.0 | 1.2 | 85.4 | 35.0 | (32.2, 37.8) | 52.2 | (48.5, 55.9) |
| 4.0 | 1.6 | 92.7 | 24.0 | (21.5, 26.5) | 37.8 | (34.2, 41.4) |
| 6.0 | 2.8 | 98.1 | 5.1 | (3.8, 6.4) | 13.8 | (11.2, 16.4) |
| 8.0 | 3.7 | 99.2 | 2.0 | (1.2, 2.8) | 6.6 | (4.8, 8.4) |
| 10.0 | 5.6 | 99.6 | 0.8 | (0.3, 1.3) | 2.9 | (1.7, 4.1) |
| \multicolumn{7}{c}{Gleason ≥ 7 cancer versus Gleason ≤ 6 or no prostate cancer} |
| 1.0 | 0.4 | 37.3 | 92.1 | (88.7, 95.5) | 95.5 | (93.0, 98.0) |
| 1.5 | 0.6 | 55.2 | 83.8 | (79.1, 88.5) | 90.9 | (87.4, 94.4) |
| 2.0 | 0.9 | 67.9 | 75.0 | (69.5, 80.5) | 79.5 | (74.6, 84.4) |
| 2.5 | 1.1 | 77.2 | 66.7 | (60.7, 72.7) | 72.0 | (66.6, 77.4) |
| 3.0 | 1.2 | 82.9 | 56.7 | (50.4, 63.0) | 67.8 | (62.2, 73.4) |
| 4.0 | 1.6 | 90.5 | 39.2 | (33.0, 45.4) | 53.0 | (47.0, 59.0) |
| 6.0 | 3.0 | 97.9 | 11.7 | (7.6, 15.8) | 19.3 | (14.5, 24.1) |
| 8.0 | 4.1 | 99.1 | 4.2 | (1.7, 6.7) | 9.5 | (6.0, 13.0) |
| 10.0 | 6.5 | 99.6 | 1.7 | (0.1, 3.3) | 4.2 | (1.8, 6.6) |
| \multicolumn{7}{c}{Gleason ≥ 8 cancer versus Gleason ≤ 7 or no prostate cancer} |
| 1.0 | 0.4 | 36.3 | 94.5 | (88.5, 100.5) | 96.3 | (92.2, 100.4) |
| 1.5 | 0.6 | 53.8 | 89.1 | (80.9, 97.3) | 96.3 | (92.2, 100.4) |
| 2.0 | 0.9 | 66.4 | 85.5 | (76.2, 94.8) | 91.4 | (85.3, 97.5) |
| 2.5 | 1.1 | 75.7 | 78.2 | (67.3, 89.1) | 87.7 | (80.5, 94.9) |
| 3.0 | 1.2 | 81.5 | 67.3 | (54.9, 79.7) | 86.4 | (78.9, 93.9) |
| 4.0 | 1.7 | 89.5 | 49.1 | (35.9, 62.3) | 64.2 | (53.8, 74.6) |
| 6.0 | 3.2 | 97.7 | 25.5 | (14.0, 37.0) | 22.2 | (13.1, 31.3) |
| 8.0 | 4.3 | 99.0 | 9.1 | (1.5, 16.7) | 13.6 | (6.1, 21.1) |
| 10.0 | 7.3 | 99.6 | 3.6 | (0.0, 8.5) | 3.7 | (0.0, 7.8) |

♣ Confidence intervals for specificities were on average within 0.9% (and at most 1.5%) of the estimates reported in the table for both finasteride and placebo. CI = confidence interval, PSA= prostate-specific antigen, PCPT = Prostate Cancer Prevention Trial.

finasteride treatment could be used to enhance detection of prostate cancer in the general population. Finasteride treatment of men with elevated PSA levels would cause the greatest fall in men with benign conditions such as benign prostatic hyperplasia while men with persistently elevated PSA levels would have a higher probability of cancer. The men with higher PSA levels in the group receiving finasteride would therefore more likely have cancer and, from the PCPT analyses, these higher PSA levels are also more likely to reflect presence of high-grade cancer *(6,10)*.

## LONG-TERM EFFECTS OF FINASTERIDE ON PSA

In the previous section, we summarized the results of Thompson, Chi, Ankerst et al. that a single PSA measure within 1 year prior to biopsy is better at predicting prostate cancer and high-grade disease when the subject is taking finasteride compared to placebo. A natural follow-up question might ask what the longitudinal pre-diagnostic PSA trajectory looks like for those who are subsequently diagnosed with prostate cancer compared to those who were cancer-free at the end of the PCPT, and what impact does finasteride have?

As previously described, initial results indicated that finasteride causes an average 50% reduction in PSA by 1 year following initiation of treatment *(4)*. This 50% reduction appeared to apply also at the individual level, leading to the "multiply by 2" rule which recommends that PSA levels in men on finasteride be doubled before being compared with standard reference ranges. Given this information, the PCPT initially adopted the "multiply by 2" rule for the purpose of interpreting annual PSA measurements in men on the intervention arm of the trial. However, on the basis of the goal of an equal percentage of interim biopsies within each study arm, the factor was changed to 2.3 in the 4th year of the study *(4)*.

The PCPT provided a unique opportunity to study the impact of finasteride in a large sample, not restricted to men with BPH, which also had some minority representation and a range of Gleason scores. The 7-year duration of the trial also allowed for the examination of the effects of finasteride on PSA levels over a much longer period of follow-up than previous studies.

Etzioni et al. *(7)* conducted an analysis to estimate the long-term effects of finasteride on PSA levels in men with and without a prostate cancer diagnosis over the course of the PCPT. Serial PSA levels from participants in the PCPT who had either an end-of-study biopsy (928 cancer cases and 8,620 men with a negative biopsy) or an interim diagnosis of prostate cancer (671 cases) were analyzed. Linear mixed effects regression models were fit to the longitudinal PSA values beginning 1 year after randomization.

To be included in the analysis, participants must have had at least two PSA measurements beyond baseline while continuously on treatment and have had either an interim diagnosis of prostate cancer or an end-of-study biopsy. Prostate cancer cases were defined as either interim cases (i.e., diagnosed as a result of a positive screening test), or end-of-study cases, i.e., detected by an end-of-study biopsy that was conducted in the absence of a positive screening test. Participants with a positive PSA test at the end of the 7th year of the study were included with the interim cases. Interim cases were further subdivided into two groups: those whose cancer was detected following a positive PSA test (PSA-detected), and those whose cancer was detected in the absence of a positive PSA test (non-PSA-detected). PSA levels below the lower limit of detectability (i.e., 0.3 ng/ml) were set to this value.

A linear, mixed-effects model was fit to the logarithm of the longitudinal PSA values beginning at 12 months following randomization. The model allowed for individual-specific baseline levels of PSA as well as individual-specific PSA velocities, thereby accounting for the correlation between serial observations from the same person. Separate models were fit to subjects with negative end-of-study biopsies (non-cases), positive end-of-study biopsies (end-of-study cases), and cases diagnosed before the end-of-study biopsies (interim diagnoses). For prostate cancer cases with more than 4 years of PSA measurements, they used data from only the last 4 years so as to focus on that part of the PSA trajectory that was most relevant to the disease process. In the models fit to interim diagnoses, the final PSA measurement was omitted, due to the biopsy recommendation being dependent on this value. Terms were included after controlling for family history to allow the effect of finasteride on PSA to differ by race (Black or other vs. White) and, for models fit to cancer cases, Gleason grade (less than 7 vs. greater than or equal to 7).

The longitudinal analysis consisted of 928 subjects with disease diagnosed at the end-of-study biopsy, 671 interim diagnoses, and 8,620 subjects with a negative end-of-study biopsy. Within each disease status group, the number of PSA measurements was balanced across study arms (data not shown – see (7) for subject characteristics). Race

Table 3
Linear Mixed-Effect Model Results. Estimates are from Linear
Regression of Log(PSA) on Treatment Group, Time, Family History,
Race, and for Those with Prostate Cancer, High-Grade Status

| Variable | Coefficient | $p$-Value |
|---|---|---|
| *Diagnosed positive at end-of-study biopsy (last 4 PSAs in 928 pts)* | | |
| Finasteride | −0.916 | < 0.0001 |
| Time | 0.048 | < 0.0001 |
| High grade | −0.059 | 0.476 |
| Family history | 0.026 | 0.717 |
| Age | 0.006 | 0.065 |
| Black race | 0.099 | 0.047 |
| Other race# | −0.095 | 0.044 |
| Time×finasteride | 0.007 | 0.450 |
| Time×high grade | 0.058 | < 0.0001 |
| *Diagnosed positive at interim biopsy (last 4 PSAs excluding final PSA in 671 pts)* | | |
| Finasteride | −0.872 | < 0.0001 |
| Time | 0.079 | < 0.0001 |
| High grade | −0.092 | 0.132 |
| Family history | −0.001 | 0.985 |
| Age | −0.006 | 0.166 |
| Black race | 0.045 | 0.355 |
| Other race# | −0.083 | 0.060 |
| Time×finasteride | 0.019 | 0.179 |
| Time×high grade | 0.086 | < 0.0001 |
| *Negative at the end of study biopsy (8620 pts)* | | |
| Finasteride | −0.596 | < 0.0001 |
| Time | 0.031 | < 0.0001 |
| Family history | 0.085 | < 0.0001 |
| Age | 0.007 | < 0.0001 |
| Black race | 0.022 | 0.255 |
| Other race# | 0.002 | 0.879 |
| Time×finasteride | −0.049 | < 0.0001 |

# Hispanic, black Hispanic, Asian or Pacific Islander, or American Indian.

did not show consistent associations with PSA levels across disease status groups. Age and family history were significantly associated with PSA level only among subjects with a negative biopsy at the end of the study.

In Table 3, PSA growth was significantly associated with grade as evidenced by significant time×high grade interaction terms in the models ($p < 0.001$ for both interim diagnoses and end-of-study cases).

Table 4 shows that in placebo group subjects, PSA levels generally increased over time ($p < 0.01$), with a median annual increase of 3% for non-cases, 6% for end-of-study cases. The increased growth rate among interim diagnoses appeared to be driven mostly by PSA-detected cases, who had a median annual PSA increase of 12%, in contrast to non-PSA-detected cases, who had a median annual PSA increase of only 6%.

PSA increased faster among men with high-grade disease than among men with low-grade disease; among interim diagnoses on the placebo arm, high-grade cases diagnosed by an increased PSA had an estimated annual increase of 17% while low-grade cases had an annual increase of 9%. Similarly, among cases on the placebo arm who were detected at the end-of-study biopsy, high-grade cases had an estimated annual increase of 11% while the annual change in low-grade cases was only 5%.

Table 4
Estimated Annual Percent Change in PSA: End-of-Study Cases, Non-cases, and
Interim Cases (Stratified by Whether There was a PSA Prompt)

| Arm | Grade | Coefficient ($b$) | Exp($b$) | Annual change (95% CI) |
|---|---|---|---|---|
| *End-of-study cases (last 4 PSAs in 928 pts)* | | | | |
| Placebo | High | 0.106 | 1.110 | 11% (8, 15) |
| Placebo | Low | 0.048 | 1.049 | 5% (4, 6) |
| Finasteride | High | 0.113 | 1.120 | 12% (7, 18) |
| Finasteride | Low | 0.055 | 1.057 | 6% (3, 9) |
| Overall placebo | – | 0.057 | 1.058 | 6% (4, 7) |
| Overall finasteride | – | 0.070 | 1.073 | 7% (4, 10) |
| *Negative on end-of-study biopsy (8620 noncases)* | | | | |
| Placebo | – | 0.031 | 1.032 | 3% (2.9, 4) |
| Finasteride | – | −0.018 | 0.982 | −2%(−2.0, −1.2) |
| *Diagnosed by increased PSA at interim biopsy (435 pts)* | | | | |
| Placebo | High | 0.159 | 1.172 | 17% (11, 24) |
| Placebo | Low | 0.089 | 1.093 | 9% (6, 12) |
| Finasteride | High | 0.211 | 1.235 | 24% (13, 35) |
| Finasteride | Low | 0.141 | 1.151 | 15% (9, 22) |
| Overall placebo | – | 0.116 | 1.123 | 12% (10, 15) |
| Overall finasteride | – | 0.184 | 1.202 | 20% (14, 27) |
| *Diagnosed by absence of increased PSA at interim biopsy (236 pts)* | | | | |
| Placebo | High | 0.081 | 1.084 | 8% (2, 15) |
| Placebo | Low | 0.058 | 1.060 | 6% (4, 8) |
| Finasteride | High | 0.027 | 1.027 | 2% (−7, 13) |
| Finasteride | Low | 0.004 | 1.004 | 0.4% (−5, 6) |
| Overall placebo | – | 0.062 | 1.063 | 6% (4, 9) |
| Overall finasteride | – | 0.010 | 1.010 | 1% (−5, 7) |

The impact of finasteride on PSA growth differed for cancer cases and subjects without cancer at the end of the study. Table 4 shows that among subjects without cancer, finasteride was associated with a general decline of approximately 2% per year in PSA levels. However, among all cancer cases on finasteride, the estimated annual change in PSA was positive; 15% for interim diagnoses (both with and without and increased PSA, data not shown), and 7% for end-of-study cases. As shown in Table 4, interim diagnoses detected by PSA had an estimated annual increase in PSA of 20%, in contrast to non-PSA-detected cases, who annual estimated change was only 1%.

The Etzioni analysis of PSA trajectories on PCPT indicates that PSA levels among men without cancer on finasteride continue, over time, to slowly diverge from those of men without cancer who are not taking finasteride. After 1 year, the median PSA level among placebo subjects without cancer is approximately twice that observed among treated subjects. However, after 7 years, the median PSA level for placebo subjects without cancer was 2.5 times that observed among treated subjects. The clinical implication of this finding is that men taking finasteride over the long-term may require a PSA adjustment factor that is greater than 2 in order to be comparable with what is generally considered to be the "normal range." These results support the PSA indexing strategy that was employed during the conduct of the PCPT; namely, that the doubling factor changed from 2.0 to 2.3 in the subject's 4th year on study.

The long-term decline in PSA levels among noncases taking finasteride contrasts with the slow increase in PSA levels among prostate cancer cases taking finasteride. Thus, in men with cancer, the increase in PSA due to disease progression overcame any decline associated with the effect of finasteride on prostate epithelium. This observation supports the previous summarized finding that PSA has greater sensitivity in the finasteride group. If a man's PSA continues to increase over time while he is on finasteride, he is more likely to have prostate cancer than a man with the same increasing PSA in the placebo group.

## REFERENCES

1. Thompson IM, Goodman PJ, Tangen CM, Lucia MS, Miller GJ, Ford LG, et al. (2003) The influence of finasteride on the development of prostate cancer. *N Engl J Med* **349**:215–224.
2. Feigl P, Blumenstein B, Thompson I, et al.(1995) Design of the Prostate Cancer Prevention Trial (PCPT). *Control Clin Trial* **16**:150–163.
3. Goodman PJ, Tangen CM, Crowley JJ, Carlin SM, Ryan A, Coltman CC, Ford LG, Thompson IM. (2004) Implementation of the prostate cancer prevention trial. *Control Clin Trial* **25**:203–222.
4. Goodman PJ, Thompson IM, Tangen CM, Crowley JJ, Ford LG, Coltman CA. (2006) The prostate cancer prevention trial: design, biases, and interpretation of study results. *J Urol* **175**:2234–2242.
5. Guess HA, Heyse JA, Gormley GG. (1993) The effect of finasteride on prostate specific antigen in men with benign prostatic hyperplasia. *Prostate* **22**:31–37.
6. Thompson IM, Chi C, Ankerst DP, Goodman PJ, Tangen CM, Lippman SM, Lucia MS, Parnes HL, Coltman CA. (2006) The effect of finasteride on the sensitivity of PSA for detecting prostate cancer. *J Natl Cancer Inst* **98(8)**:529–534.
7. Etzioni RD, Howlader N, Shaw PA, Ankerst DP, Penson DF, Goodman PG, Thompson IM. (2005*) J Urol* **174**:877–881.
8. Thompson IM, Ankerst DP, Chi C, Lucia MS, Goodman PJ, Crowley JJ, et al. (2005) Operating characteristics of prostate-specific antigen in a population with initial PSA of 3.0 ng/ml or lower. *JAMA* **294**:66–70.
9. Roehrborn CG, Boyle P, Gould AL, Waldstreicher J. (1999) Serum prostate-specific antigen as a predictor of prostate volume in men with benign prostatic hyperplasia. *Urology* **53**:581–589.
10. Handel LN, Agarwal S, Schiff SF, Kelty PJ, Cohen SI. (2006) Can effect of finasteride on prostate-specific antigen be used to decrease repeat prostate biopsy? *Urology* **68**(6):1220–1223.

# 25 The Selenium and Vitamin E Cancer Prevention Trial

*Eric A. Klein*

## Contents

## Summary

Prostate cancer is an attractive and appropriate target for primary prevention because of its incidence, prevalence, and disease-related mortality. Despite PSA-induced stage migration, a high cure rate for localized disease, and improved understanding of prostate cancer biology, most men who develop metastatic disease are still destined to die of prostate cancer. It seems self-evident that an effective prevention strategy would spare many men from this burden of diagnosis and cure. The molecular pathogenesis of prostate cancer also lends itself to a primary prevention strategy. Clinically evident prostate cancer is rare in men < 50 years old, while the precancerous lesion PIN (prostatic intraepithelial neoplasia) is apparent at autopsy in men < 30. Furthermore, the prevalence of PIN is similar in populations at much different risks of developing clinically evident cancer, suggesting that external environmental influences are important and potentially modifiable. This chapter will review the scientific and epidemiologic evidence supporting the role of selenium and vitamin E in the prevention of prostate cancer and the design of the Selenium and Vitamin E Cancer Prevention Trial.

**Key Words:** SELECT, Prostate cancer, Vitamin E, Selenium, Clinical trial, PCPT.

From: *Current Clinical Urology: Prostate Cancer Screening*, Edited by: D. P. Ankerst et al.
DOI 10.1007/978-1-60327-281-0_25 © Humana Press, a part of Springer Science+Business Media, LLC 2009

# INTRODUCTION

Despite the encouraging results seen in stage migration, high rates of cure, and mortality reduction for prostate cancer in the PSA era, the burden of therapy remains substantial. A recent study of complications after surgical therapy for localized disease in an unselected population-based cohort reported that at >18 months following radical prostatectomy, 8.4% of men were incontinent and 59.9% were impotent, while 41.9% reported that their sexual performance was a moderate-to-large problem (1). In a similarly designed study comparing outcomes after radiation to surgery, the radiation cohort reported an impotence rate of 61.5% and a substantially and statistically significantly higher incidence of bowel problems (2). While many single-institution studies have reported better results in highly selected cohorts of treated patients, it is clear that the majority of men treated for localized disease in the community pay a substantial price to be cured. While most studies have reported that most patients treated by radiation or surgery would in retrospect choose to have the same therapy again, it seems self-evident that an effective prevention strategy would spare many from this burden of cure. An effective strategy could be one which reduces the number of life-threatening, clinically evident cases or which works by causing a reduced age-dependent rate of development of the disease, i.e., the disease would become evident 5, 10, or 15 years later than it otherwise would occur.

Chemoprevention of prostate cancer is based on an understanding of the underlying molecular events which lead to neoplastic growth. A number of hypotheses regarding the pathogenesis of prostate cancer have led to several large clinical trials with oral agents meant to prevent its development. The use of nontraditional dietary supplements is widespread amongst men with prostate cancer and those who perceive themselves to be at risk, and the willingness to use such agents provides a ripe opportunity for their use in well-controlled clinical trials to determine if they are as effective as generally perceived.

In this chapter we review the epidemiologic and scientific rationale for the use of selenium and vitamin E for prevention of prostate cancer, as well as the design of the Selenium and Vitamin E Cancer Prevention Trial.

# SELENIUM

Selenium (Se) is an essential trace element occurring in both organic and inorganic forms. The organic form is found predominantly in grains, fish, meat, poultry, eggs, and dairy products and enters the food chain via plant consumption. There is marked geographic variability of Se in food related to local soil content. Typical dietary intake of Se in the USA is 80–120 μg/day, and the recommended daily allowance is 70 μg in adult men and 50 μg in adult women (3). In addition to dietary sources, Se is widely available as over-the-counter supplements and multivitamins, typically in doses of 20 μg for inorganic forms and 50–200 μg of organic Se in the form of selenized yeast or selenomethionine.

Se is widely distributed in body tissues and is an important constituent of antioxidant enzymes, including glutathione peroxidase (GPX1), selenoprotein-P, gastrointestinal glutathione peroxidase (GPX2), phospholipid hydroperoxide glutathione peroxidase (GPX4), and thioredoxin reductase. Both GPX1 and selenoprotein-P are highly expressed in the prostate. Se also subserves other functions, including thyroid hormone metabolism, where it acts as a co-factor to iodothyronine deiodinase which catalyzes the conversion of T4 to active T3, and reproductive function, where Se is important in testosterone metabolism and is a constituent of sperm capsule selenoprotein. Se deficiency can cause cardiomyopathy (Keshan disease) and arthritis (Kashin-Beck disease).

## *Epidemiology*

Many epidemiologic observations support the proposition that Se acts to protect against the development of some cancers. Shamberger and Frost were the first to observe that regional variation in cancer mortality in the USA correlates to dietary Se exposure *(4)*. Several small studies involving only a few cases of prostate cancer also suggested a protective effect based on pre-diagnostic serum Se levels *(5–7)*. Rayman observed that the increased incidence of prostate cancer in the United Kingdom in the 1990s paralleled a fall in mean blood Se levels and daily oral intake from 60 to 34 μg/d following a large-scale switch from high-Se containing wheat from the USA to Se-poor wheat from the European Union *(8)*.

Three placebo-controlled randomized trials in humans have further supported Se as an anticancer agent. In the Nutrition Intervention Trial conducted among more than 29,000 individuals aged 40–69 from the general population in Linxian, China, Se (50 μg/day) in combination with vitamin E (30 mg/day) and beta-carotene (15 mg/day) led to a 13% reduction in mortality from cancers at all sites and a 21% reduction in mortality from stomach cancer *(9)*. In the second trial, also conducted in Linxian, investigators tested the hypothesis that a multivitamin/mineral (including Se, 50 μg/day) plus beta-carotene (15 mg/day) would reduce the risk of esophageal/gastric cardia cancer in a population of more than 3,000 individuals with esophageal dysplasia *(10)*. In this population, total cancer mortality was 7% lower and esophageal cancer was 14% lower in the supplemented group. The independent effect of Se and the impact of supplementation on prostate cancers could not be evaluated in these trials because of the trial design and the small number of cases in the study population. In the third trial, Clark et al. performed a randomized, double-blinded trial in 1,312 subjects with a prior history of skin cancer to receive 200 μg/day of elemental Se in the form of selenized yeast or placebo *(11)*. With an average follow-up of 4.5 years there were no differences in rates of skin cancer. However, further analysis found that prostate cancer incidence was reduced by two-thirds among those in the Se supplemented group, with a hazard ratio (HR) of 0.35. Several other observations from this trial are also important *(12)*: (1) the effect was strongest for those participants with the lowest baseline serum Se levels; (2) the effect was strengthened when cases diagnosed within 2 years of study entry, presumed to be pre-existing, were excluded, with the HR dropping to 0.25; (3) the effect was strongest for participants < 65 years old at study entry; and (4) the effect was greater in those with low serum PSA level at study entry. There also were significant reductions in lung and colon cancer incidences in this trial. A recent update of the Clark trial added an additional 25 months of follow-up to the study cohort to reach a mean of 7.45 years *(13)*. Reanalysis of the effect of Se supplementation continues to show a marked reduction in the incidence of prostate cancer, with an HR of 0.51. As in the initial analysis, the effect was strongest for those with a PSA < 4 ng/ml and those with the lowest serum Se levels at study entry.

Several case–control studies also suggest a protective effect of Se against prostate cancer. In the Health Professionals Follow-up Study, with a mean of 7 years of follow-up, men in the highest quintile for toenail Se levels had the lowest risk of prostate cancer

(HR = 0.39), excluding those diagnosed in the first 2 years after study entry *(14)*. This trial also showed a decreased risk of advanced stage cancer, but this did not reach statistical significance. In the Honolulu Heart Program, 249 cases of incident prostate cancer were diagnosed during 12.4 years of follow-up of 9,345 Japanese–Americans. Compared to the lowest quartile, men in the highest quartile of serum Se at study entry had an HR = 0.50 for prostate cancer *(15)*. The effect was most marked for those with advanced stage disease at diagnosis, at least 5 years since study entry, and in current or former smokers. Vogt et al. reported similar protection of high serum Se levels in a study of 212 cases and 233 controls in both African-Americans and Caucasians, with a pooled HR = 0.71 *(16)*. In the Baltimore Longitudinal Study of Aging, serum Se levels were measured at a mean of 3.8 years prior to diagnosis in 52 cases and compared to 96 matched controls *(17)*. Those in the highest quartile had a markedly reduced incidence of prostate cancer compared to the lowest quartile, with an HR = 0.24. Serum Se levels were also noted to fall with age, in parallel with the increasing age-associated incidence of prostate cancer. Some large controlled studies, most notably CARET, have not found an association between blood or toenail Se and protection from prostate cancer, but none have shown an inverse risk *(18,19)*.

## *Basic Science*

Se inhibits tumorigenesis in a variety of experimental models *(20)*. Of the more than 100 reported studies in more than two dozen animal models, two-thirds have shown reductions in tumor incidence in response to Se supplementation. Se inhibits the growth of prostate cancer cell lines, including the androgen dependent lines DU-145, PC3, and the androgen independent line LnCaP *(21–23)*. There are a number of potential mechanisms proposed for the antitumorigenic effects of Se, including antioxidant effects, enhancement of immune function, induction of apoptosis, inhibition of cell proliferation, alteration of carcinogen metabolism, cytotoxicity of metabolites formed under high-Se conditions, and an influence on testosterone production *(24–28)*. As reviewed below, the most compelling evidence of Se's effects as a preventative agent come from recent observations demonstrating its effects on inducing cell cycle arrest and stimulation of apoptosis.

Ip has demonstrated that the monomethylated Se metabolite methylselenol is responsible for the antiproliferative effects of Se at the cellular level *(29)*. His work suggests that whether Se is ingested in organic or inorganic form, it must be metabolized to methylselenol to be biologically active *(30)*. Although the efficiency by which they are metabolized to methylselenol will vary, as a practical matter it is likely that any form of oral Se, including those such as selenized yeast or selenomethionine used in the Nutritional Prevention of Cancer Trial and the Selenium and Vitamin E Cancer Prevention Trial (SELECT) are likely to have similar biological effects.

Accumulating evidence suggests that Se works as a preventative agent by inhibiting important early steps in carcinogenesis. Using methylselenic acid (MSA), a rapidly metabolized precursor of methylselenol in a rat mammary cancer model, Dong has demonstrated that Se causes G1 cell cycle arrest, induction of apoptosis, and synchronous modulation of both growth-promoting and growth-inhibiting cell cycle markers including cyclins A and D1, p16 and p27 *(31)*. The net result was a reduction in the size of intraductal papillary lesions, suggesting that the combined effects inhibited clonal expansion of nascent tumors *(30)*. In another study of the effects of MSA, this group observed dose- and time-dependent growth inhibition and induction of apoptosis in the PC3 human prostate cancer cell line, and identified 12 clusters of Se-responsive genes *(32)*. MSA-induced cell cycle arrest was mediated in part by up-regulation of p19$^{INK4d}$and p21$^{WAF1}$ and down-regulation of CDK1, CDK2, and cyclin A. The proapoptotic effects of Se appeared to be modulated by up-regulation of cyclin D1, cdk5, and c-jun and down-regulation of AKT2 *(30,32)*. In similar studies, other investigators have demonstrated that (1) l-selenomethionine induces p21 and p27-mediated cell cycle arrest in the human LnCAP and PC3 cell lines and depends upon the presence of a functioning androgen receptor *(22,23)*; (2) the same compound stimulates anchorage-independent cell growth and preferentially promotes apoptosis in cancer cells compared to normal prostatic epithelium *(23)*; (3) l-selenomethionine regulates p53-dependent DNA repair mechanisms *(33)*; and (4) MSA and inorganic Se (selenite) mediate apoptosis by inhibition of NF-$\kappa$B transcription and activation *(34)*. Together these studies suggest that Se in various forms works early in the carcinogenic pathway by blocking cell proliferation and promoting cell death, and that its effects are mediated by a variety of well-defined molecular pathways.

In vivo studies also support the antitumorigenic role of Se in prostate cancer. Selenoprotein-P is an antioxidant defense protein highly expressed in prostatic epithelium and which binds a large percentage of plasma Se. Calvo has demonstrated marked down-regulation of selenoprotein-P during the carcinogenic evolution of low-grade PIN to invasive prostate cancer in a C3/Tag mouse transgenic model, low levels of selenoprotein-P in LnCAP and PC3 cell lines, and lower levels of this protein in human prostate cancers compared to normal prostatic tissue *(35)*. This work suggests that there is selective pressure during prostate carcinogenesis for loss of a protein that traps Se intracellularly, potentially allowing escape from its antiproliferative and proapoptotic effects. In a dog model, Waters demonstrated that oral Se in various forms given over 7 months as a dietary supplement resulted in lower levels of DNA damage in prostatic epithelial cells and increased intraprostatic apoptosis compared with controls *(36)*. In a study of 36 healthy men, selenized yeast with an equivalent of 247 µg Se/day taken over 9 months resulted in statistically significant increases in serum Se and glutathione levels, no change in serum testosterone and dihydrotestosterone (DHT) levels, and clinically insignificant changes in serum PSA levels *(37)*. The in vivo studies demonstrate that orally ingested Se modulates markers of oxidative stress relevant to the proposed molecular mechanisms of Se's protective effects.

In conclusion, there is robust epidemiologic and molecular evidence that Se in various forms suppresses cancer growth. The molecular evidence suggests that Se acts early in the carcinogenic process as an antiproliferative and proapoptotic agent and prevents clonal expansion of nascent tumors. These observations give strong scientific support to use of Se in the Selenium and Vitamin E Cancer Prevention Trial (SELECT).

## VITAMIN E

Vitamin E belongs to a family of naturally occurring, essential, fat-soluble vitamin compounds. Its importance in mammalian biology was first revealed by earlier fertility research *(38)*. Vitamin E functions as the major lipid-soluble antioxidant in cell membranes; it is a chain-breaking, free-radical scavenger and inhibits lipid peroxidation specifically, biologic activity relevant to carcinogen-induced DNA damage *(39)*.

The most active form of vitamin E is α-tocopherol; it is also among the most abundant and is widely distributed in nature and the predominant form in human tissues *(40,41)*.

## Basic Science

α-Tocopherol may influence the development of cancer through several mechanisms. It has a strong inherent potential for antioxidation of highly reactive and genotoxic electrophiles, such as hydroxyl, superoxide, lipid peroxyl and hydroperoxyl, and nitrogen radicals, thereby preventing propagation of free radical damage in biological membranes, and decreasing mutagenesis and carcinogenesis. Vitamin E also blocks nitrosamine formation. α-Tocopherol inhibits protein kinase-C activity and the proliferation of smooth muscle cells and melanoma cells *(42–45)*. Vitamin E also induces the detoxification enzyme NADPH:quinone reductase in cancer cell lines, and inhibits arachidonic acid and prostaglandin metabolism *(46,47)*. Effects on hormones which can increase cellular oxidative stress and proliferative activity and on cell-mediated immunity have also been reported.

Studies suggest that vitamin E can inhibit the growth of certain human cancer cell lines, including prostate, lung, melanoma, oral carcinoma, and breast, while animal experiments show prevention of various chemically induced tumors, including hormonally mediated tumors *(48–51)*. In the same studies, vitamin E has been shown to slow the growth of prostate tumors in vitro and in vivo in rats receiving various doses of chemotherapeutic agents.

## Epidemiology

The average dietary vitamin E intake among men and women in the USA is estimated to be 10 and 7 mg/day, respectively *(52,53)*. The recommended dietary allowance of the National Research Council is set at 10 mg for men and 8 mg for women daily *(54)*.

Evidence currently suggests that vitamin E status or intake is inversely related to risk of lung and colorectal cancers. Of the cohort studies of lung cancer, four of six reported that pre-diagnostic serum vitamin E level was lower in those who subsequently developed cancer compared to non-cases, and one reported no differences in baseline dietary intake between cases and non-cases, or a weakly protective association for supplemental vitamin E *(55–57)*. In two other cohorts, vitamin E intake was not associated with lung cancer *(58,59)*. Five prospective studies examined the association between serum α-tocopherol and colorectal cancer, and in general serum levels were lower in those who subsequently developed colorectal cancer as compared to non-cases: a pooled estimate of 40% lower risk has been reported for the highest as compared to the lowest category of serum α-tocopherol concentration *(60)*. By contrast, prospective studies show no association between dietary vitamin E intake and incidence of colon or colorectal cancer, although one of these among women in Iowa showed a 50% reduction in colon cancer incidence for vitamin E supplement use, and an estimated relative risk of 0.32 for the highest versus lowest quintile of vitamin E intake from diet plus supplements *(61,62)*. One case–control study conducted in Italy reported a significant inverse association for higher vitamin E intake or for ≥ 200 IU daily (versus none), while the findings from several others reveal no substantive relationship with colorectal cancer *(63–66)*.

Observational studies are inconsistent with regard to a beneficial association between serum vitamin E and prostate cancer. These studies have assessed cancer risk through estimated dietary intake or through determination of plasma or serum α-tocopherol concentrations. Of the few prospective studies having a sufficient number of prostate cancers for analysis, two reported no dose–response association, and one reported a statistically significant protective association *(67–69)*. A study of 2,974 subjects over a 17-year follow-up period found low α-tocopherol to be associated with higher prostate cancer risk *(70)*. These studies all noted lower serum or plasma vitamin E concentrations among prostate cancer cases years prior to diagnosis *(68–70)*. In a cohort analysis, the associations between prostate cancer and baseline serum and dietary α-tocopherol differed significantly according to the α-tocopherol intervention status, with the suggestion of a protective effect for total vitamin E intake among those men who also received α-tocopherol supplementation *(71)*. One case–control study reported no association between vitamin E intake and risk of prostate cancer *(72)*.

One large-scale randomized, placebo-controlled trial, the Alpha-Tocopherol, Beta-Carotene Cancer Prevention Trial (ATBC), supports the role of vitamin E in the prevention of prostate cancer. ATBC was a randomized, double-blind, placebo-controlled trial of α-tocopherol (50 mg synthetic *dl*-α-tocopheryl acetate daily) and beta-carotene (20 mg daily) (alone or in combination) among 29,133 male smokers 50–69 years old at entry *(73,74)*. During the median follow-up period of 6.1 years, there were 246 new cases and 64 deaths from prostate cancer. Among those assigned to the α-tocopherol arm ($n = 14,564$), there were 99 incident prostate cancers compared with 147 cases among those assigned to the non-α-tocopherol arm ($n=14,569$). This represented a statistically significant 32% reduction in prostate cancer incidence (95% confidence interval, 12–47%; $p = 0.002$). The observed preventive effect appeared stronger in clinically evident cases, where the incidence was decreased by 40% in subjects receiving α-tocopherol (95% confidence interval, –20 to –55%). Prostate cancer mortality data, though based on fewer events, suggested a similarly strong effect of 41% lower mortality (95% confidence interval, –1 to –64%). Although the incidence of prostate cancer was only a secondary endpoint in this trial, these findings suggest a potentially substantial benefit of α-tocopherol in reducing the risk of prostate cancer.

## SELECT – THE SELENIUM AND VITAMIN E CANCER PREVENTION TRIAL

The accumulated epidemiologic and biologic evidence that Se and vitamin E may prevent prostate cancer led to the design and launch of SELECT, The Selenium and Vitamin E Cancer Prevention Trial *(75)*. SELECT is an NCI-sponsored phase III, randomized, double-blind, placebo-controlled, population-based clinical trial designed to test the efficacy of selenium and vitamin E alone and in combination in the prevention of prostate cancer. The study has a $2 \times 2$ factorial design (Fig. 1) with a target accrual of 32,400. Eligibility criteria include age ≥ 50 years for African Americans, ≥ 55 years for Caucasians, a DRE not suspicious for cancer, serum PSA ≤ 4 ng/ml, and normal blood pressure. Randomization will be equally distributed among four study arms (selenium + placebo, vitamin E + placebo, selenium + vitamin E, and placebo + placebo). Study duration is planned for 12 years, with a minimum of 7 and a maximum of 12 years of intervention depending on the time of randomization. The study supplements consist of 200 μg of l-selenomethionine, 400 mg of racemic α-tocopheryl, and an optional multivitamin containing no selenium or vitamin E.

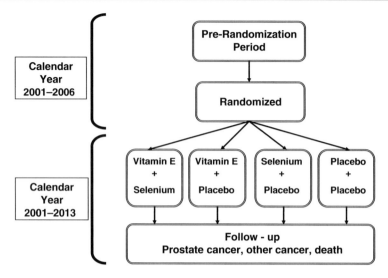

**Fig. 1.** SELECT schema.

The primary endpoint for SELECT is the clinical incidence of prostate cancer. Prostate biopsy will be performed at the discretion of study physicians according to local community standards based on abnormalities in DRE or elevations in serum PSA. Secondary endpoints will include prostate cancer-free survival, all cause mortality, and the incidence and mortality of other cancers and diseases potentially impacted by the chronic use of selenium and vitamin E. Other trial objectives include periodic quality of life assessments, assessment of serum micronutrient levels and prostate cancer risk, and studies of the evaluation of biological and genetic markers with the risk of prostate cancer. The study design will permit detection of a 25% reduction in the incidence of prostate cancer for selenium or vitamin E alone, with an additional 25% reduction for the combination of selenium and vitamin E compared to either agent alone. Since neither oral Se nor vitamin E is known to affect serum PSA, no PSA adjustments are planned.

SELECT accrued more than 35,000 men in 33 months from 428 sites throughout the USA, Puerto Rico, and Canada. SELECT was designed to be a large, simple trial that conforms as closely as possible with community standards of care for men in the SELECT age categories. The trial is expected to be complete by 2013.

## DIFFERENCES BETWEEN SELECT AND PCPT

The design of SELECT has some fundamental differences from the PCPT that impact on what will be learned from the trial about prostate cancer screening. First, neither selenium nor vitamin E is known to affect serum PSA levels, so that the adjustments in PSA necessitated by the use of 5-α-reductase inhibitors like finasteride are unnecessary in SELECT. Unlike the PCPT, where the presence or absence of prostate cancer was assessed by both "for cause" and "end of study biopsies", the primary endpoint of SELECT is the clinical incidence of prostate cancer as determined by routine clinical management. Furthermore, although acceptable PSA and DRE results were required at study entry, annual prostate cancer screening with PSA and DRE is not mandatory for SELECT participants as they were for PCPT. This design decision was made because the benefits of PSA and DRE screening were (and are) still a matter of debate and because community screening standards probably would continue to change over the 12 year course of the trial. During annual clinic visits, SELECT participants are encouraged to have PSA and DRE screening completed according to the standard of care at their study sites and their preference. This flexibility allows for prostate cancer to be diagnosed in the milieu of changing clinical practice. These changes include but are not likely to be limited to the following:

- Recent findings that prostate cancer risk is higher at lower PSA levels than previously thought *(76)*, which have altered screening standards and patterns of biopsy in the community;
- Broader use of nomograms *(77)* and risk calculators *(78)* which predict the individual likelihood of cancer on biopsy that were not available during PCPT and may lead to more selective use of biopsies by restricting them to men at the highest risk for or most worried about cancer;
- The use of new markers, such as EPCA2 *(79)* and ETS-related fusion proteins *(80)*, which may improve or replace PSA-based screening regimens;
- Results of large-scale screening trials, like the European Randomized Study of Screening for Prostate Cancer (ERSPC) *(81)*, which is expected to report initial results before SELECT reaches its primary endpoint;
- The recognition that use of finasteride improves the diagnostic accuracy of PSA *(82)*, which may change biopsy triggers in men using this drug for baldness or LUTS.

Furthermore, the performance characteristics of screening tests performed during the course of the trial will be affected by the fact that SELECT began in 2001, relatively late in the PSA era, when most men who entered the trial had already been screened at least once and after the substantial stage clinical and pathological migration induced by PSA had subsided *(83)*. Finally, it is known that African-Americans are at the highest risk world-wide of developing and dying of prostate cancer. SELECT accrual includes almost 20% African-Americans and other minority and medically underserved populations (as compared to 5% in PCPT), and will have a very large cohort of men from which to draw conclusions about the efficacy of screening in those at highest risk for prostate cancer.

## REFERENCES

1. Stanford JL, Feng Z, Hamilton AS, Gilliland FD, Stephenson RA, Eley JW, Albertsen PC, Harlan LC, Potosky AL: Urinary and sexual function after radical prostatectomy for clinically localized prostate cancer: the Prostate Cancer Outcomes Study. JAMA 2000;283:354–600.
2. Potosky AL, Legler J, Albertsen PC, Stanford JL, Gilliland FD, Hamilton AS, Eley JW, Stephenson RA, Harlan LC: Health outcomes after prostatectomy or radiotherapy for prostate cancer: results from the Prostate Cancer Outcomes Study. J Natl Cancer Inst 2000;92:1582–92.
3. National Academy of Sciences. Recommended Dietary Allowances, 10th ed. Washington, DC: National Academy Press, 217–24,1989.
4. Shamberger RJ, Frost DV: Possible protective effect of Se against human cancer. Canadian Med Association J 1969;100:682.
5. Knekt P, Aromaa A, Maatela J, et al.: Serum Se and subsequent risk of cancer among Finnish men and women. J Natl Cancer Inst 1990;82:864–68.
6. Willet WC, Polk BF, Morris JS, et al.: Prediagnostic serum Se and risk of cancer. Lancet 1983;2:130–34.
7. Coates RJ, Weiss NS, Daling JR, et al.: Serum levels of Se and retinol and subsequent risk of cancer. Am J Epidemiol 1988;128:515–23.

8. Rayman MP: Dietary Se: time to act. Brit Med J 1997;314:387.

9. Blot WJ, Li JY, Taylor PR, et al.: Nutrition intervention trials in Linxian, China: Supplementation with specific vitamin/mineral combinations, cancer incidence, and disease-specific mortality in the general population. J Natl Cancer Inst 1993;85:1483–92.

10. Li JY, Taylor PR, Li B, et al.: Nutrition intervention trials in Linxian, China: Multiple vitamin/mineral supplementation, cancer incidence, and disease-specific mortality among adults with esophageal dysplasia. J Natl Cancer Inst 1993;85:1492–98.

11. Clark, LC, Combs GF, Turnbull BW, et al.: Effects of Se supplementation for cancer prevention in patients with carcinoma of the skin. JAMA 1996;276:1957–63.

12. Clark LC, Dalkin B, Krongrad A, et al: Decreased incidence of prostate cancer with Se supplementation: results of a double-blind cancer prevention trial. British J Urol 1998;81:730–734.

13. Duffield-Lillico AJ, Dalkin BL, Reid ME, et al.: Se supplementation, baseline plasma Se status, and incidence of prostate cancer: an analysis of the complete treatment period of the nutritional prevention of cancer study group. British J Urol 2003;91:608–12.

14. Yoshizawa K, Willett WC, Morris SJ, et al: Study of prediagnostic Se level in toenails and the risk of advanced prostate cancer. J Natl Cancer Inst 1998;90:1219–24.

15. Nomura AMY, Lee J, Stemmermann GN, Combs GF: Serum Se and subsequent risk of prostate cancer. Cancer Epidemiol Biomarkers Prev 2000:9:883–7.

16. Vogt TM, Ziegler RG, Graubard BI, et al.: Serum Se and risk of prostate cancer in U.S. blacks and whites. Int J Cancer 2003;103:664–70.

17. Brooks JD, Metter EJ, Chan DW, et al.: Plasma Se level before diagnosis and the risk of prostate cancer development. J Urol 2001;166:2034–38.

18. Goodman GE, Schaffer ST, Bankson DD, et al.: Predictors of serum Se in cigarette smokers and the lack of association with lung and prostate cancer risk. Cancer Epidemiol Biomarkers Prev 2001;10:1069–76.

19. Ghardiran P, Maisonneuve P, Perret C, et al.: A case-control study of toenail Se and cancer of the breast, colon, and prostate. Cancer Detection Prevention 2000;24:305–13.

20. Combs GF Jr and Clark LC. Se and Cancer. In: Garewal H, ed. *Antioxidants and Disease Prevention*. New York: CRC Press, 1997.

21. Webber MM, Perez-Ripoli EA, James GT. Inhibitory effects of Se on the growth of DU-145 human prostate carcinoma cells in vitro. Biochem Biophys Res Commun 1985;130:603–9.

22. Venkateswaran V, Klotz LH, Fleshner N.E.: Se modulation of cell proliferation and cell cycle biomarkers in human prostate carcinoma cell lines. Cancer Res 2002;62: 2540–5.

23. Menter DG, Sabichi AL, Lippman SM: Se effects on prostate cell growth. Cancer Epidemiol Biomarkers Prev 2000;9:1171–82.

24. Ip C, Medina D. Current concepts of Se and mammary tumorigenesis. In: Medina D, Kidwell W, Heppner G, Anderson EP, eds. *Cellular and Molecular Biology of Breast Cancer*. New York: Plenum Press, 1987, p 479.

25. Kiremidjian-Schumacher L, Stotzky G. Review: Se and immune response. Environmental Res 1987;42:277–303.

26. Thompson HJ, Wilson A, Lu J, et al. Comparison of the effects of an organic and an inorganic form of Se on a mammary carcinoma cell line. Carcinogenesis 1994;15:183–6.

27. Redman C, Scott JA, Baines AT, et al.: Inhibitory effect of selenomethionine on the growth of three selected human tumor cell lines. Cancer Lett 1998;125:103–10.

28. Shimada T, El-Bayoumy K, Upadhyaya P, et al.: Inhibition of human cytochrome P450-catalyzed oxidations of xenobiotics and procarcinogens by synthetic organoSe compounds. Cancer Res 1997;57:4757–64.

29. Ip C, Thompson HJ, Zhu Z, Ganther HE: In vitro and in vivo studies of methylseleninic acid: evidence that a monomethylated Se metabolite is critical for cancer chemoprevention. Cancer Res 2000;60:2882–6.

30. Ip C, Dong Y, Ganther HE: New concepts in Se chemoprevention. Cancer Metastasis Rev 2002;21:281–9.

31. Dong Y, Ganther HE, Stewart C, Ip C: Identification of molecular targets associated with Se-induced growth inhibition in human breast cells using cDNA microarrays. Cancer Res 2002;62:708–15.

32. Dong Y, Zhang H, Hawthorne L, et al: Delineation of the molecular basis for Se-induced growth arrest in human prostate cancer cells by oligonucleotide array. Cancer Res 2003;63:52–9.

33. Seo YR, Kelley MR, Smith ML: Selenomethionine regulation of p53 by a ref1-dependent redox mechanism. Proc Natl Acad Sci USA 2002;99:14548–53.

34. Gasparian AV, Yao YJ, Lu J, et al.: Se compounds inhibit $I_kB$ kinase (IKK) and nuclear factor-$_kB$ (NF-$_kB$) in prostate cancer cells. Molec Cancer Therapeutics 2002;1:1079–87.

35. Calvo A, Xiao N, Kang J, et al.: Alterations in gene expression profiles during prostate cancer progression: functional correlations to tumorigenicity and down-regulation of Selenoprotein-P in mouse and human tumors. Cancer Res 2002;62:5325–35.

36. Waters DJ, Shen S, Cooley DM, et al.: Effects of dietary Se supplementation on DNA damage and apoptosis in canine prostate. J Natl Cancer Inst 2003;95:237–41.

37. El-Bayoumy K, Richie JP, Boyiri T, et al.: Influence of Se-enriched yeast supplementation on biomarkers of oxidative damage and hormone status in healthy adult males: a clinical pilot study. Cancer Epidemiol Biomarkers Prevention 2002;11:1459–65.

38. Evans HM and Bishop KS. On the existence of a hitherto unrecognized dietary factor essential for reproduction. Science 1922;56;650–1.

39. Burton GW, Ingold KU. Autoxidation of biological molecules. 1. The antioxidant activity of vitamin E and related chain-breaking phenolic antioxidants in vitro. J Am Chem Soc 1981;103:6472.

40. Machlin LJ. Vitamin E. In LJ Machlin, ed. Handbook of vitamins, 2nd ed. Marcel Dekker, New York, 1991.

41. Pappas AM. Vitamin E: Tocopherols and tocotrienols. In AM Pappas, ed. Antioxidant status, diet, nutrition, and health, CRC, Boca Raton, 1998.

42. Azzi A, Boscoboinik D, Marilley D, Ozer NK, Stauble B, Tasinato A. Vitamin E: a sensor and an information transducer of the cell oxidation state. Am J Clin Nutr 1995;62:1337s–46s.

43. Mahoney CW, Azzi A. Vitamin E inhibits protein kinase C activity. Biochem Biophys Res Commun 1988;154:694–7.

44. Chatelain E, Boscoboinik DO, Bartoli GM, et al. Inhibition of smooth muscle cell proliferation and protein kinase C activity by tocopherols and tocotrienols. Biochim Biophys Acta 1993;1176:83–9.

45. Ottino P, Duncan JR. Effect of alpha-tocopheryl succinate on free radical and lipid peroxidation levels in BL6 melanoma cells. Free Radic Biol Med 1997;22:1145–51.

46. Wang W, Higuchi CM. Induction of NAD(P)H:quinone reductase by vitamins A, E and C in Colo205 colon cancer cells. Cancer Lett 1995;98:63–9.

47. Traber MG, Packer L. Vitamin E: beyond antioxidant function. Am J Clin Nutr 1995;62:1501s–9s.

48. Israel K, Sanders BG, Kline K. RRR-alpha-tocopheryl succinate inhibits the proliferation of human prostatic tumor cells with defective cell cycle/differentiation pathways. Nutr Cancer 1995;24(2):161–9.

49. Kishimoto M, YanoY, Yajima S, Otani S, Ichikawa T, Yano T. The inhibitory effect of vitamin E on 4-(methylnitrosamino)-1-(3-pyridyl)-1-butanone-induced lung tumorigenesis in mice based on the regulation of polyamine metabolism. Cancer Lett 1998;126(2):173–8.

50. Sigounas G, Anagnostou A, Steiner M. dl-alpha-tocopherol induces apoptosis in erythroleukemia, prostate, and breast cancer cells. Nutr Cancer 1997;28(1):30–5.

51. Umeda F, Kato K-I, Muta K, Ibayashi H. Effect of vitamin E on function of pituitary-gonadal axis in male rats and human studies. Endocrin Japon 29:287–92, 1982.

52. USDA (U.S. Department of Agriculture). Nationwide food consumption survey continuing survey of food intake by individuals: women 19–50 years and their children 1–5 years, 4 days, 1985, Report No. 85-4, Nutrition and Monitoring Division, Human Nutrition Information Economic research Service, U. S. Department of Agriculture, Hyattsville, MD, 1987.

53. USDA (U.S. Department of Agriculture). Nationwide food consumption survey continuing survey of food intake by individuals: men 19–50 years 1 day, 1985, Report No. 85-3, Nutrition and Monitoring Division, Human Nutrition Information Economic research Service, U. S. Department of Agriculture, Hyattsville, MD, 1987.

54. National Research Council (NRC), Recommended Dietary Allowances, 10th edition. National Academy Press, Washington, D.C., 1989.

55. Comstock GW, Bush TL, Helzlsouer K. Serum retinol, beta-carotene, vitamin E, and selenium as related to subsequent cancer of specific sites. Am J Epidemiol 1992;135:115–21.

56. Shibata A, Paganini-Hill A, Ross RK, Henderson BE. Intake of vegetables, fruits, beta-carotene, vitamin C and vitamin supplements and cancer incidence among the elderly: a prospective study. Br J Cancer 1992;66:673–9.

57. Yong LC, Brown CC, Schatzkin A, et al. Intake of vitamins E, C, and A and risk of lung cancer: The NHANES I Epidemiologic Follow up study. Am J Epidemiol 1997;146:231–43.

58. Ocke MC, Bueno-de-Mesquita HB, Feskens EJ, et al. Repeated measurements of vegetables, fruits, b-carotene, and vitamins C and E in relation to lung cancer: The Zutphen study. Am J Epidemiol 1997;145:358–65.

59. Knekt P, Jarvinen R, Sepannen R, et al. Dietary antioxidants and the risk of lung cancer. Am J Epidemiol 1991;134:471–9.
60. Longnecker MP, Martin-Moreno JM, Knekt P, et al. Serum alpha-tocopherol concentration in relation to subsequent colorectal cancer: Pooled data from five cohorts. JNCI 1992;84:430–5.
61. Wu AH, Paganini-Hill A, Ross RK, Henderson BE. Alcohol, physical activity and other factors for colorectal cancer: a prospective study. Br J Cancer 1987;55:687–94.
62. Bostick RM, Potter JD, McKenzie DR, et al. Reduced risk of colon cancer with high intake of vitamin E: the Iowa Women's Health Study. Cancer Res 1993;53:4230–7.
63. Ferraroni M, La Vecchia C, D'Avanzo B, et al. Selected micronutrient intake and the risk of colorectal cancer. Br J Cancer 1994;70:1150–5.
64. Lee HP, Gourley L, Duffy SW, et al. Colorectal cancer and diet in an Asian population study among Singapore Chinese. Int J Cancer 1989;43:1007–16.
65. Freudenheim JL, Graham S, Horvath PJ, et al. Risks associated with source of fiber components in cancer of the colon and rectum. Cancer Res 1990;50:3295–300.
66. Meyer F, White E. Alcohol and nutrients in relation to colon cancer in middle-aged adults. Am J Epidemiol 1993;136:225–36.
67. Doll R, Peto R. The causes of cancer: quantitative estimates of avoidable risks of cancer in the United States. J Natl Cancer Inst 1981;66:1192–1308.
68. Comstock GW, Helzlsouer KJ, Bush TL. Prediagnostic serum levels of carotenoids and vitamin E as related to subsequent cancer in Washington County, Maryland. Am J Clin Nutr 1991;53:260S–264S.
69. Knekt P, Aromaa A, Maatala J, et al. Serum vitamin E and risk of cancer among Finnish men during a 10-year follow-up. Am J Epidemiol 1988;127:28–41.
70. Hsing AW, Comstock GW, Abbey H, Polk BF. Serologic precursors of cancer; retinol, carotenoids, and tocopherol and risk of prostate cancer. JNCI 1990;82:941–6.
71. Eichholzer M, Stahelin HB, Gey FK, et al. Prediction of male cancer mortality by plasma levels of interacting vitamins: 17-year follow-up of the prospective Basel study. Int J Cancer 1996;55:145–50.
72. Hartman TJ, Albanes D, Pietinen P, et al. The association between baseline vitamin E, selenium, and prostate cancer in the Alpha-Tocopherol, Beta-Carotene Cancer Prevention Study. Cancer Epidemiol Biomarkers Prev 1998;7:335–40.
73. The ATBC Cancer Prevention Study Group. The effect of vitamin E and beta carotene on the incidence of lung cancer and other cancers in male smokers. N Engl J Med 1994;330:1029–35.
74. Heinonen OP, Albanes D, Huttunen JK, et al. Prostate cancer and supplementation with α-tocopherol and ß-carotene: incidence and mortality in a controlled trial. JNCI 1998;90:440–6.
75. Klein EA, Thompson IM, Lippman SM, et al. The Selenium and Vitamin E Cancer prevention Trial. World J Urol 2003;21:21–7.
76. Thompson IM, Pauler DK, Goodman PJ, Tangen CM, Lucia MS, Parnes HL, et al. Prevalence of prostate cancer among men with a prostate-specific antigen level < 4.0 ng per milliliter. N Engl J Med 2004;350:2239–46.
77. Karakiewicz PI, Benayoun S, Kattan MW, Perrotte P, Valiquette L, Scardino PT, Cagiannos I, Heinzer H, Tanguay S, Aprikian AG, Huland H, Graefen M: Development and validation of a nomogram predicting the outcome of prostate biopsy based on patient age, digital rectal examination and serum prostate specific antigen. J Urol 2005;173(6):1930–4.
78. Thompson IM, Ankerst DP, Chi C, Goodman PJ, Tangen CM, Lucia MS, Feng Z, Parnes HL, Coltman CA: Assessing prostate cancer risk: results from the Prostate Cancer Prevention Trial. J Natl Cancer Inst 2006;98(8):529–34.
79. Leman ES, Cannon GW, Trock BJ, Sokoll LJ, Chan DW, Mangold L, Partin AW, Getzenberg RH: EPCA-2: a highly specific serum marker for prostate cancer. Urology 2007;69(4):714–20.
80. Laxman B, Tomlins SA, Mehra R, Morris DS, Wang L, Helgeson BE, Shah RB, Rubin MA, Wei JT, Chinnaiyan AM: Noninvasive detection of TMPRSS2:ERG fusion transcripts in the urine of men with prostate cancer. Neoplasia 2006;8(10):885–8.
81. Postma R, Schröder FH, van Leenders GJ, Hoedemaeker RF, Vis AN, Roobol MJ, van der Kwast TH: Cancer detection and cancer characteristics in the European randomized study of screening for prostate cancer (ERSPC) – Section Rotterdam a comparison of two rounds of screening. Eur Urol 2007;52(1):89–97.
82. Thompson IM, Chi C, Ankerst DP, Goodman PJ, Tangen CM, Lippman SM, Lucia MS, Parnes HL, Coltman CA: Effect of finasteride on the sensitivity of PSA for detecting prostate cancer. J Natl Cancer Inst. 2006;98(16):1128–33.
83. Dong F, Reuther AM, Magi-Galluzzi C, Zhou M, Kupelian PA, Klein EA: Pathological stage migration has slowed in the late PSA era. Urology 2007;70:839–42.

# 26 PLCO: A Randomized Controlled Screening Trial for Prostate, Lung, Colorectal, and Ovarian Cancer

*Amanda Black, Robert L. Grubb III, and E. David Crawford*

## CONTENTS

## SUMMARY

The Prostate, Lung, Colorectal, and Ovarian (PLCO) Cancer Screening Trial is an ongoing, prospective randomized controlled trial designed to determine if screening for these cancers, using the best available screening tests, reduces disease-specific mortality. PLCO has also evolved as a large epidemiologic cohort and presents a unique, comprehensive, and invaluable resource for epidemiologic, molecular, and genetic studies. This resource is being utilized by researchers who are contributing substantially to furthering our understanding of prostate carcinogenesis and progression.

From: *Current Clinical Urology: Prostate Cancer Screening*, Edited by: D. P. Ankerst et al.
DOI 10.1007/978-1-60327-281-0_26 © Humana Press, a part of Springer Science+Business Media, LLC 2009

**Key Words:** Prostate carcinoma, Randomized controlled trial, Screening, Prostate-specific antigen (PSA), Digital rectal examination (DRE), Environmental and genetic risk factors.

## PLCO TRIAL RATIONALE, DESIGN, AND METHODS

### *Rationale and Aim*

In the 1980s, medical clinics promoted transrectal ultrasound (TRUS) as an effective method of detecting prostate cancer at an early stage, with the implication that early detection would increase the probability of cure (Fig. 1) *(1)*. These claims were disputed and it was argued that, as the available evidence could not support such claims, the National Cancer Institute (NCI) was obliged to undertake investigations to determine the effectiveness and risks of such early detection practices, whether by TRUS or any other technologies. The concept for the PLCO trial began in 1989 *(1)*.

The rationale for screening for a disease is to reduce mortality and/or morbidity by successful treatment through early detection of the disease. Criteria for evaluating the efficacy and effectiveness of screening for a disease in asymptomatic individuals have been well-established *(2,3)*. It was evident that prostate cancer was of significant public health importance, had a latent phase, and acceptable screening procedures (Prostate-Specific Antigen (PSA) test and Digital Rectal Examination (DRE)). However, the criterion that screening for screen-detected prostate (P) cancer reduced prostate cancer-specific mortality was not proven. This was also the case for lung (L), colorectal (C), and ovarian (O) cancers (4). Hence, the PLCO randomized controlled trial (RCT) was designed with the primary aim of determining if screening for these cancers, using the best available screening tests, would reduce disease-specific mortality *(4)*. Secondary objectives included assessment of (1) the incidence, stage, and survival of cancer cases, (2) test operating characteristics (sensitivity, specificity, negative and positive predictive

---

PROSTATE CANCER
AND
EARLY DETECTION
Over 28,000 men die annually of Prostate Cancer.
You need not be one of them.

• The key to curing prostate cancer is early detection
• Early detection is enhanced by the new Ultrasonic Probe Test
• This ultrasonic imaging is recommended for men over 50
• A picture image of the prostate is produced from sound waves
• The test is short, painless, and inexpensive
• Most insurance companies cover the test

HIGHLY QUALIFIED UROLOGISTS & MEDICAL
STAFF TO ASSIST YOUR EVERY NEED

*Write Or Call For Brochure*

**Fig. 1.** Example of a 1980s advertisement for prostate ultrasound.

values) of each of the screening modalities, (3) costs, and (4) environmental, biomolecular, and genetic factors associated with carcinogenesis and cancer promotion *(5)*.

## STUDY DESIGN, RECRUITMENT, AND RANDOMIZATION

The PLCO Cancer Screening Trial was designed as an ongoing prospective RCT to screen 37,000 men for prostate, lung, and colorectal cancers and 37,000 women for lung, colorectal, and ovarian cancers, with an equal number of men and women undergoing usual medical care practices as control participants *(4)*. Ten screening centers (SCs) across the USA (Fig. 2 and Color Plate 13) were responsible for recruitment, screening, and follow-up of volunteer participants. The screening modalities for prostate cancer included DRE and PSA. TRUS was removed from the trial design when it was determined that it was of little added value to cancer detection beyond that of PSA and DRE *(4)*. Men aged 55–74 years at study entry were to be screened for prostate cancer by PSA at baseline and annually for the following 5 years and by DRE annually for the first 4 years. Block randomization to either the screened arm or control arm of the trial occurred subsequent to the participants signing an informed consent document. All participants were to be followed-up for a minimum of 13 years from randomization, to allow sufficient time for cancer and mortality event ascertainment, to definitively determine if screening reduces disease-specific mortality. Statistically, the trial was designed to have approximately 90% power to detect a 20% reduction in prostate cancer-specific mortality.

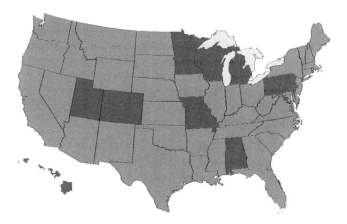

**Fig. 2.** US map showing the PLCO screening center locations (*see* Color Plate 13)

PLCO screening centers: Alabama (University of Alabama, Birmingham); Michigan (Henry Ford Health System, Detroit); Colorado (University of Colorado, Denver); Hawaii (Pacific Health Research Institute, Honolulu); Wisconsin (Marshfield Clinic Research Foundation, Marshfield); Minnesota (University of Minnesota, Minneapolis); Pennsylvania (University of Pittsburgh, Pittsburgh); Utah (University of Utah, Salt Lake City); Idaho (University of Utah/Boise, Boise) (Utah Satellite Center); Missouri (Washington University, St. Louis); Washington DC (Georgetown University, Washington).

## SCREENING AND DIAGNOSTIC FOLLOW-UP PROCEDURES

Participants were invited for a screening exam at the screening center, where the goal was to complete the screening tests for all cancers within a two hour period *(4)*. Prior to the DRE, up to 45 mL of blood was drawn for the PSA test and biorepository storage.

This sample was centrifuged and shipped to the central laboratory at UCLA where all PSA assays were performed. A PSA result of > 4 ng/mL was considered positive. A DRE was considered positive if there was nodularity or induration of the prostate gland or if the examiner judged the prostate to be suspicious based on other criteria such as asymmetry or loss of anatomic landmarks. For men who screened negative for prostate cancer, and men who had a suspicious or positive screen but for whom subsequent diagnostic evaluations did not reveal prostate cancer, a scheduling and tracking procedure was established at each SC to ensure regular attendance at repeat screens (4).

Men whose screens were positive (PSA > 4 ng/mL or suspicious DRE) received notification of their test results, as did their physicians. Men returned to their physicians for further diagnostic evaluation and treatment. The trial had no diagnostic or therapeutic algorithm and hence no direct control of these procedures following a positive screen. However, screening centers track all participants and retrieve medical record information related to any diagnostic follow-up and treatment resulting from positive screening tests. Screen and control arm participants are contacted annually to elicit health status. Therefore, data pertaining to diagnosis and treatment of individuals with a PLCO cancer are collected in both trial arms.

## DATA AND BIOSPECIMENS

Both screened and control participants were invited to complete a questionnaire at baseline to collect individual characteristics, demographics, and risk factor information including age, ethnicity, education, anthropometry, lifestyle behaviors, screening history, family history of cancer, and personal history of medical problems. In addition to the baseline questionnaire, dietary information was obtained from two dietary questionnaires and, recently, participants were invited to complete a follow-up risk factor questionnaire designed to supplement the baseline data.

The Etiologic and Early Marker Studies (EEMS) program was designed and implemented as a component of PLCO to address the secondary aims of the trial (6). PLCO maintains a biorepository of specifically processed blood products and tissue samples for molecular and genetic epidemiologic, etiologic risk assessment, and early detection research. Serial, pre-diagnostic, biological samples including serum, plasma, red blood cells with viable lymphocytes, and buffy coat have been collected and archived from consenting screened participants (4). Buccal cell DNA collected from control arm individuals is also stored. There is a current effort to create tissue microarrays (TMAs), for selected prostate cancer tumors, enhancing the unique resources and potential research opportunities that PLCO trial data present.

## PARTICIPANTS AND EXCLUSIONS

Enrollment into the trial commenced in November 1993 and the final participant was recruited in July 2001 (7). Exclusion criteria for men in PLCO included history of prostate, lung, or colorectal cancer, surgical removal of the entire prostate, participation in another cancer screening or primary prevention study, and use of finasteride in the previous 6 months. From April 1995 on, men were also excluded if they reported more than one PSA blood test in the past 3 years. In total, 154,934 individuals (76,702 males) (Fig. 3), aged 55–74 years, were randomized into the trial (7) and the final screening

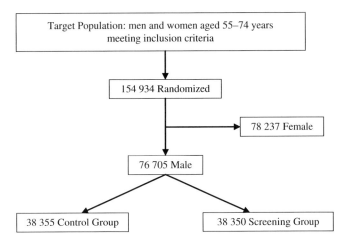

**Fig. 3.** Flow diagram of PLCO participants.

rounds were completed in 2006 (Christine D. Berg, personal communication). Participants will continue to be followed-up annually for at least 13 years from their entry into
the study.

Of 38,350 men randomized to the intervention arm, 86.2% were non-Hispanic white
*(5)*. At enrollment, all age groups were well-represented, with most men between the
ages of 55 and 64 years. About half of men in the screened arm had a college degree.
Almost one quarter of the men reported a personal history of prostate problems, 4.3%
reported a prior prostate biopsy, and 6.9% had a first-degree relative with prostate
cancer *(5)*.

The PLCO trial provides a large, high quality, and unique data resource. The main
strengths of the prostate component of PLCO are its size, prospective design, the combined use of DRE and PSA, the fact that all PSA assays were performed centrally in one
laboratory, the minimal loss to follow-up, and the comprehensiveness, diversity, and
quality of data and biospecimens collected.

## SCREENING RESULTS AND DIAGNOSTIC OUTCOMES

### Baseline PSA and DRE Screening and Diagnostic Follow-Up Results

The PLCO trial has proven to be a rich source of data on screening for prostate cancer
using serum PSA and DRE. While the results of screening with regard to the primary
outcome are awaited, numerous preliminary analyses have been performed. Andriole
et al. reported the results from the initial round of screening of the 38,350 participants
randomized to the intervention (screening) arm of the study *(5)*. The demographic characteristics of the intervention arm have been discussed above. Compliance in undergoing
PSA and DRE screening among participants was above 89% for both tests. PSA and
DRE results from the baseline screen, stratified by age are seen in Table 1. Overall,
7.9% of men had a suspicious PSA ($>4$ ng/mL) at the initial screen. There was an age-
dependent increase in the proportion of men with a suspicious PSA. Similarly, 7.5%
of men had a suspicious DRE at the baseline screen. The proportion of men with a
suspicious DRE also rose with age.

Table 1
Results of Baseline Screening Tests, Stratified by Age

| Age (years) | Suspicious DRE (%) | PSA > 4 ng/mL (%) | Both tests + (%) |
|---|---|---|---|
| 55–59 | 4.9 | 4.1 | 0.5 |
| 60–64 | 7.2 | 7.2 | 1.1 |
| 65–69 | 9.4 | 10.8 | 1.8 |
| 70–74 | 11.5 | 14.0 | 2.2 |
| All ages | 7.5 | 7.9 | 1.2 |

Adapted from (5).

Forty-one percent of the men with positive PSA screens underwent a prostate biopsy within 1 year of the screen and this increased to 64% within 3 years of a positive screen (8). Factors associated with receiving a biopsy included positive DRE, PSA > 7 ng/mL (vs. 4–7 ng/mL), and a family history of prostate cancer. Older men (≥70) were less likely to undergo a biopsy. The biopsy rates are lower than those found in the European Randomized Screening for Prostate Cancer (ERSPC) Trial (84%); which has less frequent screening and mandated follow-up (9). However, the lower biopsy rate relates to US practice; as there can be no mandated follow-up, men, on the advice of their urologist or family physician, may undergo additional diagnostic testing prior to proceeding with a biopsy. Indeed, 89% of men with a positive PSA underwent some additional diagnostic test (repeat PSA, confirmatory DRE, or biopsy) within 2 years of a positive screen (8). This indicates that men in the PLCO trial are being managed in a manner consistent with community practice, which will increase the applicability of findings in the trial to the general population.

Within 1 year of the initial screen, 556 of the 4,801 men with suspicious PSA and/or DRE screens had been diagnosed with cancer (5). This results in a positive predictive value of a positive PSA/DRE screen of 11.5%. About 1,501 biopsies were performed, indicating a 37% prostate cancer rate among men undergoing a biopsy. The overall detection rate was 1.6%, which is consistent with the detection rate of other screening studies (10).

Of the men diagnosed with prostate cancer within 1 year of the baseline screen, 83% had clinically localized (stage I or II) cancers and 10% had locally advanced or metastatic cancers (stage III or IV) (5). Among men diagnosed with PSA 4–10 ng/mL, 88% had clinically localized disease. The majority (76%) of cancers detected were Gleason score 5–7; only 12% were high-grade (Gleason 8–10). More favorable Gleason score and clinical stage distribution were seen among men diagnosed at lower PSA stratum and within each PSA stratum, those men with a non-suspicious DRE had more favorable cancers.

## REPEAT PROSTATE BIOPSY AMONG MEN UNDERGOING SERIAL SCREENING

PLCO researchers examined the outcomes of 2,761 men who had an initial negative biopsy following a positive screen. Of the men who had an elevated PSA, 43% underwent a repeat biopsy within 3 years of the initial biopsy; the proportion was much lower for men with only a suspicious DRE (13%) *(11)*. Men undergoing repeat biopsy were more likely to have had prostatic intraepithelial neoplasia (PIN) on initial biopsy (Hazard Ratio (HR) 4.8), a higher PSA (HR 1.5 for PSA 7–10 ng/mL and HR 1.8 for PSA >10 ng/mL) or a PSA velocity >1 ng/mL/year (HR 1.5). Again, the findings suggest that despite lack of a formal protocol for follow-up of abnormal tests, PLCO participants are being managed according to practices supported by experience with PSA screening.

## PSA KINETICS

The PLCO trial has spanned the evolution of understanding of the performance of PSA as a screening test. While in the early part of the PSA era, clinicians often focused on PSA as a static number, it has become increasingly apparent that the change in a man's PSA over time is a critical factor in determining his risk for prostate cancer. PLCO researchers have used the abundant data on the majority of men with a normal baseline PSA to determine the risk of developing a positive PSA over time *(12)*. About 30,495 men in the screening arm had a baseline PSA ≤ 4 ng/mL. The 5-year cumulative estimated risk of converting to a PSA > 4 ng/mL ranged from 1.5% in those men with a baseline PSA < 1 ng/mL to 79% for those men with a baseline PSA 3–4 ng/mL (Table 2). The risk of subsequent cancer diagnosis was also a function of baseline PSA. Men with a baseline PSA of 0–1 ng/mL who converted to PSA > 4 ng/mL had an 8% risk of prostate cancer being diagnosed within 2 years of their conversion, while men with a baseline PSA of 3–4 who converted to PSA > 4 ng/mL had a 22% risk of prostate cancer diagnosis. Based on the low rate of conversion to a PSA of >4 ng/mL and low rates of cancer diagnosis, investigators suggested that it might be safe to screen men with baseline PSA < 1 ng/mL every 5 years and men with baseline PSA 1–2 ng/mL every 2 years, with all others continuing annual screening. Potential delays in cancer diagnosis ranged from 5.4 to 20.9 months. While these delays seem substantial, it is unclear what their exact relationship to the lead-time factor induced by PSA screening might be or what the potential effect on treatment outcomes might be.

In addition to gaining an understanding of the outcomes of the majority of men with very low PSA values in a screening environment, examination of PLCO data has led to greater understanding of the functions of serial PSA screening, including PSA velocity. Increased PSA velocity prior to prostate cancer diagnosis has been shown to be a risk factor for more aggressive and potentially fatal prostate cancer *(13,14)*. This concept has also been examined in the PLCO trial. Outcomes of men who were diagnosed with prostate cancer and who had received ≥ 2 PSA screens were reviewed. Compared with

Table 2
Five-Year Cumulative Estimated % Converting to PSA > 4 ng/mL

| Baseline PSA (ng/mL) | Estimated % converting |
|---|---|
| 0–1 | 1.5 |
| 1–2 | 7.4 |
| 2–3 | 33.5 |
| 3–4 | 79.0 |

$N$ = 30,495 men with baseline PSA ≤ 4 ng/mL. Adapted from *(12)*.

having a PSA velocity of <0.5 ng/mL/year, men in the trial who had a PSA velocity of 1–2 ng/mL/year and >2 ng/mL/year had odds ratios of 2.2 and 2.3, respectively, of having biopsy Gleason score 7–10 *(15)*. This study examined several different models for determining PSA velocity. In contrast to the methods of D'Amico, et al. *(13)*, the PLCO authors used all PSA values rather than just the last two annual PSA levels. They found that using only the last two PSA values prior to diagnosis resulted in a higher, but more variable PSA velocity. Calculations using all PSA values resulted in a more predictive model *(15)*.

## PROSTATE CANCER RISK FACTORS

Older age, African ancestry, and a positive family history of prostate cancer have long been identified as factors associated with increased prostate cancer risk and PLCO has reported results consistent with the existing literature *(5)*. Although studies of twins have demonstrated that up to 50% of prostate cancer cases may be explained by environmental factors such as diet *(16)*, evidence for the association between prostate cancer and genetic variation, dietary and hormonal factors is somewhat mixed and inconclusive. Research utilizing PLCO data continues to contribute substantially to achieving resolution of these relationships.

## NUTRITIONAL FACTORS

Diet is estimated to account for approximately 30% of all cancers in Western countries, making it second only to tobacco as a preventable cause *(17)*.

### Nutritional Factors Associated with Decreased Prostate Cancer Risk

Antioxidants neutralize free radicals that may play a role in prostate carcinogenesis and have therefore been the focus of several investigations within PLCO as potential prostate cancer-preventive agents. To date, findings have demonstrated no overall association between prostate cancer risk and dietary intake or dietary supplementation with four major antioxidants (vitamin E, β-carotene, lycopene, and vitamin C) *(18–20)*. However, protective effects have been shown in specific sub-groups; β-carotene supplementation in men with low dietary β-carotene intake, and vitamin E supplementation in smokers were associated with a decreased risk of prostate cancer *(18,20)*. Similarly, greater serum selenium concentrations (a potential chemopreventive agent) showed no association with prostate cancer risk, except in those men who reported a high intake of vitamin E, multivitamin use, and smoking *(21)*.

### Nutritional Factors Associated with Increased Prostate Cancer Risk

Dairy product intake is suggested to increase prostate cancer risk and may act via various mechanisms including lowering the circulating, active form of vitamin D or the presence of insulin-like growth factors or estrogens in these foods *(22–24)*. Calcium may play a role in prostate carcinogenesis and promotion as extracellular calcium regulates prostate cancer cell growth *(25)*. A recent PLCO study demonstrated a modest association between greater intake of calcium and dairy products, particularly low-fat types, and increased risk of non-aggressive prostate cancer, but no relationship with aggressive disease *(26)*.

Cross et al. demonstrated an increased risk of prostate cancer associated with consuming very well done meat *(27)*. In particular, the highest quintile of 2-amino-1-methyl-6-phenylimidazo[4,5-*b*] (PhIP – a heterocyclic amine in high-temperature cooked meat) conferred a 1.2-fold increased risk of prostate cancer.

Saturated and alpha-linolenic fatty acids have also been implicated as prostate carcinogens. However, PLCO researchers reported no association with total prostate cancer risk or with prostate tumors that were defined by grade and stage *(28)*.

## HORMONAL FACTORS

Sex hormones (e.g., testosterone), insulin-like growth factors (IGF), and their associated binding proteins may play a role in prostate cancer initiation and progression. Investigators utilized PLCO data to examine the role of IGF-1 and the binding protein IGFBP-3, reporting no association with prostate cancer risk *(29)*.

## GENETIC FACTORS

The strong, consistent association between family history and prostate cancer risk suggests an important hereditary genetic component to prostate cancer etiology.

### *Sex Hormone Genes*

Genetic factors are thought to influence the regulation of sex hormones and, as mentioned previously, sex hormones have been implicated in prostate cancer carcinogenesis. This prompted researchers to use stored DNA, from PLCO prostate cancer cases and controls, to genotype 14 single nucleotide polymorphisms (SNPS) in genes involved in hormone regulation or metabolism *(30)*. This study showed an increased risk of prostate cancer associated with a common polymorphism in the sex hormone-binding globulin gene (SHBG, D356N).

### *Inflammatory Genes*

Chronic inflammation has been postulated to play a role in the etiology of prostate cancer. Evidence exists for an association between sexually transmitted diseases and prostatitis and increased prostate cancer risk, while anti-inflammatory agents (e.g., NSAIDs) have shown an inverse association with disease risk *(31–33)*. Findings for polymorphisms in inflammatory associated genes have been mixed and, despite the potential importance of inflammation in prostate carcinogenesis, no strong associations of genetic variants involved in the inflammatory pathway and prostate cancer risk have been observed in studies utilizing PLCO biorepository specimens *(34–37)*. These studies have examined polymorphisms of the following genes: (1) prostaglandin-endoperoxide synthase 2 (PTGS2), believed to play a role in the mediation of inflammation; (2) RNASEL, involved in the apoptotic response; (3) interleukin 1B (IL-1B), IL-6, IL-8, IL-10, and tumor necrosis factor-α (TNF-α), inflammatory cytokines.

Additionally, although α-Methyl-CoA Racemase (AMACR) gene variants were unrelated to prostate cancer risk, a protective effect among ibuprofen users was observed suggesting that AMACR gene variants may enhance the chemopreventive effects of ibuprofen on prostate cancer risk *(38)*.

## Chromosome 8q24

The chromosomal region 8q24 of the genome is amplified in prostate tumors and common variants in this region have been associated with prostate cancer risk. While conducting a genome-wide association study (GWAS) in the Cancer Genetic Markers of Susceptibility (CGEMS) project with 550,000 SNPs, researchers from the National Cancer Institute confirmed the association between the locus marked by rs1447295 and prostate cancer risk in men of European ancestry *(39)*. In addition, they identified a new locus within 8q24, marked by rs698267, which was estimated to confer a higher population-attributable risk than rs1447295 (21% vs. 9%). A further GWAS of 26,958 SNPs, in a case–control study in men of European ancestry, nested in the PLCO Cancer Screening Trial, confirmed the independent SNPs at 8q24 and identified multiple additional loci with moderate effects associated with susceptibility to prostate cancer *(40)*. The population-attributable risk for prostate cancer of each of seven independent loci ranged from 8 to 20%.

These studies continue to contribute to the understanding of the etiologic pathways in prostate carcinogenesis and susceptibility to disease and may facilitate prediction of high-risk in select individuals.

## CURRENT COLLABORATIONS AND SUMMARY

### Collaborative Research

In addition to individual research endeavors, PLCO is part of large collaborative research efforts including the Cohort Consortium, Pooling Project and Cancer Genetic Markers of Susceptibility (CGEMS). Further information on the PLCO cancer screening trial, collaborations, and a complete list of resulting published literature, can be found at http://www.parplco.org.

## SUMMARY

The PLCO cancer screening trial was designed as a multi-center RCT designed to determine if screening for prostate, lung, colorectal, and ovarian cancers reduces disease-specific mortality. Although final results are not expected for several years, if evidence suggests beneficial or detrimental effects from screening, these data will be made public as soon as possible. Meanwhile, the etiology of prostate cancer remains to be fully elucidated and PLCO is proving to be an indispensable resource to further our understanding of the natural history of prostate cancer, identify molecular biomarkers for early detection of disease, address potential carcinogenic and anti-carcinogenic exposures, and investigate genetic susceptibility to prostate cancer.

**Acknowledgements**   The PLCO is supported by contracts from the Division of Cancer Prevention, National Cancer Institute, NIH, DHHS. The authors thank the Screening Center investigators and staff of the Prostate, Lung, Colorectal, and Ovarian (PLCO) Cancer Screening Trial, Mr. Tom Riley and staff, Information Management Services, Inc., Ms. Barbara O'Brien and staff, Westat, Inc. Most importantly, we acknowledge the study participants for their contributions to making this study possible.

# REFERENCES

1. Gohagan JK, Prorok PC, Hayes RB, Kramer BS, Prostate, Lung, Colorectal and Ovarian Cancer Screening Trial Project Team. The Prostate, Lung, Colorectal and Ovarian (PLCO) Cancer Screening Trial of the National Cancer Institute: history, organization, and status. Control Clin Trials 2000;21: 251S–72S.
2. Kramer BS, Brown ML, Prorok PC, Potosky AL, Gohagan JK. Prostate cancer screening: what we know and what we need to know. Ann Intern Med 1993;119:914–23.
3. Kramer BS, Gohagan J, Prorok PC. NIH Consensus 1994: screening. Gynecol Oncol 1994;55:S20–1.
4. Prorok PC, Andriole GL, Bresalier RS, et al. Design of the Prostate, Lung, Colorectal and Ovarian (PLCO) Cancer Screening Trial. Control Clin Trials 2000;21:273S–309S.
5. Andriole GL, Levin DL, Crawford ED, et al. Prostate Cancer Screening in the Prostate, Lung, Colorectal and Ovarian (PLCO) Cancer Screening Trial: findings from the initial screening round of a randomized trial. J Natl Cancer Inst 2005;97:433–8.
6. Hayes RB, Reding D, Kopp W, et al. Etiologic and early marker studies in the prostate, lung, colorectal and ovarian (PLCO) cancer screening trial. Control Clin Trials 2000;21:349S–55S.
7. Andriole GL, Reding D, Hayes RB, Prorok PC, Gohagan JK, PLCO Steering Committee. The prostate, lung, colon, and ovarian (PLCO) cancer screening trial: Status and promise. Urol Oncol 2004;22:358–61.
8. Pinsky PF, Andriole GL, Kramer BS, et al. Prostate biopsy following a positive screen in the prostate, lung, colorectal and ovarian cancer screening trial. J Urol 2005;173:746,50; discussion 750–1.
9. de Koning HJ, Auvinen A, Berenguer Sanchez A, et al. Large-scale randomized prostate cancer screening trials: program performances in the European Randomized Screening for Prostate Cancer trial and the Prostate, Lung, Colorectal and Ovary cancer trial. Int J Cancer 2002;97:237–44.
10. Smith DS, Humphrey PA, Catalona WJ. The early detection of prostate carcinoma with prostate specific antigen: the Washington University experience. Cancer 1997;80:1852–6.
11. Pinsky PF, Crawford ED, Kramer BS, et al. Repeat prostate biopsy in the prostate, lung, colorectal and ovarian cancer screening trial. BJU Int 2007;99:775–9.
12. Crawford ED, Pinsky PF, Chia D, et al. Prostate specific antigen changes as related to the initial prostate specific antigen: data from the prostate, lung, colorectal and ovarian cancer screening trial. J Urol 2006;175:1286,90; discussion 1290.
13. D'Amico AV, Chen MH, Roehl KA, Catalona WJ. Preoperative PSA velocity and the risk of death from prostate cancer after radical prostatectomy. N Engl J Med 2004;351:125–35.
14. D'Amico AV, Renshaw AA, Sussman B, Chen MH. Pretreatment PSA velocity and risk of death from prostate cancer following external beam radiation therapy. JAMA 2005;294:440–7.
15. Pinsky PF, Andriole G, Crawford ED, et al. Prostate-specific antigen velocity and prostate cancer gleason grade and stage. Cancer 2007;109:1689–95.
16. Lichtenstein P, Holm NV, Verkasalo PK, et al. Environmental and heritable factors in the causation of cancer – analyses of cohorts of twins from Sweden, Denmark, and Finland. N Engl J Med 2000;343:78–85.
17. Key TJ, Allen NE, Spencer EA, Travis RC. The effect of diet on risk of cancer. Lancet 2002;360:861–8.
18. Kirsh VA, Hayes RB, Mayne ST, et al. Supplemental and dietary vitamin E, beta-carotene, and vitamin C intakes and prostate cancer risk. J Natl Cancer Inst 2006;98:245–54.
19. Kirsh VA, Mayne ST, Peters U, et al. A prospective study of lycopene and tomato product intake and risk of prostate cancer. Cancer Epidemiol Biomarkers Prev 2006;15:92–8.
20. Peters U, Leitzmann MF, Chatterjee N, et al. Serum lycopene, other carotenoids, and prostate cancer risk: a nested case-control study in the prostate, lung, colorectal, and ovarian cancer screening trial. Cancer Epidemiol Biomarkers Prev 2007;16:962–8.
21. Peters U, Foster CB, Chatterjee N, et al. Serum selenium and risk of prostate cancer-a nested case-control study. Am J Clin Nutr 2007;85:209–17.
22. Ahn J, Albanes D, Peters U, et al. Dairy products, calcium intake, and risk of prostate cancer in the prostate, lung, colorectal, and ovarian cancer screening trial. Cancer Epidemiol Biomarkers Prev 2007;16:2623–30.
23. Giovannucci E, Liu Y, Stampfer MJ, Willett WC. A prospective study of calcium intake and incident and fatal prostate cancer. Cancer Epidemiol Biomarkers Prev 2006;15:203–10.
24. Gunnell D, Oliver SE, Peters TJ, et al. Are diet-prostate cancer associations mediated by the IGF axis? A cross-sectional analysis of diet, IGF-I and IGFBP-3 in healthy middle-aged men. Br J Cancer 2003;88:1682–6.

25. Qin LQ, Wang PY, Kaneko T, Hoshi K, Sato A. Estrogen: one of the risk factors in milk for prostate cancer. Med Hypotheses 2004;62:133–42.

26. Liao J, Schneider A, Datta NS, McCauley LK. Extracellular calcium as a candidate mediator of prostate cancer skeletal metastasis. Cancer Res 2006;66:9065–73.

27. Cross AJ, Peters U, Kirsh VA, et al. A prospective study of meat and meat mutagens and prostate cancer risk. Cancer Res 2005;65:11779–84.

28. Koralek DO, Peters U, Andriole G, et al. A prospective study of dietary alpha-linolenic acid and the risk of prostate cancer (United States). Cancer Causes Control 2006;17:783–91.

29. Weiss JM, Huang WY, Rinaldi S, et al. IGF-1 and IGFBP-3: Risk of prostate cancer among men in the Prostate, Lung, Colorectal and Ovarian Cancer Screening Trial. Int J Cancer 2007;121:2267–73.

30. Berndt SI, Chatterjee N, Huang WY, et al. Variant in sex hormone-binding globulin gene and the risk of prostate cancer. Cancer Epidemiol Biomarkers Prev 2007;16:165–8.

31. Hayes RB, Pottern LM, Strickler H, et al. Sexual behaviour, STDs and risks for prostate cancer. Br J Cancer 2000;82:718–25.

32. Dennis LK, Dawson DV. Meta-analysis of measures of sexual activity and prostate cancer. Epidemiology 2002;13:72–9.

33. Mahmud S, Franco E, Aprikian A. Prostate cancer and use of nonsteroidal anti-inflammatory drugs: systematic review and meta-analysis. Br J Cancer 2004;90:93–9.

34. Danforth KN, Hayes RB, Rodriguez C, et al. Polymorphic variants in PTGS2 and prostate cancer risk: results from two large nested case-control studies. Carcinogenesis 2008;29:568–72.

35. Daugherty SE, Hayes RB, Yeager M, et al. RNASEL Arg462Gln polymorphism and prostate cancer in PLCO. Prostate 2007;67:849–54.

36. Michaud DS, Daugherty SE, Berndt SI, et al. Genetic polymorphisms of interleukin-1B (IL-1B), IL-6, IL-8, and IL-10 and risk of prostate cancer. Cancer Res 2006;66:4525–30.

37. Danforth KN, Rodriguez C, Hayes RB, et al. TNF polymorphisms and prostate cancer risk. Prostate 2008;68:400–7.

38. Daugherty SE, Shugart YY, Platz EA, et al. Polymorphic variants in alpha-methylacyl-CoA racemase and prostate cancer. Prostate 2007;67:1487–97.

39. Yeager M, Orr N, Hayes RB, et al. Genome-wide association study of prostate cancer identifies a second risk locus at 8q24. Nat Genet 2007;39:645–9.

40. Thomas G, Jacobs KB, Yeager M, et al. Multiple loci identified in a genome-wide association study of prostate cancer. Nat Genet 2008;40:310–5.

# 27 The European Randomized Study of Screening for Prostate Cancer (ERSPC)

*Tineke Wolters and Fritz H. Schröder*

## Contents

## Summary

With the introduction of the PSA test, screening for prostate cancer has become wide-spread practice. However, no evidence exists that screening for prostate cancer leads to a disease-specific mortality reduction. To provide evidence showing or excluding this mortality reduction, a large randomized trial was conducted in 1994, the European Randomized Study of Screening for Prostate Cancer (ERSPC). A total of eight centres from Europe participated in this trial and so far a total of 267,994 men are randomized: 126,219 in the screening arm, 141,775 in the control arm. No final endpoint has been reached yet and the ERSPC is still ongoing. However, up to now the ERSPC has provided much data on screening tests and protocols, biopsy outcome and predictors and early detection of prostate cancer.

This chapter describes the origin of the ERSPC, preliminary results, and the variety of aspects of screening.

**Key Words:** Screening, Screening test, Interval, Lead-time, Interval cancers, Contamination, Compliance, Overdiagnosis, Quality of life.

From: *Current Clinical Urology: Prostate Cancer Screening*, Edited by: D. P. Ankerst et al.
DOI 10.1007/978-1-60327-281-0_27 © Humana Press, a part of Springer Science+Business Media, LLC 2009

# INTRODUCTION

In this chapter, an attempt is made to describe the ongoing European Randomized Study of Screening for Prostate Cancer (ERSPC). It is written on behalf of the whole study group of the ERSPC.

# BACKGROUND

With emerging insights about the use of PSA as a screening test *(1)*, an idea of conducting a randomized controlled study of screening for prostate cancer (PC) originated in Belgium and in the Netherlands during 1990–1991 *(2,3)*. No evidence of the effectiveness of screening for prostate cancer existed at that time and the only way of obtaining such evidence seemed to be by conducting a prospective randomized controlled trial (RCT). Several uncertainties that existed related to randomization, acceptance and value of screening tests, follow-up and others. Therefore, between 1991 and 1994 a series of pilot studies were carried out in Belgium and in the Netherlands. Summaries of the results of these pilots were published in 1995 *(4,5)*. The main conclusion was that a European RCT of screening for prostate cancer seemed feasible. Yet, the expense of such a trial made international co-operation a prerequisite, as no single country could afford such a study. The ERSPC formally started on July 1, 1994 in Belgium and in the Netherlands. After the successful conduction of a pilot study *(6)*, Finland became the third partner in the ERSPC during 1995, followed by Sweden, Spain, Italy, Switzerland and France.

A publication of Adami et al. *(7)* in 1994 gave rise to a public discussion about the ethical justification of such an RTC. Some felt that prerequisites for performing screening studies, for example, knowing the natural history and effectiveness of treatment, were not met. This controversy has been the subject of an extensive discussion *(8–10)*. However, in all participating countries ethical approval was obtained and the ERSPC started in 1994.

# PURPOSE AND STRUCTURE OF THE STUDY

The main goal of the ERSPC is to show or exclude a prostate cancer mortality reduction through screening and early treatment. In this large randomized controlled trial screening is offered to the intervention group and the control group is managed according to regional health care policies. The trial aims at showing or excluding a 20% difference in prostate cancer mortality with a power of 90%. This was decided at a consensus workshop held in 1994 on the basic elements of screening in an RCT *(11)*.

During 1995 the possibility of co-operation with the National Cancer Institute RCT for Prostate, Lung, Colon and Ovary Cancer (PLCO) was explored, specifically through common analysis of both trials, as this would have the advantage of adding power to both trials. It was subsequently agreed upon *(12)*. The timing and structure of this common evaluation will depend on the time of final analyses of both trials and on an evaluation plan, which is under discussion.

Other important decisions were made at the consensus workshop, such as the determination of 4.0 ng/ml as a PSA threshold for recommending a biopsy and initially including Digital Rectal Examination (DRE) and Transrectal Ultrasound (TRUS) as screening tests. An age range of 55–70 years was determined as being the core age range on which power is calculated. Inclusion of higher or lower age ranges can be decided upon by the individual centres. Initial sample size calculations were made without consideration of possible contamination in the control arm by opportunistic PSA-based screening and it was calculated that 65,000 men per arm and a follow-up of 10 years would be needed. Re-calculations considering this contamination showed that a sample size of 85,000 men per arm would be needed *(13)*.

Furthermore, basic requirements for participation in the ERSPC and the content of the future database were discussed during this workshop. This resulted in the establishment of the following committees which run and control the ERSPC: an Epidemiology Committee, a Pathology Committee, a PSA Committee, a Quality Control Committee, a Causes of Death Committee, an independent Data Monitoring Committee (DMC) and the supervisory body of the study as a whole, the Scientific Committee (SC). All important decisions are made by the voting members of the SC, which consist of two representatives of each centre. Every participating centre has accepted the authority of the controlling committees (i.e. the Quality Control Committee and Data Monitoring Committee). Because of the relative autonomy of the participating centres, the ERSPC is conducted in a decentralized fashion. Centralized data collection is in the hands of an independent centre located in the UK (the Central Database).

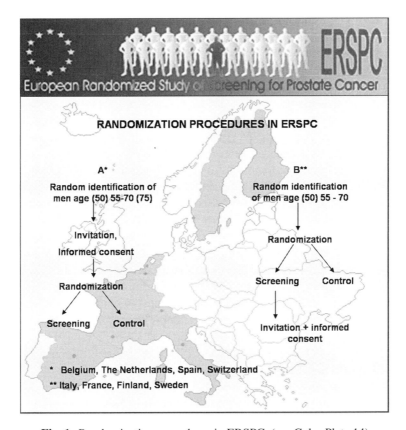

**Fig. 1.** Randomization procedures in ERSPC. (*see* Color Plate 14)

## *Randomization*

Due to differences in legal requirements for running an RCT in the participating countries, two different randomization schemes are used. In Belgium, Spain, Switzerland and the Netherlands, informed consent is required before randomization (see Fig. 1 and Color Plate 14). In the other countries, informed consent is only required for those men who are randomized to the screen arm.

## SCREENING TESTS
## *PSA, DRE and TRUS*

At the time the ERSPC started, PSA, DRE and TRUS were potential screening tests. Other screening methods, such as the use of PSA derivatives (e.g. PSA velocity, PSA density, PSA doubling time) and biomarkers are possibly proper screening tests as well, which were to be evaluated in a later phase.

Along with differences in randomization schemes, slightly different screening protocols are used across the ERSPC centres. All except one use a 4-year screening interval (Sweden uses 2 years). The general PSA level for recommending a biopsy was set at 4 ng/ml. Individual centres could lower the level or use a modified biopsy indication below this general cut-off, according to their own preferences. The core age group is 55–69 and all centres use sextant biopsies, at least initially.

For a proper screening algorithm, it is very important to find a delicate balance between sensitivity and specificity of the screening tests, as lead-time and overdiagnosis are inevitable in prostate cancer screening. Therefore, evaluation of screening procedures is an essential part of the ERSPC and prior to the initiation of the study, it was agreed that screening procedures would be adjusted one time if necessary.

The first contribution to this evaluation came from the Italian group *(14)*, and was followed by major investments made by other centres as well to clarify the role of the different screening tests. Improvements of test characteristics, potential reduction of proportions of men to be biopsied, the loss of otherwise diagnosed cancers, and the number of biopsies needed per prostate cancer were investigated and simulated by Bangma et al. *(15,16)*. These studies indicated the future direction of test evaluation: main goal was to improve specificity (avoidance of unnecessary testing and biopsies) and still maintain the detection rate of the first round (4–5%). The search for methods for improvement of specificity was continued and led to many suggestions *(17,18)*. However, great reluctance existed to change the protocol with the acceptance of the loss of a proportion of prostate cancers, whose final outcomes could not be judged. Nevertheless, a major change in the screening protocol was implemented as a result of the evaluation outcomes. From February 1996, men with a PSA value of 0–0.9 ng/ml were not further screened but advised to be re-screened 4 years later. This change was based on the observation that in 1,451 men, 174 biopsies detected 4 cancers, resulting in a positive predictive value of 2% and a cancer detection rate of 0.3% *(17)*. All centres adopted this change in protocol, saving a screening visit for 35% of the whole screening population and leading to an obvious reduction in costs of the study.

A second major change was omitting DRE and TRUS as screening tests and lowering the biopsy threshold to a PSA value of 3.0 ng/ml. This decision was based on a study from the Rotterdam centre, where the value of DRE was investigated. Ideally, sensitivity and specificity of a screening test are calculated. However, the true underlying incidence of prostate cancer is unknown. The rate at which the screening test detects the disease and truly identifies men without the disease cannot be calculated. Therefore, an estimate of the prevalence is set as the "gold standard" and used to calculate a relative sensitivity and specificity (19). Relative sensitivity and specificity of DRE were assessed in 10,523 consecutive men randomized to the screening arm of the Rotterdam section of the ERSPC, based on estimates of the predictive index (the number of cancers that would have been detected if all men had been biopsied, the "gold standard"). Of these men, 7,055 were found to have PSA values < 4.0 ng/ml. In the PSA ranges 0–0.9, 1–1.9, 2–2.9 and 3–3.9 ng/ml, positive predictive value (PPV) of a positive DRE was 4, 10, 11 and 33%, respectively. In these PSA ranges, relative sensitivities of DRE were 21, 24, 14 and 39%, respectively, and relative specificities, 94, 92, 91 and 98%, respectively. Overall PPV of DRE in the PSA range ≤3.0 ng/ml was 8.8%. Omitting DRE as a screening test in men with a PSA < 3.0 ng/ml would have missed 57 of 473 cancers actually detected (12.1%) and saved 533 biopsies (23.5%). Biopsying every man with a PSA of 3–3.9 ng/ml would have added 43 cancers and decreased the false-negative biopsy indication drastically. Furthermore, cancers detected in the PSA range < 4 ng/ml were classified as minimal, moderate, and advanced in 42, 42, and 16% in men screened during the first round in Rotterdam (20,21).

The new screening protocol, with only a PSA higher than or equal to 3.0 ng/ml as a biopsy indication, was implemented from February 1997 and a validation of this protocol was carried out on 7,943 men consecutively randomized to the screening arm of the ERSPC Rotterdam (22). It was shown that the detection rate remained almost the same (5.0% vs. 4.7% in the new protocol) and the PPV of PSA in the range ≥ 3.0 ng/ml, predicted to be 12.3%, was actually 18.0%. The proportion of men with a biopsy indication decreased from 28.2 to 19.5%. Furthermore, the overall tumour characteristics found in the new protocol differed very little from those detected in the old regimen, based on PSA, DRE and TRUS. Therefore, the new protocol seems to contribute to reaching the delicate balance between sensitivity and specificity. However, the search for an even better balance is continuing. More research on the evaluation of screening tests is being performed and definite judgments on the validity of test regimens will only be possible after the final conclusions of the trial.

## Biopsy

As for the screening regimen policy, the biopsy regimen depends on the choice of the individual screening centres. At the time the ERSPC started, a systematic sextant needle biopsy was the generally accepted biopsy regimen among urologists. In Rotterdam, a lateralized sextant biopsy scheme was chosen as the prostate cancer detection rate increases when the lateral peripheral zone is sampled (23,24). Nowadays, the trend is to obtain more than six biopsy cores, as this increases the detection rate of prostate cancer (25). Some centres adopted this more extensive biopsy regimen to assure comparability with the control group, others continue performing sextant biopsies.

## INTERMEDIATE RESULTS

### Recruitment and Cancer Detection

Randomization is concluded in all countries and the data are summarized in Table 1. A total of 267,994 men are participating in the ERSPC: 126,219 in the screening arm, 141,775 in the control arm. Randomization is unequal because Finland does not randomize in a 1:1 ratio. Of the men randomized to the screening arm, 82.2% have been

Table 1
Randomization in the Initial Screening Round in the ERSPC

| Centre | Number of men randomized | | |
|---|---|---|---|
| | Screening | Control | Total |
| **Belgium** | 5,188 | 5,171 | 10,359 |
| **Finland** | 31,970 | 48,409 | 80,379 |
| **France** | 42,827 | 42,587 | 85,414 |
| **Italy** | 7,499 | 7,478 | 14,977 |
| **Netherlands** | 21,206 | 21,163 | 42,369 |
| **Spain** | 2,416 | 1,862 | 4,278 |
| **Sweden** | 9,957 | 9,954 | 19,911 |
| **Switzerland** | 5,156 | 5,151 | 10,307 |
| **Total initial screening** | 126,219 | 141,775 | 267,994 |

Table 2
Cancer Detection in the First Screening Round in the Screening Arm of the ERSPC

| Centre | Number of men screened | Cancers detected in screening arm (%) |
|---|---|---|
| **Belgium** | 4,639 | 116 (2.5) |
| **Finland** | 23,399 | 658 (2.8) |
| **France (ongoing)** | 11,796 | 217 (1.8) |
| **Italy** | 5,727 | 98 (1.7) |
| **Netherlands** | 19,970 | 1014 (5.1) |
| **Spain** | 2,416 | 40 (1.7) |
| **Sweden (2-year interval)** | 7,429 | 209 (2.8) |
| **Switzerland** | 4,940 | 159 (3.2) |
| **Total** | 80,316 | 2511 (3.1) |

screened at least once (excluding France, still ongoing). A total of 2,294 prostate cancers have been found during the first round, leading to a detection rate of 3.3% (Table 2). Detection rates differ among the participating countries from 1.6% (Italy) to 5.1% (the Netherlands). These differences are mainly due to differences in underlying prevalence between countries and small differences in screening protocols.

During the second screening round (including the third screening round in Sweden, where a 2-year interval is used) a total of 48,968 men were screened and 1,532 prostate cancers were found. This leads to a detection rate of 3.1%. The third screening round is still ongoing in most centres.

## Distribution of Prognostic Features

For screening to be effective, a stage-shift into the direction of a more favourable distribution of prognostic factors such as local tumour extent, grading (Gleason score) and presence of metastases is a prerequisite. An early report on this issue is given by Rietbergen et al. (26), on the Rotterdam section of the ERSPC. The TNM classification of 459 screen-detected prostate cancers was compared to the TNM classification of a cohort of 4,708 men from the Amsterdam Cancer Registry. A stage-shift towards more favourable features was seen for the screen-detected cancers. Furthermore, the incidence of metastases was 24% in the cancer registry cohort, compared to 1.7% in the screen-detected series.

A recent report on the issue of metastatic disease comes from the Swedish section *(27)*. Metastatic prostate cancer incidence at diagnosis in a screened cohort was compared with a control cohort, both 10,000 men. For the control group, diagnosis of metastatic prostate cancer was monitored by using the Swedish Cancer Registry. After a follow-up of 10 years, the risk of being diagnosed with metastatic prostate cancer differed by 48.9%, decreasing from 47 cases in the control group to 24 cases in the group randomized to PSA-based screening. However, the PC incidence in the screened cohort was 1.8-fold higher than in the control group.

A comparison of all cancers found in the screening and the control arm of the Rotterdam section was performed in 2003 *(28)*. By January 1, 2003, 1,269 cancers were detected in the screening arm and 336 were detected in the control arm. A shift to more favourable clinical stage was seen in the screening arm of the trial. T1C and T2 cancers were 5.8 and 6.2 times more often diagnosed, respectively, in the screening arm than in the control arm of the trial.

A grading shift towards lower Gleason scores in screen-detected PC was reported by Postma et al. *(29)*. In radical prostatectomy specimens of the screening arm 34.6% of the cancers had a Gleason score equal to or higher than 7, a significantly lower proportion as compared to the 53.5% of cancers in the control arm. Furthermore, the median tumour volume was significantly smaller in the screened population (1.0 ml vs. 3.9 ml).

These studies suggest that the prerequisite for effective screening, i.e. the shift towards more favourable prognostic features, can be met.

## SCREENING INTERVAL

### *Lead-Time*

All centres, except for Sweden, have adopted a screening interval of 4 years. This was based on the estimations of lead-time available at the beginning of the ERSPC. Lead-time was estimated to be 6–10 years, based on serum banks used for PSA-determinations and the subsequent diagnosis of clinical prostate cancer *(30,31)*. Of course, data that could confirm the correctness of this relatively long interval were highly desirable.

A first evaluation of lead-time came from Finland *(32)*. Auvinen et al. defined lead-time as the duration of follow-up needed to accrue the same expected number of incident prostate cancer cases in the absence of screening as detected in the initial screening round. Expected numbers were calculated using an age-cohort model. Based on findings among 10,000 men screened in 1996–1997 with 292 screen-detected cancers, lead-time was estimated as approximately 5–7 years. With the assumption that the cancers are detected on average at the midpoint of the detectable preclinical phase, this detectable preclinical phase was estimated to be 10–14 years.

In the Netherlands, a microsimulation model (MISCAN) was used to estimate lead-time *(33)*. Simulation models are based on results of the Rotterdam section, which enrolled 42,376 men and in which 1,498 cases of prostate cancer were identified, and on baseline prostate cancer incidence and stage distribution data. The models were used to predict mean lead-times, overdetection rates, and ranges. Mean lead-times and rates of overdetection depended on a man's age at screening. For a single screening test, the estimated mean lead-time was 12.3 years at age 55 and 6 years at age 75. For a screening program with a 4-year screening interval from age 55 to 67, the estimated mean lead-time was 11.2 years (range 10.8–12.1 years), and the overdetection rate was 48% (range 44–55%). This screening program raised the lifetime risk of a prostate cancer diagnosis from 6.4 to 10.6%.

These studies seem to confirm the appropriateness of an inter-screening interval of at least 4 years.

## Distribution of Prognostic Factors at Re-screening

For a screening interval to be appropriate, characteristics of tumours found at re-screen should be favourable for curative treatment.

The incidence of potentially advanced malignancies in the second screening round of the Rotterdam section was evaluated by Postma et al. *(34)*. Potentially advanced malignancy was defined as a biopsy Gleason score of 7 or higher. During the second screening round, 503 prostate cancers were detected in 11,210 screened men, of which 30 (6.0% of cancers) had features of potentially advanced malignancy. Curative treatment was offered to 26 men, 12 men were treated with radical prostatectomy (RP). Of these 12 RP specimens, 11 showed organ-confined disease. This study shows that potentially advanced disease is a rare finding in the second screening round, but is still potentially curable in most men.

Furthermore, other studies demonstrated a shift towards more favourable tumour characteristics in the second screening round, compared to the initial round *(35,36)*. In Sweden, where screening is performed with a 2-year interval, stage distribution showed a trend towards a lower stage at the second screening (an increase in T1 lesions from 60 to 74% in the second round) as well as lower PSA in men diagnosed with cancer *(35)*.

First and second round findings from the Rotterdam section were evaluated as well *(36)*. In the second screening round, the mean PSA value was lower (5.6 vs. 11.1 ng/ml), advanced clinical stage T3–T4 was 7.1-fold less common, and 76.4% versus 61.5% of the biopsy Gleason scores were less than 7. In the first screening round, 13 regional and 9 distant metastases were detected. In the second round, two cases with distant metastasis were found. Overall, a shift towards more favourable tumour characteristics was seen for the second round of screening. These results support the screening methods used and the inter-screening interval of 4 years.

## Interval Cancers

The rate of interval cancers is an important parameter in determining the sensitivity of the screening procedure and screening interval. In the Swedish centre, 5,854 men participated in the first screening round and 145 prostate carcinomas were detected. During the second screening round, 2 years later, 5,267 men participated and 111 cancers were found. Nine interval carcinomas were diagnosed (10.6% of the control group prevalence) *(35)*. Of these, three men had metastatic disease, the others seemed confined to the prostate gland and were detected through opportunistic screening or because of urinary symptoms.

In the Rotterdam section, interval carcinomas were studied in a cohort of 17,226 men (8,350 in the screening arm, 8,876 in the control arm), enrolled consecutively on the ERSPC *(37)*. During the first screening round, 412 prostate cancers were detected. During the following 4-year interval, 135 cancers were found in the control group, and 25 cancers were diagnosed in the screened arm (18.5% of the control group prevalence). Of these 25, 7 men had refused a recommended biopsy in the initial screening round. The remaining 18 prostate cancers were all classified as T1 or T2A and none were poorly differentiated or metastatic. These data, which show a low interval carcinoma rate, suggest that the 4-year screening interval is reasonable.

## CONTAMINATION

### *Contamination and Effective Contamination*

PSA contamination, i.e. the opportunistic PSA-based screening in the control arm of the study, can jeopardize the power of the ERSPC. With increasing contamination during the early years of the study, the power decreases, leading to higher numbers of participants needed in both the screening and control arm (as described previously in the section on structure of the study). Therefore, the extent of contamination has been carefully studied in several participating centres *(38–41)*.

However, it is important to realize that "effective" contamination cannot be determined by assessing the number of PSA tests only. It is necessary to evaluate the number of men who were PSA-tested and who subsequently had a biopsy if indicated by the PSA level.

Such an analysis of "effective contamination" in the Rotterdam area was reported by Otto et al. *(41)*. During a period of 2.9 years, 1,981 of 14,052 men (14.1%) in the screening arm were PSA-tested outside the regular screening protocol and 2,895 of 14,349 men (20.2%) in the control arm were PSA-tested. The proportion of men in the control arm with a PSA $\geq$ 3.0 ng/ml followed by a biopsy and prostate cancer was 7–8 and 3%, respectively (3 and 0.4–0.6 % in the screening arm). Therefore, although the PSA testing rate in the control arm is high, this was not followed by a substantial increase in prostate biopsies. Especially when one takes into account that in the first screening round 20% of men presented with a PSA $\geq$ 3.0 ng/ml and were biopsied. The effective PSA contamination is relatively small and may not jeopardize the power of the trial. Furthermore, the rate of effective contamination was in line with the predicted contamination rate of 20% used in adjusting the initial sample size *(13)* (see section on "Purpose and structure").

### *Adjustment for Contamination and Non-compliance*

Next to contamination, another process that may dilute the effects of the ERSPC is non-compliance. Non-compliers are participants randomized to the screening arm, who are not screened or do not participate in the whole screening regimen. When during the final analysis of the ERSPC, an adjustment could be made for contamination and non-compliance, the unbiased effect of screening could be determined for those who are willing to participate in a screening program. A method for this adjustment has been described by Cuzick et al. *(42)*.

Roemeling et al. reported on a feasibility study in which the impact of non-compliance on the results of the Rotterdam centre was simulated using the method described by Cuzick et al. *(43)*. Endpoints in the analysis were simulated prostate cancer mortality reductions. In the Rotterdam centre, a total of 5,083 men in the screening arm (24.0%) did not comply with the PSA determinations. Furthermore, 655 men in the screening arm (3.1%) with a biopsy indication based on the PSA level were not biopsied. This gives a total rate of non-compliance of 27.1%. In the control arm, 30.7% of the men had undergone a PSA test and this rate was considered the contamination rate. Under a hypothetical endpoint of 6.7% mortality reduction in an intention-to-screen setting, the secondary, adjusted, analysis resulted in a decrease of 16.1% for those actually screened. This study showed that adjustment for contamination and non-compliance was feasible, although contamination was defined as a PSA test only. A secondary analysis on the final results of the ERSPC will be carried out to provide accurate information for those men actually screened.

## OVERDIAGNOSIS

Overdiagnosis is the detection of prostate cancer that would never have been diagnosed without screening. Those cases of prostate cancer would not have led to symptoms or death during life and therefore would not have been diagnosed clinically. However, if such a carcinoma is found through screening, adverse psychological and physical effects may arise. This would in particular be the case under invasive treatment for prostate cancer, which would not have been clinically relevant, but would have possible harmful side effects.

Using the microsimulation (MISCAN) model, the extent of overdiagnosis in the Rotterdam section of the ERSPC was estimated *(33)*. A 100% attendance rate for each screening program was assumed. Obviously, overdiagnosis leads to a rise in prostate cancer incidence. This was reflected in the observed data from the Rotterdam centre: the first-round detection rate in the screened arm was almost 30 times as high as baseline detection rates (54 vs. 1.86 cases per 1,000 man-years). In the control arm, 3.18 cases per 1,000 man-years were detected in the first round.

Screening men aged 55–67 years with a 4-year screening interval detects 41 irrelevant cancers in 1,000 men. This corresponds with an overdiagnosis rate of 48% (range 44–55%). Furthermore, the lifetime prostate cancer risk increases from 64 to 106 per 1,000, a relative increase of 65%.

This amount of overdiagnosis may be unacceptable in population-based screening, for both healthcare providers and policy makers. Reduction of overdiagnosis by increasing specificity, i.e. through individualizing screening programs and new markers, will be of great importance during the years to come *(44)*.

Another approach focuses on identification of potentially indolent cancers. A recently developed nomogram *(45)* can be used to identify 20–30% of screen-detected PC as "potentially indolent" depending on the probability level chosen (70–80%). This may make screening as a healthcare policy more acceptable.

## QUALITY OF LIFE

The evaluation of quality of life in relation to screening and treatment aspects of prostate cancer has been considered essential from the start of the ERSPC. Therefore, next to mortality reduction, quality adjusted life years (QUALYs) will be calculated. Unfortunately, only in one of the centres (Rotterdam) a truly systematic study of quality of life has been conducted and is still ongoing. So far, only short-term effects could be analyzed and final conclusions about the impact of prostate cancer screening on quality of life will only become clear after the final analysis of the ERSPC.

Up to now, it has been shown that prostate cancer screening induced no important short-term health status effects, with some exceptions of high levels of anxiety in sub-groups (46). Health-related quality of life (HRQoL) was related to tumour stage and the detection method (screen vs. clinically detected PC) (47). Furthermore, the type of post-treatment HRQoL impairments was dependent on treatment modality (prostatectomy or radiotherapy). Patients with screen-detected or clinically diagnosed PC reported similar post-treatment HRQoL (48).

Prostate cancer diagnosis was shown to worsen mental and self-rated overall health immediately after diagnosis in screened patients. However, 6 months later, health status scores improved and no longer differed significantly from pre-diagnosis scores (49).

If prostate cancer screening proves to be effective, some cases will be prevented from reaching the advanced stage. In order to evaluate a screening program thoroughly, it is important to quantify course, care and accompanying costs of advanced disease. Data on these factors are reported in (50). Together with the effects of advanced prostate cancer on quality of life, these data will be used for the evaluation of prostate cancer screening.

## PREDICTIONS OF OUTCOMES

Several studies described in this chapter show promising results for the validity of screening tests and distribution of prognostic factors in a screening setting. Moreover, the ERSPC has shown so far that a large scale RCT on screening is possible in Europe. Furthermore, understanding of screening procedures, prostate biopsy outcomes and pre-dictors, and methods to study contamination has improved due to the ERSPC. These findings have been related to public health, contributing to better understanding of early detection and the problems of opportunistic screening.

However, the primary aim of the ERSPC is to show or exclude a mortality reduction in prostate cancer through screening and early treatment. Data are collected and evaluated in a centralized way, by the independent data centre and by the DMC. These data are confidential, the DMC functioning as the "ethical watchdog" of the ERSPC. Predictions of the outcomes are continuously monitored by the microsimulation system (MISCAN). Any information on the final outcomes of the ERSPC is unknown to the participating centres and the public until the DMC decides a final endpoint has been reached.

### Power and Time Frame

Estimates of power and time frame were reported by De Koning et al. (13). The pur-pose was to calculate the power of the trial, determining what point in time statistically significant differences in prostate cancer mortality can be expected. Data at recruitment and initial screening were collected from the screening centres. The expected number of prostate cancer deaths in each follow-up year was calculated, based on national statistics and expected rate in trial entrants. Different assumptions on intervention effects, partic-ipating rates and contamination were used to calculate power (see Fig. 2 and Color Plate 15). With an assumed 25% intervention effect in men actually screened and a 20% contamination rate, the trial will reach a power of 0.86 in 2008. The ERSPC trial has suf-ficient power to detect a significant difference in prostate cancer mortality between the 2

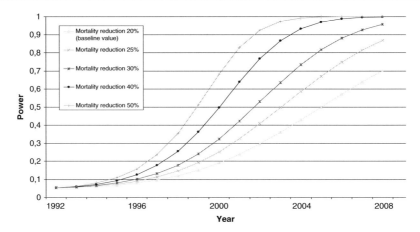

**Fig. 2.** Effect of different assumptions on the power of the ERSPC trial by follow-up year. (*see* Color Plate 15)

(Source: H. de Koning (2002). International Journal of Cancer 98: 268–73.)

arms if the true reduction in mortality by screening is 25% or more or if contamination remains limited to 10% if the true effect is 20% or more.

## FUTURE PROSPECTS

In the ERSPC, no final endpoint has been reached yet, though final data are expected within the coming years. Whether the final analysis will lead to a recommendation for screening or not, the ERSPC has provided much information on prostate cancer and screening for this malignancy. This is very important, as screening for prostate cancer will be performed by general practitioners and urologists, independently of the final recommendations of the ERSPC. Therefore, attention should be drawn to optimizing the screening regimen. The use of new biomarkers, nomograms and features of the individual screening participant may play a role in this search for optimal future screening programs.

## REFERENCES

1. Catalona WJ, Smith DS, Ratliff TL, Dodds KM, Coplen DE, Yuan JJ, Petros JA, and Andriole GL. Measurement of prostate-specific antigen in serum as a screening test for prostate cancer *N Engl J Med* 1991;**324**:1156–61
2. Schröder FH. (1993) Prostate cancer: to screen or not to screen? *BMJ* **306,** 407–8.
3. Schröder FH, and Boyle P (1993). Screening for prostate cancer- necessity or nonsense? *Eur J Cancer* **29A,** 656–61.
4. Schröder FH, Damhuis RAM, Kirkels WJ, De Koning HJ, Kranse R, Nijs HGT and Blijenberg BG (1996). European randomized screening for prostate cancer – The Rotterdam pilots *Intern J Cancer* **65,**145–51.
5. Schröder FH, Denis LJ, Kirkels WJ, De Koning HJ and Standaert B. (1995) European randomized study of screening for prostate cancer: Progress report of Antwerp and Rotterdam pilot studies *Cancer* **76,**129–34.
6. Auvinen A, Tammela T, Stenman U-H, Uusi-Erkkilä I, Schröder FH and Hakama M. (1996) Screening for prostate cancer using serum prostate-specific antigen; a randomized, population-based pilot study in Finland *Br J Cancer* **74,** 568–72

7. Adami HO, Baron JA, and Rothman KJ. Ethics of a prostate cancer screening trial *Lancet* 1994;343:958–60

8. Schröder FH. Screening for prostate cancer (letter to the editor). (1993) *Lancet* **343**, 1438–9.

9. Schröder FH. (1995) Detection of prostate cancer, screening the whole population has not yet been shown to be worth while (letter to the editor).*BMJ* **310**, 140–1.

10. Denis L, and Standaert B. Contributors Chapter Prostate Cancer. (Döbrössy L ed.) (1995) Prevention in primary care. Recommendations for promoting good practice. Copenhagen, *SHO regional office for Europe,* 139–45.

11. Denis LJ, Murphy GP, and Schröder FH. (1995) Report of the consensus workshop on screening and global strategy for prostate cancer *Cancer* **75**, 1187–207.

12. Auvinen A, Rietbergen JBW, Denis LJ, Schröder FH, and Prorok PC. (1996) Prospective evaluation plan for randomized trials of prostate cancer screening *J Med Screen* **3**, 97–104.

13. De Koning HJ, Liem MK, Baan CA, Boer R, Scröder FH, and Alexander FE. (2002) Prostate cancer mortality reduction by screening: power and time frame with complete enrollment in the European Randomized Study of Screening for Prostate Cancer *Int J Cancer* **98**, 268–73.

14. Ciatto S, Bonardi R, Mazzotta A, Lombardi C, Santoni R, Cardini S, and Zappa M. (1995) Comparing two modalities of screening for prostate cancer: digital rectal examination and transrectal ultrasonography vs. prostate specific antigen *Tumori* **81**, 225–9.

15. Bangma CH, Kranse R, Blijenberg BG, and Schröder FH. (1995) The value of screening tests in the detection of prostate cancer. Part I: Results of a retrospective evaluation of 1726 men*Urology* **46**, 773–778.

16. Bangma CH, Kranse R, Blijenberg BG, and Schröder FH. (1995) The value of screening tests in the detection of prostate cancer. Part II: Retrospective analysis of free/total prostate specific analysis ratio, age-specific reference ranges, and PSA density *Urology* **46**, 779–784.

17. Beemsterboer PMM, Kranse R, De Koning HJ, Habbema JDF, and Schröder FH. (1999) Changing role of 3 screening modalities in the European Study of Screening for Prostate Cancer (Rotterdam) *Int J Cancer* **84**, 437–41.

18. Kranse R, Beemsterboer PMM, Rietbergen JBW, Habbema D, Hugosson J, and Schröder FH. (1999) Predictors for biopsy outcome in the European Study of Screening for Prostate Cancer (Rotterdam region) *The Prostate* **39**, 316–22.

19. Schröder FH, Alexander FE, Bangma CH, Hugosson J, and Smith DS. (2000) Screening and early detection of prostate cancer *Prostate* **44**, 255–63.

20. Schröder FH, van der Maas P, Beemsterboer P, Kruger AB, Hoedemaeker R, Rietbergen J, Kranse R. (1998) Evaluation of the digital rectal examination (DRE) as a screening test for prostate cancer *JNCI* **90**, 1817–23.

21. Schröder FH, Van der Cruijsen-Koeter I, De Koning HJ, Vis AN, Hoedemaeker RF, and Kranse R. (2000) Prostate cancer detection at low prostate specific antigen *J Urol* **163**, 806–12.

22. Schröder FH, Roobol-Bouts MJ, Vis AN, Van der Kwast ThH, and Kranse R. (2001) PSA-based early detection of prostate cancer – validation of screening without rectal examination *Urology* **57**, 83–90.

23. Stamey TA. (1995) Making the most out of six systematic sextant biopsies. *Urology* **45**, 2–12.

24. Eskew LA, Bare RL, and McCullough DL. (1997) Systematic 5 region prostate biopsy is superior to sextant method for diagnosing carcinoma of the prostate *J Urol* **157**, 199–202.

25. Aus G, Ahlgren G, Hugosson J, Pedersen KV, Rensfeldt K, and Söderberg R. (1997) Diagnosis of prostate cancer: optimal number of prostate-specific antigen and findings on digital rectal examination *Scand J Urol Nephrol* **31**, 541–4.

26. Rietbergen JBW, Hoedmaeker RF, Boeken Kruger AE, Kirkels WJ, and Schröder FH. (1999) The changing pattern of prostate cancer at the time of diagnosis: characteristics of screen detected prostate cancers in a population-based screening study *J Urol* **161**, 1191–8.

27. Aus G, Bergdahl S, Lodding P, Lilja H, and Hugosson J. (2007) Prostate cancer screening decreases the absolute risk of being diagnosed with advanced prostate cancer- results from a prospective, population-based randomized controlled trial *Eur Urol* **51**, 659–64.

28. Van der Cruijsen-Koeter IW, Vis AN, Roobol MJ, Wildhagen MF, De Koning HJ, Van der Kwast TH, and Schröder FH. (2005) Comparison of screen-detected and clinically diagnosed prostate cancer in the European Randomized Study of Screening for Prostate Cancer, section Rotterdam *J Urol* **174**, 121–5.

29. Postma R, Van Leenders GJ, Roobol MJ, Schröder FH, and Van der Kwast ThH. (2006) Tumour features in the control and screening arm of a randomized trial of prostate cancer *Eur Urol* **50**, 70–5.

30. Stenman UH, Hakama M, Knekt P, Aromaa A, Teppo L, and Leinonen J. (1994) Serum concentrations of prostate-specific antigen and its complex with $\alpha$1-antichymotrypsin before diagnosis of prostate cancer *Lancet* **334**, 1594–8.

31. Parkes C, Wald NJ, Murphy P, George L, Watt HC, Kirby R, Knekt P, Helzlsouer KJ, and Tuomilehto J. (1995) Prospective observational study to assess value of prostate-specific antigen as a screening test for prostate cancer *BMJ* **311**, 1340–3.

32. Auvin A, Määttänen L, Stenman UH, Tammela T, Rannikko S, Aro J, Juusela H, and Hakama M. (2002) Lead-time in prostate cancer screening (Finland) *Cancer Causes Control* **13**, 279–85.

33. Draisma G, Boer R, Otto SJ, van der Cruijsen IW, Damhuis RA, Schröder FH, and de Koning HJ. (2003) Lead-time and overdetection due to prostate-specific antigen screening: estimates from the European Randomized Study of Screening for Prostate Cancer *JNCI* **95**, 868–78.

34. Postma R, Roobol MJ, Schröder FH and Van der Kwast TH. (2004) Potentially advanced malignancies detected by screening for prostate carcinoma after an interval of 4 years *Cancer* **100**, 968–75.

35. Hugosson J, Aus G, Lilja H, Lodding P, Pihl C-G, and Pileblad E. (2003) Prostate specific antigen based biennial screening is sufficient to detect almost all prostate cancers while still curable *J Urol* **169**, 1720–3.

36. Van der Cruijsen-Koeter IW, Roobol MJ, Wildhagen MF, Van der Kwast TH, Kirkels WJ and Schröder FH. (2006) Tumour characteristics and prognostic factors in two subsequent screening rounds with four-year interval within prostate cancer screening trial, ERSPC Rotterdam *Urology* **68**, 615–20.

37. Van der Cruijsen-Koeter IW, Van der Kwast TH, and Schröder FH. (2003) Interval carcinomas in the European Randomized Trial of Screening for Prostate Cancer (ERSPC) – Rotterdam *JNCI* **95**, 1462–6.

38. Lujan M, Paez A, Pascual C, Angulo J, Miravalles E, and Berenguer A. (2006) Extent of prostate-specific antigen contamination in the Spanish section of the European Randomized Trial of Screening for Prostate Cancer (ERSPC) *Eur Urol* **50**, 1234–40.

39. Paez A, Lujan M, Llanes L, Romero I, de la Cal MA, Miravalles E, and Berenguer A. (2002) PSA-use in a Spanish industrial area *Eur Urol* **41**, 162–6.

40. Beemsterboer PM, de Koning HJ, Kranse R, Trienekens PH, van der Maas PJ, and Schröder FH. (2000) Prostate specific antigen testing and digital rectal examination before and during a randomized trial of screening for prostate cancer: European Randomized Study of Screening for Prostate Cancer, Rotterdam *J Urol* **164**, 1216–20.

41. Otto SJ, van der Cruijsen IW, Liem MK, Korfage IJ, Lous JJ, Schröder FH, and de Koning HJ. (2003) Effective PSA contamination in the Rotterdam section of the European Randomized Study of Screening for Prostate Cancer *Int J Cancer* **20**, 394–9.

42. Cuzick J, Edwards R, and Segnan N. (1997) Adjusting for non-compliance and contamination in randomized clinical trials *Stat Med* **16**, 1017–122.

43. Roemeling S, Roobol MJ, Otto SJ, Habbema DF, Gosselaar C, Lous JJ, Cuzick J, and Schröder FH. (2007) Feasibility study of adjustment for contamination and non-compliance in a prostate cancer screening trial *Prostate* **67**, 1053–60.

44. Bangma CH, Roemeling S, and Schröder FH. (2007) Overdiagnosis and overtreatment of early detected prostate cancer *World J Urol* **25**, 3–9.

45. Steyerberg EW, Roobol MJ, Kattan MW, Van der Kwast ThH, De Koning HJ, and Schröder FH. (2007) Prediction of indolent prostate cancer: validation and updating of a prognostic nomogram *J Urol* **177**, 107–12.

46. Essink-Bot ML, De Koning HJ, Nijs HGT, Kirkels WJ, Van der Maas PJ, and Schröder FH. (1998) Short-term effects of population-based screening for prostate cancer on health-related quality of life *JNCI* **12**, 925–31.

47. Madalinska JB, Essink-Bot ML, De Koning HJ, Kirkels WJ, Van der Maas PJ, and Schröder FH. (2001) Health-related quality of life in patients with screen-detected versus clinically diagnosed prostate cancer preceding primary treatment *Prostate* **46**, 87–97.

48. Madalinska JB, Essink-Bot ML, De Koning HJ, Kirkels WJ, Van der Maas PJ, and Schröder FH. (2001) Health-related quality-of-life effects of radical prostatectomy and primary radiotherapy for screen-detected or clinically diagnosed localized prostate cancer *J Clin Oncol* **19**, 1619–28.

49. Korfage IJ, De Koning HJ, Roobol MJ, Schröder FH, and Essink-Bot ML. (2006) Prostate cancer diagnosis: the impact on patient's mental health *Eur J Cancer* **42**, 165–70.

50. Beemsterboer PMM, De Koning HJ, Birnie E, Van der Maas PJ, and Schröder FH. (1999) Advanced disease in prostate cancer, course, care and cost implications *The Prostate* **40**, 970–104.

# Index